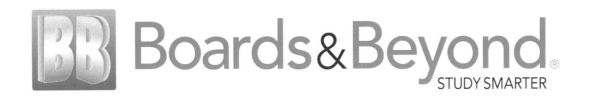

Boards & Beyond:
Basic Pharmacology Slides

Color slides for USMLE Step 1 preparation
from the Boards and Beyond Website

Jason Ryan, MD, MPH

2022 Edition

Boards & Beyond provides a virtual medical school curriculm used
by students around the globe to supplement their education and
prepare for board exams such as USMLE Step 1.

This book of slides is intended as a companion to the videos for
easy reference and note-taking. Videos are subject to change
without notice. PDF versions of all color books are available via the
website as part of membership.

Visit www.boardsbeyond.com to learn more.

Table of Contents

Enzymes

Enzymes
Jason Ryan, MD, MPH

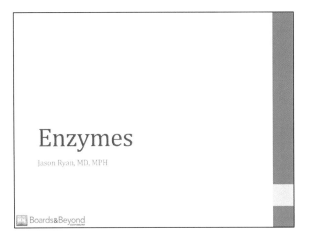

Enzymatic Reactions

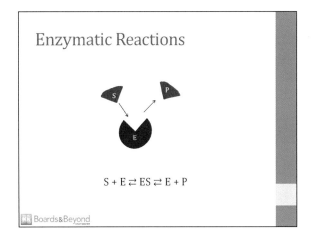

$$S + E \rightleftharpoons ES \rightleftharpoons E + P$$

Enzymatic Reactions

$$S + E \rightleftharpoons ES \rightleftharpoons E + P$$

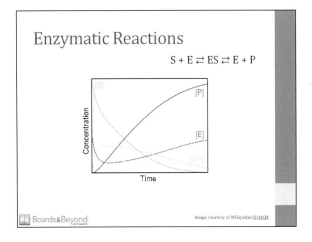

Image courtesy of Wikipedia/U+003F

Michaelis-Menten Kinetics

V = Reaction velocity
Rate of P formation

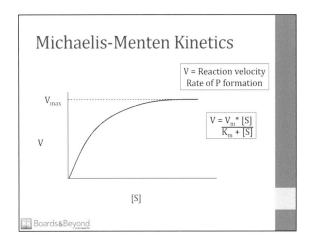

$$V = \frac{V_m * [S]}{K_m + [S]}$$

Michaelis-Menten Kinetics

- Adding S → More P formation → Faster V
- Eventually, reach Vmax

Michaelis-Menten Kinetics

- At Vmax, enzymes saturated (doing all they can)
- Only way to increase Vmax is to add enzyme

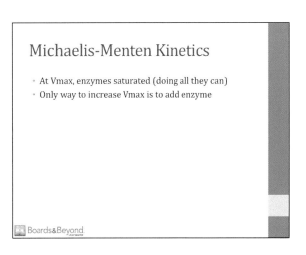

1

Enzyme Kinetics

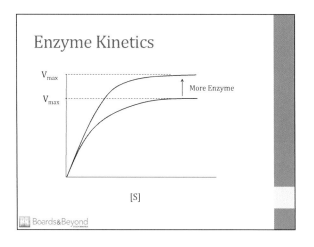

Michaelis-Menten Kinetics

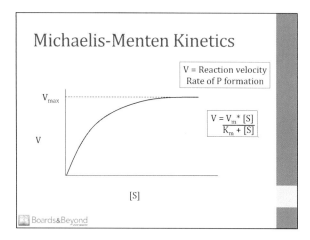

V = Reaction velocity
Rate of P formation

$$V = \frac{V_m * [S]}{K_m + [S]}$$

Michaelis Constant (Km)

$$V = \frac{V_m * [S]}{K_m + [S]}$$

Key Points:
1. Km has same units as [S]
2. At some point on graph, Km must equal [S]

Michaelis Constant (Km)

$$V = \frac{V_m * [S]}{[S] + [S]} = \frac{V_m * [S]}{2 [S]} = \frac{Vm}{2}$$

When $V = V_m/2$
$[S] = K_m$

Michaelis Constant (Km)

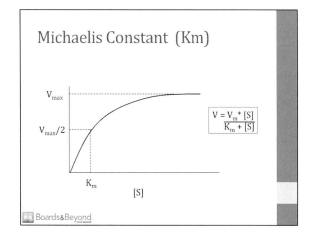

$$V = \frac{V_m * [S]}{K_m + [S]}$$

Michaelis Constant (Km)

- Small Km → Vm reached at low concentration [S]
- Large Km → Vm reached at high concentration [S]

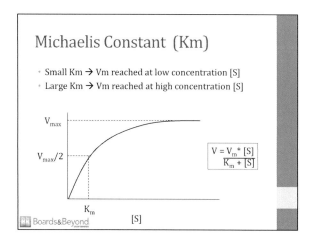

$$V = \frac{V_m * [S]}{K_m + [S]}$$

Michaelis Constant (Km)

- Small Km → Substrate binds easily at low [S]
  - High affinity substrate for enzyme
- Large Km → Low affinity substrate for enzyme

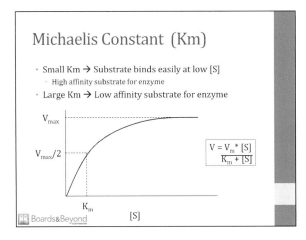

$$V = \frac{V_m * [S]}{K_m + [S]}$$

Key Points

- Km is characteristic of each substrate/enzyme
- Vm depends on amount of enzyme present
- Can determine Vm/Km from
  - Michaelis Menten plot V vs. [S]
  - Lineweaver Burk plot 1/V vs. 1/[S]

Lineweaver Burk Plot

$$V = \frac{V_m * [S]}{K_m + [S]}$$

$$\frac{1}{V} = \frac{Km + [S]}{Vm\ [S]} = \frac{Km}{Vm\ [S]} + \frac{[S]}{Vm[S]}$$

$$\frac{1}{V} = C * \frac{1}{[S]} + \frac{1}{Vm}$$

Lineweaver Burk Plot

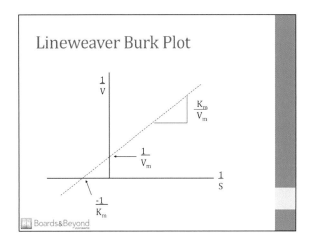

3

Enzyme Inhibitors

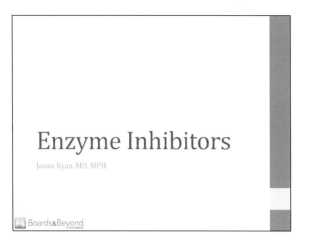

Enzyme Inhibitors

Jason Ryan, MD, MPH

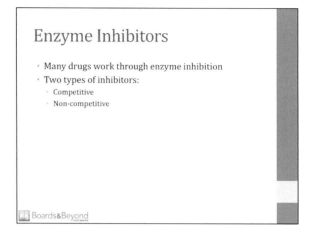

Enzyme Inhibitors

- Many drugs work through enzyme inhibition
- Two types of inhibitors:
  - Competitive
  - Non-competitive

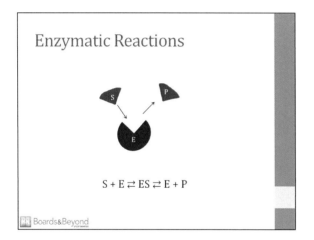

Enzymatic Reactions

$$S + E \rightleftarrows ES \rightleftarrows E + P$$

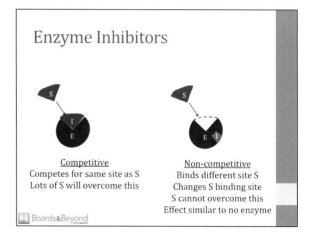

Enzyme Inhibitors

Competitive
Competes for same site as S
Lots of S will overcome this

Non-competitive
Binds different site S
Changes S binding site
S cannot overcome this
Effect similar to no enzyme

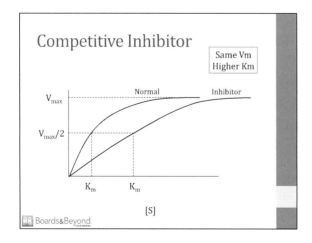

Competitive Inhibitor

Same Vm
Higher Km

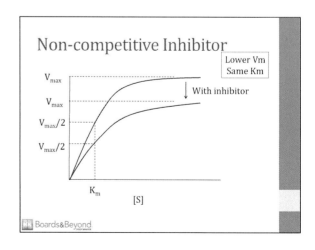

Non-competitive Inhibitor

Lower Vm
Same Km

Competitive Inhibitor

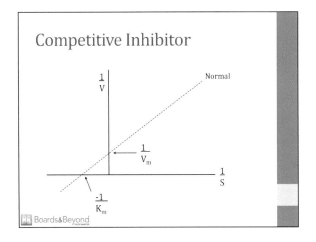

Competitive Inhibitor

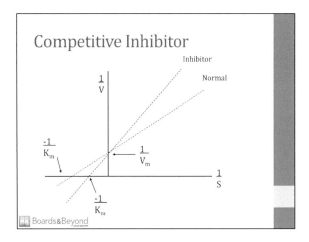

Non-competitive Inhibitor

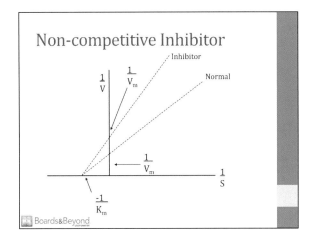

Inhibitors

Competitive	Non-competitive
Similar to S	Different from S
Bind active site	Bind different site
Overcome by more S	Cannot be overcome
Vm unchanged	Vm decreased
Km higher	Km unchanged

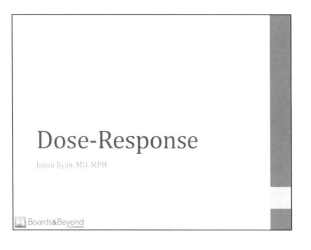

Dose-Response

Jason Ryan, MD, MPH

Efficacy

- Maximal effect a drug can produce
  - Morphine is more efficacious than aspirin for pain control

Potency

- Amount of drug needed for given effect
  - Drug A produces effect with 5mg
  - Drug B produces same effect with 50mg
  - Drug A is 10x more potent than drug B
- More potent not necessarily superior
- Low potency only bad if dose is so high it's hard to administer

Pain Control

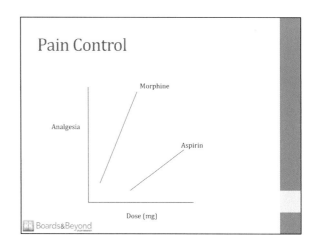

Dose-Response

- For many drugs we can measure response as we increase the dose
- Can plot dose (x-axis) versus response (y-axis)

Dose-Response

- Graded or quantal responses
- Graded response
  - Example: Blood pressure
  - Can measure "graded" effect with different dosages
- Quantal response
  - Drug produces therapeutic effect: Yes/No
  - Example: Number of patients achieving SBP<140mmHg
  - Can measure "quantal" effect by % patients responding to dose

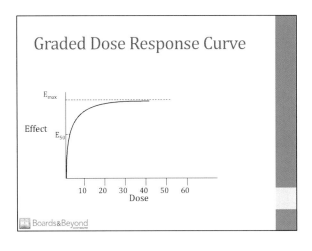

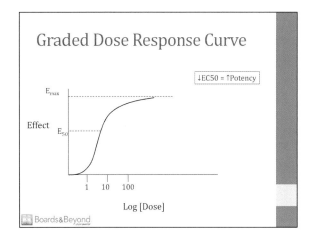

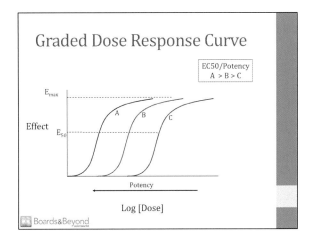

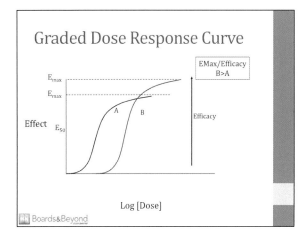

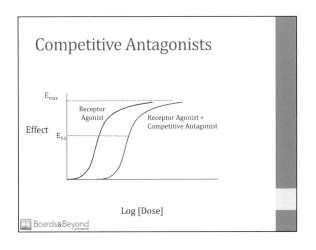

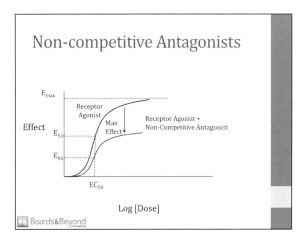

Spare Receptors

- "Spare" receptors: Activate when others blocked
- Maximal response can occur even in setting of blocked receptors
- Experimentally, spare receptors demonstrated by using irreversible antagonists
  - Prevents binding of agonist to portion of receptors
  - High concentrations of agonist still produce max response

Spare Receptors

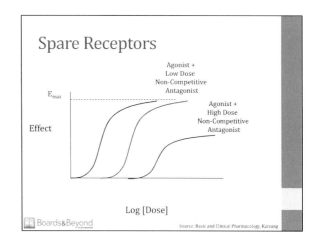

Partial Agonists

- Similar structure to agonists
- Produce less than full effect

Partial Agonists
Agonist or Partial Agonist Given Alone

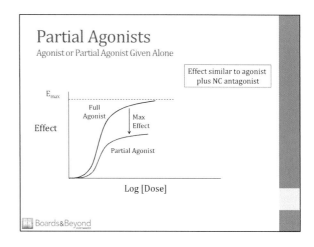

Partial Agonist
Single Dose Agonist With Increasing Partial Agonist

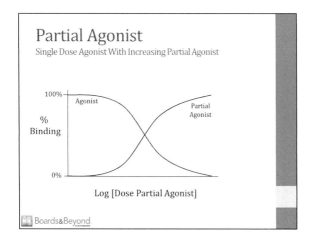

Partial Agonist
Single Dose Agonist With Increasing Partial Agonist

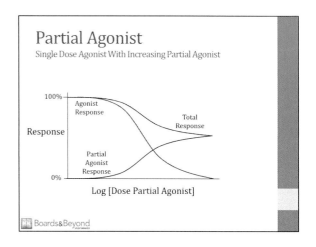

Partial Agonists

- Pindolol/Acebutolol
  - Old anti-hypertensives
  - Activate beta receptors but to less degree that norepinephrine
  - "Intrinsic sympathomimetic activity" (IMA)
  - Lower BP in hypertensive patients
  - Can cause angina through vasoconstriction
- Buprenorphine
  - Partial mu-opioid agonist
  - Treatment of opioid dependence
- Clomiphene
  - Partial agonist of estrogen receptors hypothalamus
  - Blocks (-) feedback; ↑LH/FSH
  - Infertility/PCOS

Quantal Dose Response Curve

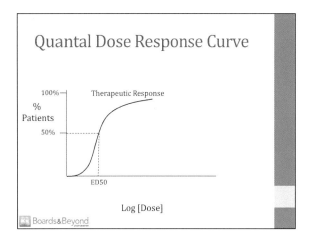

Quantal Dose Response Curve

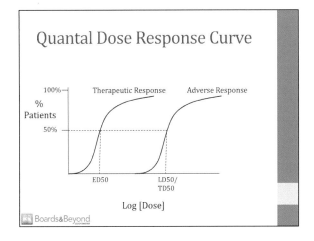

Therapeutic Index

- Measurement of drug safety

$$\text{Therapeutic Index} = \frac{LD_{50}}{ED_{50}}$$

Therapeutic Window

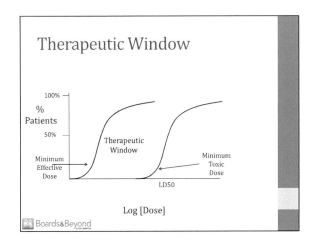

Low TI Drugs

- Often require measurement of levels to avoid toxicity
- Warfarin
- Digoxin
- Lithium
- Theophylline

Drug Elimination

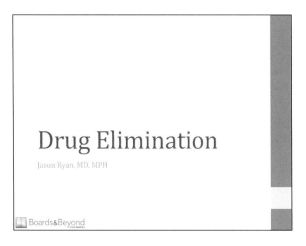

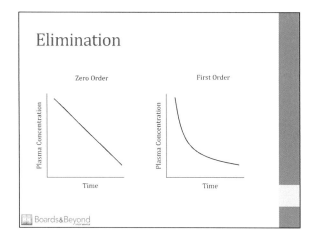

Zero Order Elimination

- Constant rate of elimination per time
- No dependence/variation with [drug]
- No constant half life

$$Rate = 5 * [Drug]^0$$

- Ethanol
- Phenytoin
- Aspirin

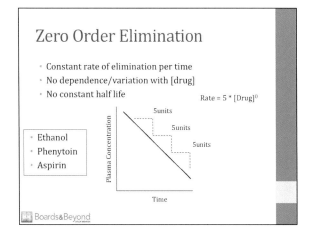

First Order Elimination

- Rate varies with concentration of drug
- Percent (%) change with time is constant (half life)
- Most drugs 1st order elimination

$$Rate = C * [Drug]^1$$

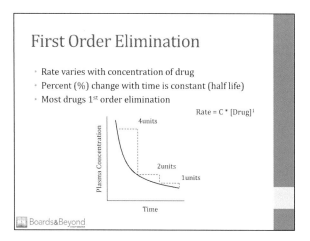

Zero Order Elimination

Time (hr)	Amount (g)	Change (g)	%
0	20		100
1	15	5	75%
2	10	5	50%
3	5	5	25%

First Order Elimination

Time (hr)	Amount (g)	Change (g)	%
0	10		100
1	5	5	50
2	2.5	2.5	25
3	1.25	1.25	12.5

Special Types of Elimination

- Flow-dependent
- Capacity-dependent

Boards&Beyond

Flow-dependent Elimination

- Some drugs metabolized so quickly that blood flow to organ (usually liver) determines elimination
- These drugs are "high extraction" drugs
- Example: Morphine
- Patients with heart failure will have ↓ clearance

Boards&Beyond

Capacity-dependent Elimination

- Follows Michaelis-Menten kinetics
- Rate of elimination = $V_{max} \cdot C / (K_m + C)$
- "Saturatable" → High C leads to V_{max} rate
- When this happens zero order elimination occurs
- Three classic drugs:
  - Ethanol
  - Phenytoin
  - Aspirin

Boards&Beyond

Urine pH

- Many drugs are weak acids or weak bases

Weak Acid: HA <-> A$^-$ + H$^+$

Weak Base: BOH <-> B$^+$ + OH$^-$

Boards&Beyond

Urine pH

- Drugs filtered by glomerulus
- Ionized form gets "trapped" in urine after filtration
- Cannot diffuse back into circulation

Weak Acid: HA <-> A$^-$ + H$^+$

Weak Base: BOH <-> B$^+$ + OH$^-$

Boards&Beyond

Urine pH

- Urine pH affects drug excretion
- Weak acids: Alkalinize urine to excrete more drug
- Weak bases: Acidify urine to excrete more drug

Weak Acid: HA <-> A$^-$ + H$^+$

Weak Base: BOH <-> B$^+$ + OH$^-$

Boards&Beyond

Examples

- Weak acid drugs
  - Phenobarbital, aspirin
  - Sodium bicarbonate to alkalinize urine in overdose
- Weak base drugs
  - Amphetamines, quinidine, or phencyclidine
  - Ammonia chloride (NH_4Cl) to acidify urine in overdose
  - Historical: Efficacy not established, toxicity severe acidosis

Drug Metabolism

- Many, many liver reactions that metabolize drugs
- Liver "biotransforms" drug
- Usually converts lipophilic drugs to hydrophilic products
  - Creates water-soluble metabolites for excretion
- Reactions classified as Phase I or Phase II

Phase I Metabolism

- Reduction, oxidation, or hydrolysis reactions
- Often creates active metabolites
- Two key facts to know:
  - Phase I metabolism can slow in elderly patients
  - Phase I includes cytochrome P450 system

Cytochrome P450

- Intracellular enzymes
- Metabolize many drugs (Phase I)
- If inhibited → drug levels rise
- If induced → drug levels fall

Cytochrome P450

- Inhibitors are more dangerous
  - Can cause drug levels to rise
  - Cyclosporine, some macrolides, azole antifungals
- Luckily, many P450 metabolized drugs rarely used
  - Theophylline, Cisapride, Terfenadine
- Some clinically relevant possibilities
  - Some statins + Inhibitor → Rhabdo
  - Warfarin

P450 Drugs
Some Examples

Inducers	Inhibitors
Chronic EtOH	Isoniazid
Rifampin	Erythromycin
Phenobarbital	Cimetidine
Carbamazepine	Azoles
Griseofulvin	Grapefruit juice
Phenytoin	Ritonavir (HIV)

Phase II Metabolism

- Conjugation reactions
  - Glucuronidation, acetylation, sulfation
- Makes very polar inactive metabolites

Slow Acetylators

- Genetically-mediated ↓ hepatic N-acetyltransferase
- Acetylation is main route isoniazid (INH) metabolism
- Also important sulfasalazine (anti-inflammatory)
- Procainamide and hydralazine
  - Can cause drug-induced lupus
  - Both drugs metabolized by acetylation
  - More likely among slow acetylators

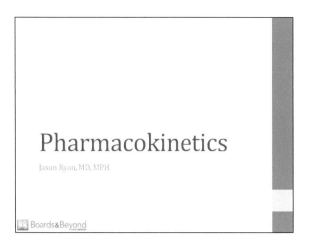

Pharmacokinetics

Jason Ryan, MD, MPH

Pharmacokinetics

- Absorption
- Distribution
- Metabolism
- Excretion
- All impact drug's ability to achieve desired result

Drug Administration

- Enteral
  - Uses the GI tract
  - Oral, sublingual, rectal
- Parenteral
  - Does not use GI tract
  - IV, IM, SQ
- Other
  - Inhalation, intranasal, intrathecal
  - Topical

Bioavailability (F)

- Fraction (%) of drug that reaches systemic circulation unchanged
- Suppose 100mg drug given orally
- 50mg absorbed unchanged
- Bioavailability = 50%

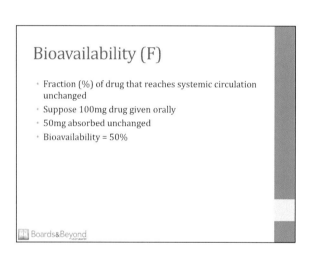

Bioavailability (F)

- Intravenous dosing
  - F = 100%
  - Entire dose available to body
- Oral dosing
  - F < 100%
  - Incomplete absorption
  - First pass metabolism

First Pass Metabolism

- Oral drugs absorbed → liver
- Some drugs rapidly metabolized on 1st pass
- Decreases amount that reaches circulation
- Can be reduced in liver disease patients

Bioavailability (F)

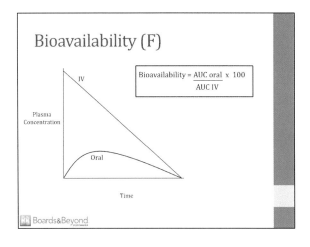

$$Bioavailability = \frac{AUC\ oral}{AUC\ IV} \times 100$$

Volume of Distribution (Vd)

- Theoretical volume a drug occupies
- Determined by injecting known dose and measuring concentration

Determining Fluid Volume

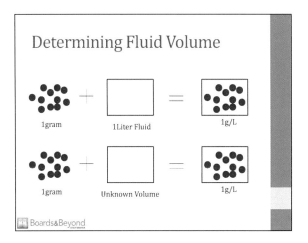

1gram + 1Liter Fluid = 1g/L

1gram + Unknown Volume = 1g/L

Volume of Distribution (Vd)

$$Vd = \frac{Total\ Amount\ In\ Body}{Plasma\ Concentration}$$

$$Vd = \frac{10g}{0.5g/L} = 20L$$

Volume of Distribution (Vd)

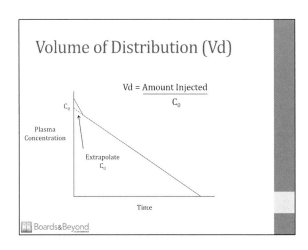

$$Vd = \frac{Amount\ Injected}{C_0}$$

Volume of Distribution (Vd)

- Useful for determining dosages
- Example:
  - Effective [drug]=10mg/L
  - Vd for drug = 10L
  - Dose = 10mg/L * 10L = 100mg

Fluid Compartments

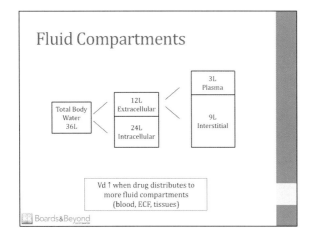

Vd ↑ when drug distributes to more fluid compartments (blood, ECF, tissues)

Volume of Distribution (Vd)

- Drugs restricted to vascular compartment: ↓Vd
  - Large, charged molecules
  - Often protein bound
  - Warfarin: Vd = 9.8L
- Drugs that accumulate in tissues: ↑↑Vd
  - Small, lipophilic molecules
  - Often uneven distribution in body
  - Chloroquine: Vd = 13000L

Protein Binding

- Many drugs bind to plasma proteins (usually albumin)
- This may hold them in the vascular space
- Lowers Vd

Hypoalbuminemia

- Liver disease
- Nephrotic syndrome
- Less plasma protein binding
- More unbound drug → moves to peripheral compartments
- ↑Vd
- Required dose of drug may change

Clearance

- Volume of blood "cleared" of drug
- Volume of blood that contained amount of drug
- Number in liters/min (volume flow)

$$C_x = \frac{\text{Excretion Rate}}{P_x}$$

Clearance

- Mostly occurs via liver or kidneys
- Liver clearance
  - Biotransformation of drug to metabolites
  - Excretion of drug into bile
- Renal clearance
  - Excretion of drug into urine

Clearance

- In liver or kidney disease clearance may fall
- Drug concentration may rise
- Toxicity may occur
- Dose may need to be decreased

Clearance

- Can also calculate from Vd
- Need elimination constant (Ke)
- Implications:
  - Higher Vd, higher clearance
  - Supposed 10g/hour removed from body
  - Higher Vd → Higher volume holding 10g → Higher clearance

$$C_x = Vd * Ke$$

Clearance

$$C_x = Vd * Ke$$

$$Ke = \frac{C_x}{Vd}$$

Clearance

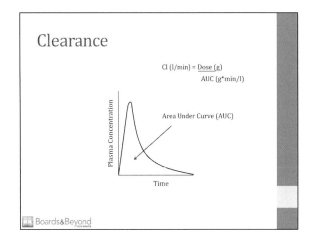

$$Cl\ (l/min) = \frac{Dose\ (g)}{AUC\ (g*min/l)}$$

Area Under Curve (AUC)

Plasma Concentration

Time

Half-Life

- Time required to change amount of drug in the body by one-half
- Usually time for [drug] to fall 50%
- Depends on Vd and Clearance (CL)

$$t_{1/2} = \frac{0.7 * Vd}{CL}$$

Half-life

No. Half Lives	% Remaining
0	100
1	50
2	25
3	12.5
4	6.25
5	3.12
6	1.56

Steady State

- Dose administered = amount drug eliminated
- Takes 4-5 half lives to reach steady state

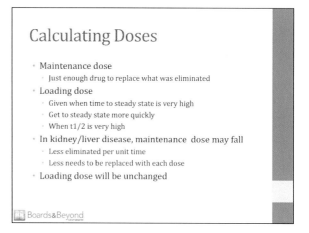

Calculating Doses

- Maintenance dose
  - Just enough drug to replace what was eliminated
- Loading dose
  - Given when time to steady state is very high
  - Get to steady state more quickly
  - When t1/2 is very high
- In kidney/liver disease, maintenance dose may fall
  - Less eliminated per unit time
  - Less needs to be replaced with each dose
- Loading dose will be unchanged

Maintenance Dose

$$\text{Dose Rate} = \text{Elimination Rate}$$
$$= [\text{Drug}] * \text{Clearance}$$

$$\text{Dose Rate} = [5g/l] * 5L/min$$
$$= 25 \text{ g/min}$$

Maintenance Dose

- * If Bioavailability is <100%, need to increase dose to account for this

$$\text{Dose Rate}_{oral} = \frac{\text{Target Dose}}{F}$$

$$\text{Target Dose} = 25g/min$$
$$\text{Bioavailability} = 50\%$$
$$\text{Dose Rate} = 25/0.5 = 50g/min$$

Loading Dose

- Target concentration * Vd
- Suppose want 5g/l
- Vd = 10L
- Need 5 * 10 = 50grams loading dose
- Divide by F if bioavailability <100%

$$\text{Loading Dose} = \frac{[\text{Drug}] * Vd}{F}$$

Steady State

- Dose administered = amount drug eliminated
- Takes 4-5 half lives to reach steady state

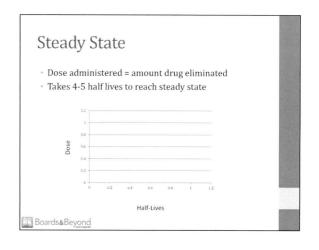

Key Points

- Volume Distribution = Amt injected / [Drug]
- Clearance = 0.7 * Vd / t12
- 4-5 half lives to get to steady state
- Maintenance dose = [Steady State] * CL / F
- Loading dose = [Steady State] * Vd / F

Boards&Beyond

Made in United States
Orlando, FL
07 January 2023

28378527R00015

COMPARING
STATE POLITIES

COMPARING STATE POLITIES

A Framework for Analyzing 100 Governments

Michael J. Sullivan III

Contributions in Political Science, Number 369

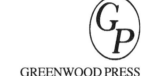

GREENWOOD PRESS
Westport, Connecticut • London

JF
51
S85
1996
NVTGC

Library of Congress Cataloging-in-Publication Data

Sullivan, Michael J.
    Comparing state polities : a framework for analyzing 100
governments / by Michael J. Sullivan III.
        p.   cm. — (Contributions in political science, ISSN 0147–1066 ;
no. 369)
    Includes bibliographical references and index.
    ISBN 0–313–29395–3 (alk. paper)
    1. Comparative government.   2. Post-communism.   I. Title.
II. Series.
    JF51.S85   1996
    320.3´09´045—dc20   95–41692

British Library Cataloguing in Publication Data is available.

Library of Congress Catalog Card Number: 95–41692
ISBN 0–313–29395–3
ISSN 0147–1066

First published in 1996

Greenwood Press, 88 Post Road West, Westport, CT 06881
An imprint of Greenwood Publishing Group, Inc.

Printed in the United States of America

The paper used in this book complies with the
Permanent Paper Standard issued by the National
Information Standards Organization (Z39.48–1984).
10   9   8   7   6   5   4   3   2   1

To Jeremy and Alexandra

**In the hope that they may live in a
more humanely governed world**

Contents

Exhibits

FORMATS

EXCERPTS

Introduction

Since the end of the Cold War, the world has seen more than a score of new countries come into being, and a similar number of new wars break out. The end of the Cold War did not bring about the "end of history" as some predicted (Fukuyama, 1989), but instead has resulted in new forms of politics and government for which Cold War paradigms have proved inadequate.

This book provides a comparative framework for understanding governance in today's world. It is based upon the model put forth in Chapter 5 of my earlier book, *Measuring Global Values* (Sullivan, 1991), which analyzed five "world order" values (peace, economic well-being, ecological balance, social justice, and political participation) in 162 states. Since that time, although the number of countries in the world has expanded to more than 185, the focus of my comparative political analysis has been purposely narrowed to the arbitrarily round number of 100. This figure was consciously chosen to exclude from consideration some 48 "ministates," each with fewer than 2 million people, and 39 other states from among the 68 countries with populations between 2.0 and 10.3 million people (Population Reference Bureau, 1995).

The purpose of this compression of scope in numbers of states studied is to identify, among the myriad nationalities and polities competing for attention in today's world, those countries worthy of greater investigation. This introductory chapter will explain why these 100 states have been selected; the rest of the book will provide a comparative political analysis of their governing structures. It will also highlight 50 of these states as being particularly prone to ethnic-based problems, and 33 of them as beset by violent domestic conflict. As such, this work should be of interest not only to the general reader trying to understand governing regimes in the post–Cold War world, but also to students of comparative politics interested in a broader, more global conceptual focus than that found in traditional textbooks.

Three points implied in the previous paragraphs need further elaboration. First, the number of states to be studied, while only about half the number of sovereign political entities in the world today, is much larger than the half-dozen or so archetype states often presented for detailed analysis in the typical books on comparative politics (Gamer, 1994; Mahler, 1995; Curtis, 1993; Hauss, 1994). Second, the focus of this study is on governing structures, purposely omitting many non-governmental, societal, economic, and private organizations which are considered in more comprehensive approaches to "political systems" (Dahl, 1989; Jacobs and Shapiro, 1994). This is because of the third matter: the author's continuing interest in measurement, not only of the output of government policies in the achievement of societal values (the focus of his earlier work), but also in this study of some of the modes of government itself.

Two traditional areas of inquiry—demography and geography—help to further define the scope and method of this work.

1 DEMOGRAPHY: POPULATIONS

The first variable to consider if one is attempting to understand today's global political world is population: States with more people are generally more important than those with fewer inhabitants (Fornos, 1988; Brown and Jacobson, 1986; United Nations Population Fund, 1990). **Table I.1** lists—in order of population in the five geographic zones to be described in the next section—all 187 states currently in the United Nations or (in the cases of Switzerland and Taiwan) of enduring political significance.

Table I.1 is further divided into five clusters of states based upon categories of population size. In the first tier is the top group of 10 "super-sized" states with more than 100 million people each; next are presented 21 "significant-sized" powers of between 31 and 99 million people, and 45 "middle-sized" countries of between 9.6 and 30 million. These 76 states, although representing only 41 percent of the world's sovereign political entities, command more than 93.5 percent (or 5.332 billion) of the world's population of 5.702 billion people (Population Reference Bureau, 1995). Since politics concerns the way *people* order their societal power relations, the states on this first half of Table I.1 obviously represent most of those worthy of further study; 74 of these 76 states (all except Belarus and Malawi, indicated in smaller print on the table) will be among the 100 states whose political systems will be analyzed in this book.

The second half of **Table I.1** displays, in two parts, the remaining 111 states (those with populations less than that of greater New York City, about 10 million). In the lowest cluster are 48 "ministates," defined here as those having less than 2 million people (and portrayed in this table and frequently throughout this book in small type). None of these ministates is chosen for further comparative analysis of its governing structure because, although some

Table I.1
Populations (mid-1995, in millions)

Europe	Islamic Zone	Africa	Asia	West. Hemisphere
more than 100 million (Super-Sized States), n=10				
			China-1,218.8	
			India-930.6	
				US-263.2
Russia-147.5			Indonesia-198.4	Brazil-157.8
			Pakistan-129.7	
			Japan-125.2	
		Nigeria-101.2	Bangladesh-119.2	
31 to 99 million (Significant-Sized States, pop.>*California*=31 mil.), n=21				
Germany-81.7			Vietnam-75.0	Mexico-91.8
UK-58.6	Egypt-61.9		Philippine I.-68.4	
France-58.1	Turkey-61.4		Thailand-60.2	
Italy-57.7	Iran-61.3	Ethiopia-56.0		
Ukraine-52.0				
		Zaire-44.1	S.Korea-44.9	
Spain-39.1		South Africa 43.5	Myanmar-44.8	Colombia-37.7
Poland-38.6				Argentina-34.6
9.6 to 30 million (Middle-Sized States), n=45				
	Morocco-29.2			Canada-29.6
	Algeria-28.4	Tanzania-28.5		
	Sudan-28.1	Kenya-28.3	N.Korea-23.5	Peru-24.0
Romania-22.7	Uzbekistan-22.7		Nepal-22.6	
	Iraq-20.6	Uganda-21.3	Taiwan 21.2	Venezuela-21.8
	Saudi A.-18.5		Malaysia-19.9	
		Ghana-17.5	Afghanistan-18.4	
	Kazakhstan-16.9	Mozambique-17.4	Sri Lanka-18.2	
Netherlds.-15.5			Australia-18.0	
	Syria-14.7	Madagascar-14.8		Chile-14.3
Yugoslavia-10.8		Ivory Coast-14.3		
Greece-10.5	Yemen-13.2	Cameroon-13.5		
Czech.Rep.-10.4				
-Belarus-10.3		Angola-11.5		Ecuador-11.5
Hungary-10.2		Zimbabwe-11.3		Cuba-11.2
Belgium-10.2		Burkina Faso-10.4	Cambodia 10.6	Guatemala-10.6
Portugal-9.9		-Malawi 9.7		
------	------	------	------	------
TOT., p.1 17	12	16	19	12 (76)
643.9 mil.	376.8 mil.	433.6 mil.	3,167.6 mil.	710.0 mil. (5.3 bil.)

(n=76 states > ~9.6 mil. pop.; n=110 states less than *Greater New York City* in pop. on next page.)

Notes: *Italics* = Two US states' populations for comparison.
   smaller print = non-ministate alternatives to 100 states selected for further study (n=2).

Table I.1 *(continued)*

2.0 to 9.5 million, (most states), n=63

Sweden-8.9	Somalia-9.3	-Mali-9.4		
Bulgaria-8.5	Tunisia-8.9	-Niger-9.2		
-Austria-8.1	Azerbaijan-7.3	Zambia-9.1		Dom.Rep.-7.8
-Switzerland-7.0		Senegal-8.3		Bolivia-7.4
	-Chad-6.4	Rwanda-7.8		Haiti-7.2
-Slovakia-5.4	Tajikistan-5.8	Guinea-6.5		
Denmark-5.2	Israel-5.5	-Burundi-6.4		
-Finland-5.1	Georgia-5.4			El Salv.-5.9
-Croatia-4.5	Libya-5.2	-Benin-5.4		-Honduras-5.5
-Norway-4.3			-Laos-4.8	
-Moldova-4.3	-Turkmenistan-4.5			-Paraguay-5.0
	-Kyrghyzstan-4.4	-Sierra Leone-4.5		
-Lithuania-3.7	Jordan-4.1	-Togo-4.4	-Papua NG-4.1	Nicaragua-4.4
Ireland-3.6				
-Bosnia-3.5	-Armenia-3.7		-New Zealand-3.5	Costa Rica-3.3
-Albania-3.5	-Lebanon-3.7	-C.Af.R.-3.2		-Uruguay-3.2
	-Eritrea-3.5	Liberia-3.0	Singapore-3.0	
-Latvia-2.5		-Congo-2.5		Panama-2.6
-Macedonia-2.1	-Mauritania-2.3		-Mongolia-2.4	Jamaica-2.4
-Slovenia-2.0	-Oman -2.2	-Lesotho-2.1		
Subtot: 17:4+13	16:8+8	14:5+9	5:1+4	11:8+3 (63)

less than 2.0 million (ministates), n=48

	UAE-1.9	Namibia-1.5		
Estonia-1.5	Kuwait-1.5	Botswana-1.5		Trinidad-1.3
		Gabon-1.3		
		Mauritius-1.1		Guyana-0.8
		Guinea Bissau-1.1	Fiji-0.8	
	Cyprus-0.7	Gambia-1.1	Bhutan-0.8	Suriname-0.4
	Djibouti-0.6	Swaziland-1.0		Bahamas-0.3
	Bahrain-0.6	Comoros-0.5	Solomons-0.4	Barbados-0.3
Luxmbrg.-0.4	Qatar-0.5	Equat. Guinea-0.4	Brunei-0.3	Belize-0.2
Malta-0.4		CapeVerde-0.4	Maldives-0.3	St.Lucia-0.1
Iceland-0.3			Vanuatu-0.2	St.Vincent-0.1
Andorra-0.05			W.Samoa-0.2	Grenada-0.1
Monaco-0.03		STP-0.1	Micronesia-0.1	Antigua-0.1
Liechten.-0.03		Seychelles-0.1	Marshalls-0.1	Dominica-0.1
San Marino-0.02			Palau-0.02	St.Chris.-0.04
n=8	n=6	n=12	n=10	n=12 (48)

TOT.,p.2: 25	22	26	15	23 (111)
TOTAL: n= 42	34	42	34	35 (187)
~Pop. TOT:		(~720m. w/ n.AF)		(~5.7bil.)
~ 680 mil	~460 mil.	~590 mil.	~3.2 bil.	~770 mil.

Source: Population Reference Bureau (1995); includes debatable estimates for Somalia, Saudi Arabia, Yemen.

Notes: smaller print = non-ministate alternatives to 100 states selected for further study (n=37).
ministates not in UN: Vatican City, Kiribati, Tonga, Tuvalu, Nauru.

of them are of geostrategic importance—and, indeed, have been the location of wars and other interesting political activity in recent years (e.g., Estonia, Kuwait, Namibia, Fiji, and Grenada, to cite one from each zone)—they are ultimately dependent in their politics on decisions made elsewhere, generally by a larger neighbor or ideological patron (Jackson, 1991). It might also be noted that all of these minstates combined total fewer than 40 million people, about the population of Spain or South Africa (slightly more than that of California) on page 1 of **Table I.1**.

On the top half of page 2 of **Table I.1** is the largest of the five clusters of countries based upon population size, with 63 states of between 2.0 and 9.5 million people each. Fewer than half these states (26 of 63) are selected for further consideration in this book. The criteria for inclusion are elaborated upon in the next (geographic) section of this chapter, and relate to the fact that the types of political–cultural systems being excluded can generally be accommodated by a study of one of the other states under discussion (e.g., Germany is chosen rather than Austria, Saudi Arabia for Oman, Zaire for Congo, Australia for New Zealand, El Salvador for Honduras, again citing examples from each zone). The 26 countries chosen from this tier of Table I.1 for further study are displayed in normal-size print, whereas the 37 states excluded are in the small print of the ministates.

One final point must be made before leaving this macroanalysis of global population. There is not always a "comfortable fit" between the governmental machinery of these 187 states and the political allegiance of the nationalities living within their boundaries (Gottlieb, 1993; Brass, 1992). This is particularly true in the case of the states with larger populations, from which most subsequent examples in this study will be drawn. In these countries, various political institutions—from apparently benign civilian constructs (such as federalism, bicameral representative assemblies, and affirmative-action electoral schemes), to more repressive military measures (such as house arrests, disappearances, and forced evacuations)—will be employed to accommodate or eliminate recalcitrant national minority populations.

Even some of the smaller states listed among the lower clusters of **Table I.1**, and omitted from extensive mention later in this book, have not succeeded in establishing in their political structures an acceptable nation/state mix (e.g., Bosnia, Chad, Togo, Laos, and Guyana, from the respective zones). In the case of Burundi, to cite one example of a state excluded from this study's selected 100, its politics are so intertwined with that of its slightly larger neighbor Rwanda that, throughout this text (particularly in Chapters 4 and 5), the designation Rwanda/Burundi often will be used and the linked pair treated virtually as one. Similar situations of close identification of national and political destiny might be found in the cases of Russia and Belarus, Syria and Lebanon, Vietnam and Laos, and the small states of the English-speaking Caribbean.

Before leaving **Table I.1**, one other aspect of its methodology might be noted. Within the columns, countries are "clustered" so as to facilitate comparison of states of similar population size across the five zones. This method of comparing will be employed in many of the 54 tables found throughout this book.

2 GEOGRAPHY: ZONES AND REGIONS

The second variable which will be an important part of the methodology of this book is geography: the physical size and (especially) location of the 100 states to be studied. **Table I.2a** divides the world's 187 countries into five zones and about (depending on how north America is treated) fifteen regions. Any such geographic groupings inevitably reflect political and pedagogical assumptions (Magstadt, 1994; Ward, 1992; Gyohten, 1992; Wallerstein, 1991), and an attempt will be made here to make them explicit.

The zones generally represent certain obvious continental divisions (Europe, Africa, Asia, Western Hemisphere), in which some state placements are admittedly arguable, especially on the fringes of the fifth, Islamic, zone, which stretches from Morocco and Mauritania in northwest Africa to the five new central Asian states which emerged from the old Soviet Union in 1991. One reason for having five zones is to have an approximately equal number of states (about 35 to 40) in each zone in order to make more meaningful zonal comparisons where this is appropriate (Sullivan, 1991:5). This framework also expands the Cold War paradigm of "three worlds" (two of which were largely European)—the Western capitalist democracies, the Eastern communist bloc, and the Third World—to a broader perspective which provides more equitable treatment of all of the world's major civilizations, a matter of rising relevance in the contemporary era (Arnold, 1993; Huntington, 1993).

Sixteen states whose zonal placement might be questionable are annotated Δ in **Table I.2a**. These "shatterbreak" states (Cohen, 1991) include Cyprus, a state which is geographically in west Asia close to Turkey, but culturally and politically part of southern Europe (Greece); Mauritania, Chad, Sudan, Eritrea, Djibouti, and Somalia, whose populations are often black African, but which are placed in the north African region of the Islamic zone rather than in the African zone because their political systems are generally dominated by Islamic (and often Arab) factions; and Mali, Niger, and Burkina Faso, which are placed in the African zone (western region), because though similar to the countries just mentioned, they relate more to the politics of the sub-Saharan black African states to their south. Also, the Indian Ocean island ministates of Seychelles and Maldives represent the division between the African and Asian continents, respectively. Similarly, Afghanistan and Pakistan are considered the dividing line between the Islamic and Asian zones; although both states have Islamic governments and Muslim populations, their modern histories make their politics (especially Pakistan's) more akin to that

Table I.2a
Comparative Government: Zones and Regions (187 states)

Europe	Islamic Zone	Africa	Asia	West.Hemisph.
northern (11)	west Asia (11)	western (15)	south (8)	south Am.(12)
Iceland	Cyprus^Δ	Cape Verde	AfghanistanΔ	Suriname
Ireland	TURKEY	Guinea Bissau	PakistanΔ	Guyana
UNITED KINGDOM	Georgia^	Senegal	INDIA	
FRANCE	Armenia^	Gambia		BRAZIL
Belgium	Azerbaijan	Guinea	Nepal	Paraguay
Luxembourg	Kazakhstan	Sierra Leone	Bhutan	Uruguay
Netherlands	Kyrgyzstan	Liberia	Bangladesh	Argentina
Denmark	Tajikistan	Ivory Coast		Chile
Norway	Uzbekistan	Ghana	Sri Lanka	Bolivia
Sweden	Turkmenistan	Togo		Peru
Finland	IRAN	Benin	MaldivesΔ	Ecuador
		Burkina FasoΔ		Colombia
southern(17)		MaliΔ		Venezuela
Monaco		NigerΔ	east,mainland(10)	
Andorra	Arabian peninsula (12)	NIGERIA	Myanmar	cent./n.Am.(8+2*)
Spain	Iraq		Thailand	Panama
Portugal	Kuwait	central-eastern(13)	Laos	Costa Rica
Malta	Bahrain	Cameroon	Cambodia	Nicaragua
ITALY	U.A.Emirates	Equat.Guinea	Vietnam	Honduras
San Marino	Qatar	SaoTome&Principe		El Salvador
Greece	Oman	Gabon	CHINA	Guatemala
Albania	Yemen	Congo		Belize
Slovenia	SAUDI ARABIA	Cent.Afr.Republic	Mongolia	MEXICO
Croatia	Jordan	ZAIRE	N.Korea	
Bosnia	Syria	Burundi	S.Korea	(n.America (2*))
Yugoslavia	Lebanon	Rwanda	Taiwan	UNITED STATESΔ
Macedonia	ISRAEL^	Uganda		CanadaΔ
Bulgaria		ETHIOPIA		
Romania	north Africa(11)	Kenya	offshore (16)	Caribbean/n.Am(13+2*)
Moldova	EGYPT	Tanzania	JAPAN	Bahamas
	Libya		Philippines	Cuba
central (14)	Tunisia	southern(14)	Brunei	Jamaica
Hungary	Algeria	Zambia	Malaysia	Haiti
Austria	Morocco	Angola	Indonesia	
Liechtenstein	MauritaniaΔ	Namibia	Singapore	Domin.Republic
Switzerland	ChadΔ	Botswana		St. Chris.-Nevis
GERMANY	SudanΔ	SOUTH AFRICA	Australia	Antigua-Barbuda
Czech.Rep.	EritreaΔ	Lesotho	Papua New Guinea	Dominica
Slovakia	DjiboutiΔ	Swaziland	Solomon I.	St. Lucia
Poland	SomaliaΔ	Zimbabwe	Vanuatu	St.Vincent & G.
Lithuania		Malawi	Fiji	Barbados
Latvia		Mozambique	W.Samoa	Grenada
Estonia		Comoros	Micronesia	Trinidad-Tobago
Belarus		Madagascar	Marshall I.	
Ukraine		Mauritius	Palau	
RUSSIA		SeychellesΔ	New Zealand	
n=42	n=34	n=42	n=34	n=35 (TOT.187)

n=187: United Nations' 185 (w/ 12/94 Palau admission); + Switzerland and Taiwan.

Notes: Δ = zonal shatterbreak states (n=16): Cyprus; Mauritania-thru-Somalia in north Africa; Mali, Niger,
  Burkina Faso; Seychelles, Maldives; Afghanistan, Pakistan; US and Canada.
^ = Islamic in geography, not ethnicity (n=4).   * = US and Canada in two regions.
Capital letters = most important state(s) in region (see Chapter 2d), n=20.

of the Indian subcontinent than to that of the ex-Soviet republics or Iran. (Other Islamic states like Indonesia, Bangladesh, and Malaysia are not in the Islamic zone for reasons of geographic contiguity.)

Finally, the case could be made for placing the United States and Canada in the European zone because their political structures draw largely from the ideas of that civilization (Sullivan, 1991); however, with the end of the Cold War in Europe, and with the rise of the North American Free Trade Zone (to be expanded in the future into South America) and of the Pacific Rim as areas of national economic ambition for both the north American states, it has been decided to place them in the Western Hemisphere (Oman, 1994).

The five zones are further broken down into three regions in each zone. This division draws upon the author's successful experience in teaching Comparative Government courses in which students are required for their term projects to compare a "reasonable" number (Collier, 1991) of "related" countries. The regional clusters of states proposed here represent historical–cultural groupings within the five overarching zones, each of which will be associated with particularly important dominant states (capitalized in **Table I.2a**) and, more to the point of this study, distinctive polity types.

In creating the fifteen regions, an attempt has been made to break up contemporary political blocs (generally formed for reasons of foreign policy), such as the North Atlantic Treaty Organization (NATO), the Arab League, the Organization of African Unity (OAU), the Association of South East Asian Nations (ASEAN), and the Organization of American States (OAS). Rather, the goal here is to embed this analysis of comparative (largely domestic) political structures in a more enduring geographic and cultural foundation. This technique will keep the focus on the diversity of governmental types within relatively small geographic regions and thus enhance the quality of the comparative analysis.

The three divisions of the European zone evoke echoes of earlier religious traditions with the northern region roughly reflecting the impact of the Protestant Reformation, and the divisions within the southern and central areas corresponding to an earlier western (Roman Catholic) and eastern (Orthodox Christian) breakdown (Harbison, 1955; Geanakoplos, 1966).

The *northern* region is the birthplace of parliamentary democracy, the site not only of the "mother of parliaments" (Great Britain), but also of the first parliament (in Iceland in A.D. 930). It also includes France, a regional shatterbreak country (see **Table I.2b**), whose distancing away from southern and central Europe has been more episodic. The *southern European* region encompasses those European states bordering on the Mediterranean, Adriatic, and Black Seas. It can be divided politically into two camps—the "western" (Greco-Roman-Iberian) states, and the "eastern" (Byzantine, Balkan) countries. As such, this region remains a legatee to the Roman empire and its religious remnants. *Central Europe* refers to those nations at the heart of the continent dominated by Germany and Russia, whose struggles for influence have defined the international politics of this region for the past century, resulting in two world wars, a forty-five-year "Cold War," and the destruction of four empires (Russian, Prussian, Austro-Hungarian, and Soviet).

Religion is the obvious dominant factor in the Islamic zone, often called the "Middle East," a phrase with colonial overtones which made sense when London ruled most of the world. That term will not be used in this work, but two of the three regions in this zone do indeed represent bridges, or "midway passages," between Europe and other continents. A case could be made that this is the most conflict-ridden of the five zones (twelve of the thirty-three wars identified in Chapter 5), and religious differences are at the heart of many of its political disputes. The inclusion of non-Islamic Israel, Cyprus, Georgia, and Armenia within this zone (each annotated ^ on **Table I.2a**) explains, almost by definition, the central political difficulties facing these four countries. Even among the Muslim states, the differences between Shi'ite and Sunni Islam, as well as between secular and fundamentalist Muslims, undergirds much political struggle (Lewis, 1988).

The *west Asian* region includes most of the old Silk Route between southern Europe and China, and also represents a bridge from these two continents into the Arab world. Turkey and Iran have historically vied with Russia (and Britain) for political influence in this region (Menashi, 1994). The *Arabian peninsula,* on the other hand, includes the Arab heartland—the birthplace of the Prophet Mohammed, never violated by European colonialism and dominated today by the Saudi monarchy (Polk, 1991)—as well as states farther north and west (to the Mediterranean coast) which have had considerable interaction with European society, Israel being the extreme example. Finally, *north Africa* represents a second bridge from Europe, this time into the African continent; it is dominated demographically and historically by Egypt and includes other states which have had historic connections with (and substantial populations from) black Africa.

The divisions within the black African zone reflect not so much traditional cultural (i.e., tribal) differences as the more recent history of European imperialism. The divide-and-conquer tactics of this era were carried into the 1958 to 1980 decolonization experience which created an inordinately large number of states (42) in a relatively small geographic area. The result today is many weak countries with only rudimentary political structures and continued dependence on either the former metropolitan power or their larger neighbors (Asiwaji, 1985).

Western Africa is the site of the old slave coast; just as the Europeans carved up the region in furtherance of that evil institution in the seventeenth and eighteenth centuries, so too in the colonial nineteenth and twentieth centuries the divisions resulted in 15 states today, many too small and resource poor to be economically viable. Nigeria is the notable exception, though it may be too large (also a function of British colonialism) to be politically stable. *Central and eastern Africa*, a region with 90 percent of the world's

HIV infection (Economic Research Service, 1994), reflects a similarly dispiriting "Heart of Darkness," as Conrad called the area in his novel about penetrating the Congo River (the northern boundary of today's Zaire). Even in the east, where the core of Ethiopia was the only part of this zone not conquered by European imperialism, the political situation today is primitive in terms of the institutional standards to be discussed in this book. In *southern Africa*, the European presence lingered the longest and, in some respects, still dominates the newly multiracial South Africa.

The division of the Asian zone into south, east, and offshore regions reflects, in turn, the presence of India, China, and Japan, three historic civilizations whose current polities comprise 40 percent of humankind.

The *south As.·.* of the Indian subcontinent south of the Himalayan mountains is a highly heterogenous region, culturally and politically. The huge state of India alone contains more than a dozen sizable nations within it. Historically influenced by Hinduism, Buddhism, and Islam, and more recently by Great Britain, today the region has an interesting political mix of party systems heavily militarized to contain the myriad ethnic and religious differences found within it (Wriggins et al., 1992). The *east Asia* mainland includes China and the states on its periphery, which historically were in tributary relationship to the Chinese Middle Kingdom; the political influence of the world's largest culture continues to dominate the region (Kim, 1992; Rozman, 1993). *Offshore and oceanic Asia* includes two subregions: In the first are Japan and five of the six states of ASEAN, an economic–political entity which today effectively approximates the offshore goals of Japan's World War II East-Asia Co-Prosperity Sphere (Halliday and McCormack, 1973); in the second are grouped ten states of the south Pacific, an oceanic buffer zone for Asia vis-à-vis European and American sea power and the site of much of the fighting in that war. Today, the entire region is often referred to as part of the Pacific Rim and is still an area of shared ambition between Japan and the United States.

Finally, in the Western Hemisphere, the legacy of Spain and Portugal continues to challenge the immediacy of the United States. Even the manner of the Iberian colonial withdrawal from *south America* in the early nineteenth century has left its mark: the Portuguese departure resulting in one large state (Brazil); the more violent Spanish exit leaving several smaller republics in its wake. In both cases, however, the tradition of independence has put more distance between this region and that of the other two regions in this zone vis-à-vis the *north American* colossus (Smith, 1994). With the possible periodic exception of Mexico, the banana republics of *central America* have been particularly subject to intervention by the dominant neighbor to the north. The *Caribbean,* on the other hand, reflects more the interplay of other colonial powers (Britain, France, and, in the notable case of Cuba, Spain) with that of the United States (Watson, 1994).

Moving down from this global overview of the world's 187 countries, **Table I.2b** displays the 100 states chosen for further analysis in this book in the zones and regions defined above. As with the zones, the shatterbreak concept of states placed on the fringe of one region rather than another is also present in the demarcation of these regions. A Δ annotates some of the more debatable placements: Denmark and Finland in northern Europe despite their historic ties to Germany and Russia, respectively, in central Europe; France, whose large size and strategic location places it at the nexus of the northern, southern, and central regions; Moldova, which is designated in southern Europe related to Romania as opposed to in central Europe with Ukraine and Russia; Iraq, which is placed in the Arabian peninsula (to which it possibly aspired in its move into Kuwait in 1990) rather than in non-Arab west Asia; Cameroon, whose smaller, former English-speaking areas in the west now seem more thoroughly oriented to the franczone in former French Equatorial (i.e., central) Africa; land-locked Zambia, whose 1960s Chinese-built railroad to the east through Tanzania has not succeeded in redirecting trade and influence away from the southern routes through South Africa; and Myanmar (Burma), which has been isolated from both south Asia and southeast Asia for most of the past generation, but seems to be coming out in the southeast in the 1990s. Finally, the two states of north America (United States and Canada) are placed in Table I.2b in *both* central America and the Caribbean, as indicative of their dominance of both these regions.

Also in **Table I.2b**, in smaller print, are the names of all the non-ministate countries with more than 2 million population which will be "represented" in subsequent discussion by more significant prototype states in their regions. In addition to geographic and cultural propinquity, most states have similar polity types (as these will be defined in Chapter 1) to their surrogates. Listed below are the 39 excluded states, along with their "representatives" and the common polity types (using abbreviations explained in Chapter 1).

Excluded State	Representative
Norway, Finland	Sweden, Denmark—mpr, CO
Moldova	Romania—excom—>1pd
Albania, Croatia, Bosnia, Macedonia, Slovenia	Yugoslavia, Bulgaria—excom—> 1pd/mil°
Austria, Switzerland	Germany—mpr, federal
Latvia, Lithuania, Belarus, Slovakia	Russia, Ukraine, Czech Republic —excom—>1pd/~mpr
Armenia	Azerbaijan—excom —>mil°
Turkmenistan, Kyrgyzstan	Uzbekistan, Kazakhstan—excom—>1pd
Lebanon	Syria—mil^
Oman and four other Arab Persian Gulf states	Saudi Arabia—mon
Mauritania, Chad, Eritrea	Morocco, Sudan, Somalia—mon/mil°
Togo, Benin, Mali, Niger, Sierra Leone	Ghana, Burkina Faso—mil^*

Table I.2b
Comparative Government: Zones and Regions (100 states, with non-ministate alternatives in parentheses after prototypes)

Europe	Islamic Zone	Africa	Asia	West.Hemisph.
northern (7)	west Asia (7)	western (7)	south (6)	south Am. (8)
Ireland	TURKEY	Senegal	Afghanistan	BRAZIL
UNITED KINGDOM	Azerbaijan(Armenia)	Guinea	Pakistan	(Parag.,Urug.)
				Argentina
Sweden(Nor.,Fin.Δ)	Georgia	Liberia (S.Leone)	INDIA	Chile
DenmarkΔ		Ivory Coast		Bolivia
	Kazakhstan(Kyrgyz.)	Ghana(Togo)	Nepal	Peru
Netherlands	Uzbekistan(Turkmn.)	NIGERIA	Bangladesh	Ecuador
Belgium		Burkina Faso		Colombia
FRANCEΔ	IRAN	(Mali,Niger,Benin)	Sri Lanka	Venezuela
southern (7)	Arabian peninsula(6)	central-east (7)	east,mainland(8)	cent./n.Am.(6+2*)
Portugal	IraqΔ	CameroonΔ	MyanmarΔ	Panama
Spain	SAUDI ARABIA		Thailand	Costa Rica
ITALY	(Oman + 4 Gulf states)	ZAIRE(Congo,CAF)	Cambodia	Nicaragua
Greece		Rwanda(Burundi)	Vietnam(Laos)	(Honduras)
	Yemen			El Salvador
Bulgaria		Uganda	CHINA(Mongolia)	Guatemala
Romania(Mold.Δ)	Jordan	ETHIOPIA		
Yugoslavia	Syria(Lebanon)	Kenya	N.Korea	MEXICO
(Croatia,Bosnia,...		Tanzania	S.Korea	
Macedon.,Sloven.)	ISRAEL		Taiwan	UNITED STATESΔ
(Albania)				CanadaΔ
central (6)	n. Africa(7)	southern(6)	offshore (6)	Carib./n.Am.(4+2*)
Hungary	EGYPT	ZambiaΔ	JAPAN	CanadaΔ
GERMANY	Libya	(Malawi)		UNITED STATESΔ
(Austria,Switz.)	Tunisia	Zimbabwe	Philippines	
Czech. (Slovakia)	Algeria			Cuba
		SOUTH AFRICA	Malaysia	
Poland	Morocco		Singapore	Jamaica
Ukraine	(Mauritania)	Angola		(+ n=9 black Engl.-sp.)
(Latv.,Lith.,etc.)	Sudan(Chad)	Mozambique	Indonesia	
RUSSIA		(Lesotho)	(Papua N.Guinea)	Haiti
(Belarus)	Somalia(Eritrea)	Madagascar	Australia(N.Z.)	Dominican Rep.
				(TOT.100)
n=20	n=20	n=20	n=20	n=20
w/14 alternates	w/8+ alternates	w/10 alternates	w/ 4 alternates	w/ 3+ alternates

Notes: Δ =regional shatter-break states (n=10):
France, Denmark, Finland, Moldova; Iraq; Cameroon, Zambia; Myanmar; US, Canada.
Capital letters = most important state(s) in region (see Chapter 2d).   *= US and Canada in two regions.
smaller print = 39 non-ministate alternatives to 100 states for further study.

Congo, Central African Republic, Burundi	Zaire, Rwanda—mil°
Malawi	Zimbabwe, Zambia—1p-other/ 1pdom/~mpr
Lesotho	Madagascar, Mozambique—mil*^°
Mongolia, Laos	China, Taiwan, Vietnam —excom——>1pd/other
Papua New Guinea, New Zealand	Australia—mpr
Paraguay, Uruguay, Honduras	Brazil, Argentina, El Salvador, Nicaragua—*mpr
Nine black English Caribbean states	Jamaica, Dominican Republic —~mpr/mpr

Finally, it might be noted that, in both **Tables I.2a** and **I.2b**, are 20 states in capital letters representing the most important states in each region: the United Kingdom, France, Italy, Germany, and Russia in Europe; Turkey, Iran, Saudi Arabia, Israel, and Egypt in the Islamic zone; Nigeria, Zaire, Ethiopia, and South Africa in sub-Saharan Africa; India, China, and Japan in Asia; and Brazil, Mexico, and the United States in the Western Hemisphere. (The phenomenon of regional hegemony will be discussed at greater length in Chapter 2d.)

In any event, the arbitrary limits of 100 total states, and 20 in each zone, force the analyst to make priority choices among states worthy of further focus. Combined with the desirability of limiting the number of similar states to be compared to a reasonable number, the regional clusters of 6 to 8 states presented in Table I.2b are judged to be the optimum groupings for the purposes of making a balanced, global comparative study of the political systems of the world.

3 STUDYING THE "NATION-STATE" IN THE 1990S

Students of comparative government face a new world in the wake of the Cold War. The global community is no longer so protective of the territorial integrity of states, even if changes to some are brought about by force: witness its acceptance of the redrawing of the map of former Yugoslavia, of the emergence of Eritrea after the Ethiopian civil war, and even of a "protective zone" of autonomy for Kurds in northern Iraq. Accordingly, the demography and geography parameters introduced in this introductory chapter can be expected to be under periodic challenge as subnational groups within states whose governmental legitimacy is in question push for greater expressions of self-determination. This book will feature three significant **Tables** (1a, 4b, and 5b) which will endeavor to portray this phenomena, as well as *Formats* for the orderly display of data related to states of particular polity types, and *Excerpts* from the Data Bank of comparative information associated with this research.

Chapter 1's **Table 1a**—the Comparative Government Spread Sheet (CGSS)—lists (for the 100 states identified earlier) their current political types, divided into ten categories. Five civilian political systems (page 1 of Table 1a) will be studied in Chapter 3; 5 military polities (page 2 of Table 1a) will be covered in Chapter 6. Between these two chapters, the phenomena of nationalism and militarism in the 100 selected states will be analyzed in Chapters 4 and 5.

Chapter 4's **Table 4b**—Categories of Ethnic Analysis—will specify 50 of the 100 states as having the most significant ethnic or nationalistic challenges to their legitimacy. Chapter 5's **Table 5b**—Major Current (Violent, Domestic) Conflict—will list 33 of the 100 countries as sites where the most serious military challenges to governing legitimacy are currently being waged. (There is a signficant overlap between the states on these two tables, reflecting the fact that ethnic strife underlies most [25 of 33 in 1995] of the resorts to violence in the contemporary era (Sullivan, 1995).

One purpose of this study will be to investigate whether adoption of the political modalities and institutions of the civilian polities to be studied in Chapter 3 might help some of the culturally divided and conflict-ridden states, listed on Tables 4b and 5b and discussed in Chapter 6, accommodate their political systems to the ethnic and militaristic challenges to their legitimacy (Smouts, 1995).

A second significant methodological feature used throughout this study will be the various *Formats* to be presented. By providing for a regularized manner of collecting and displaying information on the 100 states, these *Formats* allow for the easy generation of tables of comparative data based upon the formatted information.

For example, in Chapter 2 (section 2f), the *Format* will identify five dimensions along which power can be measured in any political system. In Chapter 3, *Formats* will be proposed for comparing states in the two types of multiparty systems, the two forms of one-party systems, as well as the former communist states evolving toward either the multiparty or the one-party prototype. In Chapter 4, a system for ranking the salience of ethnicity within states will be suggested; and in Chapter 5, a framework for analyzing contemporary violent conflict will be proposed. Finally, Chapter 6's *Formats* will provide a means for measuring participation in each of the five militarized systems.

The third methodology to enhance this work involves **Excerpts** from the Data Bank associated with this research, carefully culled to represent states of particular polity types in proportion to their number among the 100 states selected for further study. All told, Data Bank **Excerpts** from 60 of the 100 states will be displayed; 12 from each of the five zones, chosen to highlight the most interesting and politically significant states.

In Chapter 2, **Excerpts** from 19 states will be presented to illustrate the various modes of power sharing; the data shown here are generally more permanent in nature than those displayed in the two chapters where the main forms of political systems are covered. These are Chapter 3, where 17 civilian polities will be excerpted, and Chapter 6, where 14 militarized political systems are shown. The Data Bank *Excerpts* in these two chapters are some-what more transitory in nature than those in Chapter 2 as regards which parties or personalities or institutions are most powerful at any point in time; but the *Format* for analyzing each of these factors is relatively enduring. Finally, by way of example of how the data in Chapter 4 can be used in Chapter 2's power-sharing *Format,* and how the data in Chapter 5 can be used in Chapter 6's *Format,* token numbers of *Excerpts* are displayed in Chapter 4 (8 states), and Chapter 5 (5 states).

The 60 states thus excerpted are selected to reflect geographic balance (12 from each zone), and to include the most important countries among the 100 on the CGSS. Among the states not excerpted, considered relatively less sig-nificant than the first 60, are the following 8 in each zone: Ireland, Sweden, Belgium, Portugal, Romania, Yugoslavia, Czech Republic, and Ukraine in Europe; Azerbaijan, Uzbekistan, Tajikistan, Iraq, Yemen, Libya, Morocco, and Somalia in the Islamic zone; Ghana, Guinea, Ivory Coast, Cameroon, Uganda, Tanzania, Zambia, and Madagascar in Africa; Afghanistan, Nepal, Bangladesh, Vietnam, Cambodia, North Korea, Singapore, and Australia in Asia; and Chile, Colombia, Peru, Ecuador, Costa Rica, Guatemala, Dominican Republic, and Canada in the Western Hemisphere. (Some of these countries may seem important and worthy of more consideration, but they are either in a state of transition and the data for them is dubious at the present time [e.g., Yugoslavia, Nigeria], or they are deemed less significant than the prototype state chosen to illustrate its political system in the *Excerpts* for this book (e.g., Russia for Ukraine, China for Vietnam, the United Kingdom for Canada).

Throughout this work, the combination of **Tables** for the comparative dis-play of countries' political, ethnic, and conflict systems; *Formats* for analyz-ing power along several dimensions within the different political systems; and *Excerpts* from the Data Bank to illustrate particular polities will provide the student of comparative politics with the analytic and conceptual tools to understand politics and government in the complex, new post–Cold War world of the twenty-first century.

REFERENCES

Arnold, G. (1993) *The End of the Third World.* New York: St. Martin's Press.

Asiwaji, A. I. (ed.) (1985) *Partitioned Africans: Ethnic Relations Across Africa's International Boundaries 1884–1984.* New York: St. Martin's Press.

Brass, P. R. (1992) *Ethnicity and Nationalism.* Thousand Oaks, CA: Sage.

Brown, L. R. and J. L. Jacobson (1986) *Our Demographically Divided World.* Washington, DC: Worldwatch Institute.

Cohen, S. B. (1991) "Global Geopolitical Change in the Post-Colonial World Era," *Annals of the Association of American Geographers,* 81(4): 551–580.

Collier, D. (1991) "The Comparative Method: Two Decades of Change," Chapter 2 in *Comparative Political Dynamics: Global Research Perspectives,* ed-ited by D. K. Rustow and K. P. Erickson. New York: HarperCollins.

Curtis, M. (ed.) (1993) *Introduction to Comparative Government*. New York: HarperCollins.

Dahl, R. A. (1989) *Democracy and Its Critics*. New Haven, CT: Yale University Press.

Economic Research Service of the United States Department of Agriculture (1994) "Africa and the Middle East."

Fornos, W. (1988) *Gaining People, Losing Ground*. Washington, DC: The Population Institute.

Fukuyama, F. (1989) "The End of History," *The National Interest*, 16(Summer): 3–18.

Gamer, R. E. (1994) *Government and Politics in a Changing World*. Madison, WI: Brown and Benchmark.

Geanakoplos, D. J. (1966) *Byzantine East and Latin West*. New York: Barnes and Noble.

Gottlieb, G. (1993) *Nation against State: A New Approach to Ethnic Conflicts and the Decline of Sovereignty*. New York: Council on Foreign Relations Press.

Gyohten, T. (1992) *Regionalism in a Converging World: A Report to the Trilateral Commission*. New York: Trilateral Commission.

Halliday, J. and R. McCormack (1973) *Co-Prosperity in Greater East Asia: Japanese Imperialism Today*. New York: Monthly Review Press.

Harbison, E. H. (1955) *The Age of Reformation*. Ithaca, NY: Cornell University Press.

Hauss, C. (1994) *Comparative Politics: Domestic Response to Global Challenges*. Minneapolis–St. Paul, MN: West.

Huntington, S. (1993) "The Clash of Civilizations," *Foreign Affairs*, 72(3, Summer): 22–49.

Jackson, R. H. (1991) *Quasi-States: Sovereignty, International Relations, and the Third World*. New York: Cambridge University Press.

Jacobs, L. R. and R. Y. Shapiro (1994) "Studying Substantive Democracy," *PS: Political Science and Politics*, 27(1): 9–16.

Kim, S. S. (1992) "China as a Regional Power," *Current History* 91(566): 247–252.

Lewis, B. (1988) *The Political Language of Islam*. Chicago: University of Chicago Press.

Magstadt, T. M. (1994) *Nations and Governments: Comparative Politics in Regional Perspective*. New York: St. Martin's Press.

Mahler, G. S. (1995) *Comparative Politics: An Institutional and Transitional Approach*. Englewood Cliffs, NJ: Prentice-Hall.

Menashi, D. (ed.) (1994) *Central Asia Meets the Middle East*. Portland, OR: Frank Cass.

Oman, C. (1994) *Globalisation and Regionalisation: The Challenge for Developing Countries*. Paris: OECD Publications.

Polk, W. R. (1991) *The Arab World Today*. Cambridge, MA: Harvard University Press.

Population Reference Bureau (1995) *World Population Data Sheet, 1995*. Washington, DC: Population Reference Bureau.

Rozman, G. (ed.) (1993) *The East Asian Region: Confucian Heritage and Its Modern Adaptation.* Princeton, NJ: Princeton University Press.

Smith, P. H. (1994) *Latin America in Comparative Perspective: New Approaches to Methods and Analysis.* Boulder, CO: Westview Press.

Smouts, M.-C. (1995) "The Meanings of Violence and Its Role in Legitimation," *Mershon International Studies Review* 39: 111–115.

Sullivan, M. J., III (1991) *Measuring Global Values: The Ranking of 162 Countries.* Westport, CT: Greenwood Press.

——— (1994) "Ethnicity and War in the Post–Cold War Era." Paper presented at the 49th Annual Convention of the New York State Political Science Association, April 28–29, New York.

United Nations Population Fund (1990) *The State of the World Population 1990.* New York: United Nations Publications.

Wallerstein, I. (1991) *Geopolitics and Geoculture: Essays on the Changing World System.* New York: Cambridge University Press.

Ward, M. D. (ed.) (1992) *The New Geopolitics.* New York: Gordon and Breach.

Watson, H. (ed.) (1994) *The Caribbean in the Global Political Economy.* Boulder, CO: Lynne Rienner.

Wriggins, W. H., F. G. Gause, T. P. Lyons, and E. Colbert (1992) *Dynamics of Regional Politics: Four Systems in the Indian Ocean Rim.* New York: Columbia University Press.

1

Frameworks of Analysis

1a POLITICAL SYSTEM (COMPARATIVE GOVERNMENT) TYPES

This book will analyze the governing structures in the 100 selected states by dividing them into two main polity types: civilian and military. **Table 1a**—the Comparative Government Spread Sheet, which appears on pages 21 and 22—has two parts. On its first page are listed (in their respective zones) 50 states divided into five civilian political systems; on its second page are displayed 50 countries divided into five militarized political systems.

The most salient factor in accounting for the ten different political systems is political parties—whether there are any at all, and what their strength and number is. While interest groups exist for various specific purposes, the political party is considered in this book as the essential organizing tool for seizing the machinery of government to make public policy in a state (Panebianco, 1988; Farrell, Holliday, and Janda, quarterly).

On page 1 of the CGSS are 50 states in which it will be argued that the civilian party is the most significant political institution. For the 50 countries on page 2 of the CGSS, civilian parties may exist, but the presence of organized force and violence (i.e., military might) is a more significant determinant of the political fortunes of the state.

It is a main contention of this work that the presence of at least two civilian parties (one running the government and one in opposition) is essential for a mature political system to exist (Weiner and Huntington, 1994). The vibrant functioning of the second or oppositional party, with a genuine opportunity to come to power if the governing party's policies prove to be unpopular with the citizenry, is necessary to provide a counter to unbridled governing power (Moore, 1966). As a corollary, if one or the other of these parties fails in its

Table 1a
Comparative Government Spread Sheet (p. 1)

Europe	Islamic Zone	Africa	Asia	West.Hemisph.

MPR = **Multiparty Republics** (n=25: 13+12)
3a. mpr = **multiparty republics** (n=13)

			Australia	Jamaica
UK,Ireland				Canada
Belgium,Nethrlds.				United States
Denmark,Sweden				Costa Rica
Germany, France				
Sbtot: 8			1	4 (13)

3b. ~mpr = **weak multiparty republics** (n=12)

			Japan	
Italy,Greece				Ecuador
Spain,Portugal				Venezuela
Czech.,Hungary				Dom.Rep.
Poland,Bulgaria				
Sbtot: 8			1	3 (12)
Tot.mpr: 16			2	7 (25)

****

3c. ex-com = **ex-communist** (n=19)
Czech.,Hung.,Pol.,Bulg.----->~mpr (n=4)
Rom.,Russ,Ukr.,Kazak.,Uzbek.----> 1pdom (n=5)
Yugo.,China,N.Korea,Vietnam,Cuba----> 1p-other (n=5)
Ga.,Azerb.,Tajik.,Afghan.,Cambodia----> mil°(n=5)

****

1PP = **One-Party Polities** (n=2 5:13+12)
3d. 1pdom = **one-party dominant** (n=13)

Romania		Senegal		
Russia		Cameroon		
Ukraine	Uzbekistan	Kenya,Zambia	Malaysia	
	Kazakhstan	S.Africa	Taiwan	Mexico
Sbtot: 3	2	5	2	1 (13)

3e. 1p-oth = **other one-party** (n=12)

Yugoslavia	Egypt	Ivory Coast	Singapore	
	Tunisia	Tanzania	China	
	Iran	Zimbabwe	Vietnam	
			N.Korea	Cuba
Sbtot: 1	3	3	4	1 (12)
Tot.1P: 4	5	8	6	2 (25)

****

TOT.CIV.: 20	5	8	8	9 (50)
Tot.mil: 0	15	12	12	11 (50)
TOTAL: 20	20	20	20	20 (100)

Notes:
MPR = more than one party has chance of gaining power, but this does not happen often in weak (~) mprs;
1PP = one party dominates political process, either through "structuring" (1pdom) or repression (1p-oth);
ex-com = former one-party communist state now in transition;
3a,3b,3c,3d,3e = sections of text (Chapter 3) where this polity type is discussed.

Table 1a
Comparative Government Spread Sheet (p. 2)

Europe	Islamic Zone	Africa	Asia	West.Hemisph.

MILP* = **Militarized Party Systems** = *s: (n=2 0: 20+0)
6a. *mpr = **militarized multiparty republic** (n=20)

			India,Pakistan	
			Nepal,Bangladesh	Arg.,Brazil,Chile
	Israel	Madagascar	Sri Lanka	Bolivia,Colombia
	Turkey		Thailand	Guatemala,El Sal.
			S.Korea, Phil. I.	Nicaragua,Panama

6b. *1pd = **militarized one-partydominant** (n=0)

Tot.*MILP:	2	1	8	9	(20)

****

MIL^o = **Military Regimes** (n=30: 14 +13 +3)
6c. mil^ = **moderating military** (n=14)

	Syria	Ghana, Guinea	Indonesia	Peru
	Iraq	Burkina Faso, Zaire		
	Yemen	Ethiopia,Uganda		
	Libya	Mozambique		Haiti

Sbtot:	4	7	1	2	(14)

6d. mil° = **entrenched military** (n=13)

	Georgia,Tajikistan	Liberia	Afghanistan	
	Azerbaijan	Nigeria		
	Algeria,Sudan	Rwanda	Myanmar	
	Somalia	Angola	Cambodia	

Sbtot:	6	4	3		(13)

6e. mon^o = **monarchies** (n=3)

| | Jordan,Morocco | | | |
| | Saudi Arabia | | | |

Sbtot:	3				(3)
Tot.MIL^o:	13	11	4	2	(30)

****

TOT:MIL: 0	15	12	12	11	(50)
Tot.civ.: 20	5	8	8	9	(50)
TOTAL: 20	20	20	20	20	(100)

XXXXXXXXXXXXXXXXXXXXXXXXXXXXXXXXXXXXXXXXXXXXXXXXXXXXXXXXXXXXXXXXXXXXXXXXXXX

6f. **Important Colonies/Aspirant Nation-States** (n=13)

	Palestine		Kashmir	
	Kurdistan	s.Sudan	Tamil Eelam	Puerto Rico
	W.Sahara		E.Timor	
	N.Cyprus		Tibet	Quebec
	Ngorno-Karabakh		Hong Kong	

	5	1	5	2	(13)

Notes:
MILP* = party states with heavy military influence (n=20): 20*mpr plus 0 *1pdom;
mil^ = moderating mil. regimes where military controls executive branch, but sometimes allows parties to run and be represented in a weak assembly (n=14);
mil° = entrenched mil. regimes, party activity is minimal/non-existent, civil war (n=13);
6a, 6b, 6c, 6d, 6e, 6f = sections of text (Chapter 6) where this polity type is discussed.

opportunity to gain power, it must know that it can remain organized and have another chance at power at a later date (Dahl, 1971; Lipset, 1990).

In the first part of the CGSS, five civilian polity types are identified and stratified based, more or less, on the existence and strength of one or more oppositional political parties. On the second page of the CGSS, five polity types are listed in descending order of the strength of political parties in these states vis-à-vis organized centers of military force and violence.

The division of the CGSS's 100 states into precisely 50 civilian and 50 military is somewhat arbitrary and intentionally so. Also suspiciously "round" are the numbers of 25 multiparty (MPR) and 25 one-party states (1PP), 20 militarized party states (MILP*), and 30 military regimes (MIL^o). There could be some disagreement as to the placement of certain states within these four major classes of polity types. In fact, on the boundaries of all ten polity categories can be found shatterbreak states, which arguably might belong in a higher or lower category.

Although precise definitions of these various political systems must await more extensive elaboration, a brief identification of some of these countries on the boundaries of the four major polity categories (separated by asterisks on **Table 1a**) might be made at this point. By so doing, some preliminary understanding of the way the CGSS will be used throughout this book to compare different countries and polity types will be gained.

For example, as between the multiparty republics and the one-party polities, Bulgaria, Poland, Hungary, or the Czech Republic might be moved further down the CGSS, page 1, and Romania, Russia, or Ukraine might be moved higher up. As regards the multiparty and militarized party category on the CGSS, page 2, Venezuela or the Dominican Republic might deserve to be moved lower, to the second page, whereas Israel, Turkey, India, or Colombia might be placed higher, on the first page.

On CGSS, page 2, military regimes such as Indonesia or Peru might be considered more multiparty than their current placement would indicate, whereas Madagascar, Thailand, or Nepal might be judged to be less so. As regards the lower halves of both pages of the CGSS, the civilian one-party states of Yugoslavia, Iran, China, North Korea, or Cuba might be deemed as more appropriately military, whereas Georgia, Syria, or Iraq might be considered less so.

The exact placement of particular states is not the essential item in this CGSS framework for analysis of government. What is more important is the argumentation behind any individual state-assignment, and whether the definition and data resulting in such judgment is sound.

The justifications of these decisions in the pages to follow will be more substantive and sophisticated than that which occurred during the Cold War, when there was a tendency to divide all polities into two types (democracies and totalitarians). In addition to parties and military institutions as independent variables in the determination of a state's polity type, this work will study other structures of government to see how those two main actors are being accommodated within their respective systems. The focus of analysis, however, is on processes and institutions, not on more abstract concepts like freedom, human rights, or democracy, which require a different methodology from that of this book (Bunce, 1990; Dahl, 1979; Freedom House, 1994).

Within the defined scope of its inquiry, however, this study will provide the conceptual tools to compare 100 countries and, by extension, all of today's 187 sovereign political entities as well as any others to emerge in the future. Data for confirming or updating the judgments for state placements in each of the ten polity types are readily available in numerous regularly published reference books on political systems (Banks, Clements, Europa, U.S. Central Intelligence Agency, U.S. Department of State, etc.) and on parties (Ameringer, 1992; Day and Degenhardt, 1988; Delury, 1987; Fukui, 1985; McHale, 1983).

With these tools of methdology and data collection, the conclusions drawn with respect to the 100 selected states for the period of the mid-1990s can be confirmed or contested, regularly updated, or applied to larger or smaller groups of states of interest to the individual reader. As such, this work is a worthy addition to the literature of comparative political analysis (Bebler and Seroka, 1990; Cantori and Ziegler, 1988; Chilcote, 1994). At this point, it is appropriate to look more deeply into the two basic divisions of states under scrutiny.

i Five Civilian Polities

Civilian polities will be defined as those in which most political power is in the hands of civilians. All governments are ultimately buttressed by some institutional military establishment, but in the civilian political systems, the control of the military by civilian policy makers is traditionally respected. The key leaders and decision makers are politicians with backgrounds in business, law, parties, or interest groups. The rule of law is respected.

A list and brief definitions of the five civilian polity types follow. Each is introduced with an indication of the section in which it is covered in this book (e.g., 3a through 3e), along with its abbreviation (mpr through 1p-oth), as these section numbers and abbreviations appear on the first page of the CGSS. Mention of some exemplar states in each category is also made. More extensive definitions can be found in the relevant sections of the later chapters.

3a. Multiparty republic (mpr)—two or more political parties participate; more than one has a credible chance of gaining power in a free and fair election (n = 13: e.g., United Kingdom, Australia, United States).

3b. *Weak* multiparty republic (~mpr)—two or more political parties participate; more than one has a credible chance of coming to power; but the structure of the system is weak, because either one party has ruled almost every year since start of this study (n = 2: e.g., Italy, Japan), the state is relatively new to mpr category, having been moved up within the past generation from a more militarized party system (n = 6: e.g., Spain, Ecuador), or from the one-party category where the state was dominated by a communist system (n = 4: e.g., Poland).

3c. Ex-communist state (ex-com)—formerly one-party communist states (i.e., one vanguard party directing the government and economy, and controlling the country's cultural life) now in transition; may be evolving into weak multiparty (if Communist Party has lost power in a multiparty election [n = 4, ex-com—>~mpr: e.g., Hungary]), or into a one-party dominant system (if the Communist Party, perhaps under a new name, has never relinquished power despite holding multiparty elections [n = 5, ex-com—>1pdom: e.g., Ukraine]). Such states could also be modifying their Marxist economic policies while retaining Leninist one-party systems (n = 5, ex-com—>1p-other: e.g., China), or could be hanging on to power in a state which has degenerated into civil war (n = 5, ex-com—>mil°: e.g., Tajikistan).

3d. One-party dominant (1pdom)—two or more political parties participate and have representation in the non-administrative branch of government, but the political system is structured (i.e., rigged) so that only one dominant party has a credible chance of gaining executive power in an election (n = 13: e.g., Malaysia, Mexico).

3e. Other one-party (1p-oth)—extremely limited civilian one-party rule due to fact that other parties (if allowed at all) are so restricted that they achieve only minimal (if any) representation in the non-executive branch of government (n = 7: e.g., Zimbabwe, Singapore), or the ruling party retains its commitment to Leninism and tolerates no opposition parties or even dissident factions within the vanguard party (n = 5: e.g., North Korea).

ii Five Military Polities

In military polities, the key political actors are military (or former military) officers. The state, moreover, has a record of governance by society's institutional military forces, or a history of civil warfare against some important segment of the population which has militarized significantly the country's political life. For these reasons, the rule of law is often suspended and replaced by martial law (or other forms of states of emergency). Signs of contemporary militarism (like heavy military spending or large percentages of the able-bodied population being members of military or paramilitary forces) are also prominent.

A list and brief definitions of the five military polity types follows. Each is introduced with an indication of the section in which it is covered in this book (e.g., 6a through 6e) and its CGSS abbreviation (*mpr through mon°). Exemplar states are also noted. Further discussion is found in the relevant sections of the later chapters.

6a. Militarized multiparty (*mpr)—a multiparty republic with a high degree of military influence over the system, owing generally to either a history of military coup rule, the impact of civil war or lesser forms of insurgency, or both (n = 20: e.g., Argentina, India, Turkey).

6b. Militarized one-party dominant (*1pd)—a one-party dominant system with a high degree of military influence for the reasons noted in the previous paragraph; at the time of publication, there are no such states, but in the recent past Madagascar, Bangladesh, Taiwan, or Sri Lanka might have qualified, and arguments could be made that Indonesia, Syria, or Iraq might belong there now.

6c. Moderating military regime (mil^)—the military controls the executive branch of the government, but allows parties to compete in elections and be represented in a weak assembly (n = 14: e.g., Yemen, Ghana, Guinea).

6d. Entrenched military regime (mil°)—political system beset by civil war, coup regime where party activity is minimal to nonexistent, or both (n = 13: e.g., Azerbaijan, Nigeria, Myanmar).

6e. Monarchy (mon°)—leader of state chosen from (and by) members of a royal family whose roots go back to some past military conquest (n = 3: e.g., Saudi Arabia).

As section 3 of the Introduction indicated, one reason for such militarism to be prominent in one-half of the 100 states selected for further scrutiny is the sub-national component present in many of today's 187 "nation-states." Most of these political entities have no signficant fit between the nation and the state, and are increasingly no longer held together by the structural contraints of the Cold War system. The result is domestic warfare, due to the presence of some ethnic group within the state which does not accept the legitimacy of the ruling regime.

Chapter 4 will analyze this phenomenon from the perspective of the culture match, or mismatch, between the purported "nation" and the "state." Chapter 5 will study force and violence in state politics and whether an ethnic/national component is a significant variable. Taken together, these two chapters will provide the foundation, and many substantiating data, for the selection of the 50 countries to go on page 2 of the CGSS and to be covered in Chapter 6.

But ethno-nationalistic conflict is not the only source of turmoil and illegitimacy in a state. Despite the end of the Cold War, there still can be political conflict over the proper organization of the economy, even in a 100 percent ethnically homogeneous society. It is to this second source of conflict—economic ideology—that this chapter next turns its attention, because differences in economic beliefs are often the reasons for the formation of many of the parties found in the civilian and military political systems (Hanley, 1994; Shaw and Bell, 1994).

1b ECONOMIC (AND OTHER IDEOLOGICAL)TYPES

i The Spectrum, inTheory and in Domestic Politics

The issue of economic ideological systems is often difficult to understand because the use of the words "liberal" and "conservative" is not consistent across different philosophic and political contexts (Susser, 1995) and there is often confusion between economic and political concepts. **Table 1b.i** attempts to clarify these matters by identifying some points along an ideological spectrum divided into economic, political, and "composite" parts.

This study posits an economic spectrum between socialism and capitalism, where socialism is defined as government macro-management of the economy, and capitalism refers to an economy controlled by private concentrations of wealth (i.e., transnational corporations [TNCs] and multinational corpora-

Table 1b.i
Economic (and Other) Ideologies

Spectrums
economic:
Govt.own/control/redistrib............private(TNC)own/control.................Govt.regulate/favor
            SOCIALISM----MIXED----LIBL./CAPITALISM----MIXED----CONS./PROTEC./FEUD.
"Names"   Marx   A. Smith
values: redistribute   cooperate   compete   protect/enhance
                help/care/share   every man for himself

            COMMUNISM-----------DEMOCRACY-----------FASCISM-----------MILIT./MON
political: 1 party.....................multiparty.......................1 party.......................NO party
"Names"   Lenin   Jefferson

            Composite economic-political spectrum, abbreviations
f-l=far left;   l=left;   l-c=left center;   c=centrist;   r-c=right-center;   r=right;   f-r=far right
    comm.............soc...........soc-dem.............libl..............cons..............fasc...........ethnic/theoc.
anarch.   (capitalism)   libertar.

Short ideological definitions:
communism = vanguard party controls redistributive economy, government, politics, and culture.
socialism = government controls macromanagement of economy, including social welfare programs; politics
    may be more or less pluralist.
soc.-democracy/dem.-socialism = govt. involved in economic regulation for social purposes; pluralist politics.
liberalism = "free" economy; minimal govt. redistribution/regulation/protection (i.e., capitalism).
capitalism = economy controlled by private concentrations of wealth (i.e., corporations, esp. TNC/MNCs);
    politics may be more or less pluralist.
conservatism=(multiparty) govt. protects private power concentrations in economy (esp. church).
fascism = (1-party, nationalist) govt. protects private power concentrations in the economy.
ethnic/theocratic= govt. protects/advances interests of a special (ethnic, religious, regional) group.

---

tions [MNCs]). Socialism is usually associated with the writings of Karl Marx—especially his *Communist Manifesto* (1848) and *Das Kapital* (1867)—and is often portrayed on the "left" of the U.S. domestic political spectrum. Capitalism relates to the writings of Adam Smith—especially his *Wealth of Nations* (1776)—and is typically considered to anchor the "right" wing of the American ideological spectrum.

However, it will be argued here that this bipolar division of economic systems is oversimplified. Capitalism, as defined by Smith, is more properly labelled *liberalism,* whose root is drawn from the Latin word *liber* (free), and means freedom (i.e., minimal government interference) in the economy. In the real world, there has never been an absolute "invisible" hand of no government policies and only market forces guiding an economy. All governments intervene to some extent to manage, guide, and regulate their economies; the essence of politics is determining the character and degree of intervention—for whose economic interest and on whose economic behalf.

If the government makes policies (i.e., intervenes) in a way which protects existing (i.e., status quo) private power concentrations in society, then that government can be said to have *conservative* economic policies. If the government intervenes for purposes of redistributing to (or favoring) the less powerful sectors of a society, then that government can be said to have *socialist* (not liberal) economic policies, particularly if socialism is defined (as by Marx) to include programs relating to the health, education, or general social welfare of its weakest members (e.g., the old, the young, the sick, the poor, and other typically marginalized groups).

In short, in most of the world the opposite of conservative is not liberal, as is often claimed in American political discourse, but socialist. Liberalism, in its classical sense as developed in eighteenth- and nineteenth-century industrial Europe, can be said to occupy a mid-point in the economic continuum, in recognition of the fact that all governments intervene in the economy. What defines much of politics are questions of "to what extent" and "to what purpose" (i.e., on whose behalf), that of the rich and powerful or that of the poor and dispossessed). As a result, all economies are mixed, to the extent that government intervention takes the form of regulating, or favoring, certain industries (Freeman, 1989) and of ignoring other economic activities. In many countries, politics centers around the issue of what these industries should be (e.g., aviation, atomic energy, health, education, coal, steel, transportation, communications, etc.), not whether the government ought to be in the business of making decisions about them in the first place.

Liberalism, then, if taken to mean total economic freedom from government control, is an archetype which does not exist (and never has existed) anywhere in the world. Its opposite in terms of government control would be *communism,* as defined by Lenin—writing in *Imperialism* (1895), and in *What Is to Be Done* (1905)—to mean total control of the economy (and of government, politics, and the wider culture) by a single, elite vanguard party.

This party not only would lead the revolution to overthrow the capitalist system controlled by private concentrations of wealth, but would then manage the economy for the purposes of the general welfare.

Like liberalism, however, communism is an archetype which has never existed for any length of time in its complete, totalistic form (though it came close to being practiced during the Stalinist period in the USSR and under Mao in China). The twentieth-century historical record of communist control of society—especially of the culture and of its Marxist redistributive economic goals—is that it does not survive the first generation of the revolution which overthrows capitalism in a given country.

One reason for the failure of communism in its ideal form, some have asserted, is that it does not conform to basic values found in human nature. As idealized by Marx, economic socialism had a redistributive ethic based upon all members of a society sharing and cooperating to help and care for each other. Capitalism, on the other hand, assumes human beings are naturally competitive and would act first to protect and enhance their own interests. In fact, both instincts can be found in the individual, and it is the realm of politics, not economics, that determines which aspect of humankind's nature will be appealed to as the basis for public policy.

It is when political terms become intermingled with economic ones that confusion ensues, particularly where the words liberal and conservative have been debased in the popular culture's need for shorthand code words. A similar confusion has perhaps already been created here with the use of the word communism, an essentially political concept referring to Lenin's theory of single-party government, as a kind of shorthand to refer to Marxism–Leninism, the combination of Lenin's one-party political ideology with Marx's redistributive socialist economic philosophy.

In this respect, on **Table 1b.i** the political opposite of Lenin's one-party idea is the *multiparty* philosophy illustrated by Thomas Jefferson's writing in the *Declaration of Independence* (1776) and the *U.S. Constitution* (1789). Although political parties are not explicitly mentioned in either of these documents, the idea of "government by the consent of governed" carries with it the implicit acceptance of an opposition (i.e., second) party to the group in charge of the polity at any particular time, and the ability of that party to change the government.

But just as socialism and capitalism do not exhaust all options in the economic realm, the two choices of one-party and multiparty are not the only possibilities in the political arena. To begin with, there is the situation of *no parties*, a common choice of many regimes, particularly those under the control of the military or other unrepresentative groups (monarchs, minority ethnic parties, etc.) as in the case of at least the last 30 states on the Comparative Government Spread Sheet.

Moreover, a single party can be applied not only to Marxist redistributive ends (i.e., communism), but rather to enhance and protect the wealth and privileges of the most powerful sectors of society. *Fascism* (as practiced in Mussolini's Italy, Hitler's Germany, and many developing nations in the contemporary era) is the most appropriate name to apply to what is essentially a "one-party–political, capitalist–economic" system reinforced by brutal methods of policy implementation (and appeals to nationalism) beyond those found in merely conservative societies.

A similar mix of political and economic forms comes in the case of *democratic socialism,* or social(ist) democracy, as it is sometimes called. Here there can be many parties in the political arena (i.e., pluralism), but the government is under the control of parties more committed to the redistribution of wealth (i.e., social welfare programs) than to the preservation of the status quo. Finally, the term *liberal democracy* can now be put in its proper context as liberalism (i.e., capitalism) in the economic arena and democracy (i.e., multiparty government by the consent of the governed) in the political sector.

The above terms are all combined and displayed on a spectrum from far-left to far-right in the final composite economic–political spectrum of **Table 1b.i.** Also included there, on the fringes, are a few more political philosophies: anarchism, libertarianisn, and ethnic–theocratic rule. The first two are extreme expressions of the desire for no government at all, reflecting respective leftist and rightist inclinations. Ethnic–theocratic rule is a narrower version of fascism wherein the favored group is an even smaller entity than that encompassed by the nation.

Understanding of the above words is necessary in order to have an appreciation of the way political–economic ideological terms will be used to describe the parties to be analyzed in Chapters 3 and 6. The designation *right* will be applied to states and political parties committed to the smooth functioning, and enhancement, of the global capitalist system. The designation *left* is reserved for those states and political parties which are trying to ameliorate the effects of the operation of this system by having government intervene to regulate and control the system, and perhaps even to redistribute some of its benefits.

Understanding these terms is particularly important in a world where traditional political identifications are increasingly challenged by the workings of the global capitalist economy. It is this relatively new phenomenon of international political economy, schematically summarized in **Table 1b.ii,** to which this chapter next turns.

ii The International Economic Reality

In today's global capitalist economy, there is significant government intervention despite a rhetoric of classical liberalism. The main challenger to this economic system—Marxist–Leninist socialist–communism, which at the height of its strength was embraced by about only a dozen states—is in retreat everywhere

Table 1b.ii
International Political Economy

Main State-Actor Groups:
G7 (core) = Group of Seven: US, Japan, Germany, France, Italy, UK, Canada.
OECD 25 = G7 + Western Europe, Australia, New Zealand, & (1994) Mexico.
NIC=New-Industrializing Semi-Periphery, n=~25:   Czech.,Poland, Hungary,Russia;
Egypt,Morocco,Saudi A.,Turkey,Israel,Iran;   S.Africa,Nigeria;
India,China,Taiwan,S.Korea,Singapore,Thailand   Brazil,Argentina,Chile,Mexico.
Periphery = remaining ~135 "developing" states.

Non-State Citadels of Capitalism and their *Functions:*
MNC/TNCs (n=1000s) = multinational/transnational corporations = *investments.*
World Bank/Intl. Monetary Fund(n=179) = make *loans* to enhance capitalist system.
GATT/WTO (n=123) = regulating regime for free (i.e., low tariff) international *trade.*
OECD DAC (Development Assistance Committee) (n=18) = monitors economic *aid* (1%
    GNP/yr. target)

---

around the world (Heilbroner, 1989). Bare subsistence, or illegal, "off-the-books" economic activity outside the reaches of formal capitalism, is also a waning phenomenon as the dominant system has expanded in recent decades to virtually every spot on the globe.

What remains as the most significant economic activity in the world is a capitalist system tightly managed and controlled by its central actors. It is summarized on **Table 1b.ii**, and it can be visualized by thinking of expanding concentric circles. At its core is that handful of wealthy states known as the "Group of Seven" (G7) leading capitalist countries—in descending order of economic output, they are the United States, Japan, Germany, France, Italy, the United Kingdom, and Canada—whose leaders meet annually in "economic summits" to coordinate policies and set goals for the following year (Putnam and Bayne, 1984; Williamson and Miller, 1987). Through their weighted voting rights, these states control the four main non-state citadels of the world capitalist system: the World Bank, the International Monetary Fund (IMF), the Organization of Economic Cooperation and Development's Development Assistance Committee (OECD DAC), and the World Trade Organization (WTO) (until recently known as the General Agreement on Tariffs and Trade [GATT]) (North–South Roundtable, 1995).

At a ring just beyond the inner core is a group of eighteen other rich countries (mainly European, plus Australia, New Zealand, and, added in 1994 pursuant to the North American Free Trade Agreement, Mexico) which together with the first seven form the OECD. Before the Group of Seven was formed in 1974, this was the main organization in which the leading capitalist nations of the core of the world system met to coordinate policy among themselves and to standardize measures for national accounting systems (Organization for Economic Cooperation and Development, annual).

Most countries in the world are on the periphery of this system, and are probably destined never to reach the level of development, industrialization, and modernization of the states in the core. The planet simply does not have the resources to sustain 2 billion Chinese and Indians (not to mention the populations of Africa, Latin America, and the rest of Asia) at the level of electricity, oil, and steel consumed by the average European today (Brown, 1981; Kane and Brown, 1995; Kennedy, 1993; O'Connor, 1994). Moreover, the states at the center, which make the rules according to which capitalism operates, are running the system not for the purpose of making underdeveloped coutries developed, but in such a way as to protect their own status and investment in the system (Sullivan, 1991: 99–100; Seligson and Passé-Smith, 1993).

There are perhaps another 25 countries (including the large, resource-rich states of Russia, Brazil, India, China, and several states in east Asia) which could be deemed to be on the "semi-periphery" of the capitalist core, with some chance of industrializing and attaining a quality of life somewhat comparable to the 25 rich states (Harris, 1987). But for the remaining 135 or so of the world's states, the rules of the system are not designed to bring them a better economic life (Adams, 1993; Arrighi and Drangel, 1986).

Table 1b.iii—Gross Domestic Product—provides a graphic look at this stratified world as of 1993, the latest year for which data are available (World Bank, 1995). At the bottom of the display are 35 economies from among the 100 CGSS states, each totalling less than $10 billion a year in economic output, a figure which is some sixty times less than that of the United States ($6,260 billion). At the top of the page are highlighted ten countries whose GDPs are more than $425 billion each, a listing which reveals that there is some question as to Canada's position among the Group of Seven. Since that institution was formed in 1974, Spain has overtaken Canada in output, and even more recently the former communist economy of China which today is so unregulated that some sources (e.g., the U.S. CIA; see ! on Table 1b.iii) estimate its GDP to be more than five times that reported by the World Bank.

To maintain the smooth running of this global capitalist system, the leaders of the Group of Seven meet each year in July in a summit of their heads of government to set various targets and guidelines for economic growth, investment, savings, consumption, inflation, unemployment, and the like within the system. Through the multilateral citadels of the capitalist system, the general policies which they agree upon each summer are given specific implementation throughout the rest of the year via a multitude of multilateral organizations which the seven core nations dominate to the point of virtual control.

These institutions are functionally specific as regards the main means by which the capitalist system operates and expands to encompass the rest of the world (viz., through aid, trade, loans, and investments). A synopsis of these instruments, discussed next, can be found in **Table 1b.ii**—International Political Economy: Non-State Citadels.

Table 1b.iii
Gross Domestic Product, 1993 (US$ billions)

Europe	Islamic Zone	Africa	Asia	West. Hemisph.
			Japan $4214.2	US $6259.9
Germany $1910.8			!China 2,350('93,CIA)	
France 1215.7				
Italy 991.4				
UK 819.0				
Spain 478.6				Canada 477.5
			!China 425.6	Brazil $444.2

\-----world's Top 10 economies > $400 bil./yr.-----/

Europe	Islamic Zone	Africa	Asia	West. Hemisph.
Russia 329.4			S.Korea 330.8	Mexico 343.5
Netherlands 309.6			Australia 289.4	
			India 225.4^	Argentina 255.6
Belgium 210.6			Taiwan 220.7^	
Sweden 166.7	Turkey $156.4			
Denmark 117.6	Saudi A. 121.5		Indonesia 144.7	
Ukraine 109.1			Thailand 124.9	
	Iran 107.3	S.Africa 105.6		
Poland 85.9				
Portugal 85.7	Israel 69.7		Malaysia 64.4	Venezuela 60.0
Greece 63.2			Singapore 55.2	
			Philippines 54.1	Colombia 54.1
Ireland 43.0	Syria 41.5e^			
Hungary 38.1	Algeria 39.8		Pakistan 46.4	Chile 43.7
	Egypt 35.0		Myanmar 45.8e	Peru 41.1
Czech Rep. 31.6	Libya 31.1^	Nigeria 31.3		
	Morocco 26.6		Bangladesh 24.0	Cuba 21.5^
Romania 26.0	Kazakhstan 24.7		N.Korea 19.9e^	
	Uzbekistan 20.4			
	Iraq 17.5e^			
Bulgaria 10.4	Tunisia 12.8		Vietnam 12.8	Ecuador 14.4
Yugo. 10.0^	Yemen 12.0	Cameroon 11.4		Guatemala 11.3

\----------$10 billion Cut-Off: Top 65/Bottom 35 Economies----------/

Europe	Islamic Zone	Africa	Asia	West. Hemisph.
		Zaire 8.4e^	Sri Lanka 9.4	Dom.Rep. 9.5
		Ivory Coast 8.1		
		Ghana 6.1		El Salvador 7.6
		Ethiopia 5.8		Costa Rica 7.6
	Sudan 5.6^	Senegal 5.7		
	Azerbaijan 5.0	Zimbabwe 5.0		Panama 6.6
		Kenya 4.7		
	Jordan 4.4	Angola 4.4e^		Bolivia 5.4
		Zambia 3.7	Nepal 3.6	
		Guinea 3.2		Jamaica 3.8
	Georgia 3.0	Madagascar 3.1		
		Uganda 3.0	Afghanistan 3.0e^	
	Tajikistan 2.5	Burkina F. 2.7		
		Tanzania 2.1	Cambodia 2.2^	Haiti 2.1e^
		Rwanda 1.4		Nicaragua 1.8
		Mozambique 1.4		
	Somalia .740e^	Liberia 1.4e^		
n=20	n=20	n=20	n=20 + 1!	n=20 (100)

Source: World Bank, *World Development Report 1995* for 1993 data, Table 3; plus ^US Arms Control & Disarmament Agency (ACDA), *World Military Expenditures and Arms Transfers (WMEAT) 1995* for 1993 data (GNP for Yugo.,Syria,Libya,Sudan,Iraq,Som.,Zaire,Liberia,Taiwan,NK,Myanmar,Afgh.,Camb.,Cuba,Haiti).
Notes: ! = widely varying estimates for China.   e=extrapolated data from ACDA, WMEAT.

Investments are largely the prerogative of multinational and transnational corporations, which are generally beyond the control of most governments (even the Core Seven) (MNCs/TNCs), except for some modest and rare taxation and regulation encumbrances. In fact, many would say that governments are significantly influenced by, and often do the bidding of, MNCs and TNCs nominally within their jurisdiction (Barnet and Cavanagh, 1994; Jenkins, 1987; Moran, 1985).

Loans are also in the purview of a subset of MNC/TNCs, commercial banks. But because loans to many areas on the periphery of the capitalist system can not be counted on to produce a profit (i.e., to be repaid with interest), the core states have set up quasi-governmental lending agencies such as the World Bank, several regional development banks (Culpeper, 1995), and the International Monetary Fund, which make loans not for profit but for the purpose of stimulating and enlarging the global capitalist system. Controlling votes over the policies of these institutions are based on the amount of capital contributed to them, with the lion's share of the power held by the Group of Seven nations and the other rich OECD states.

Trade is governed by the World Trade Organization, a body set up as the General Agreement of Tariffs and Trade in the late 1940s, with the goal of reducing tariff barriers around the world and promoting Adam Smith's idealized liberal capitalist system. The fact that this entity is still engaged, fifty years after its inception, in arguing for the reduction of national barriers to an open global trading system on a product-sector by product-sector basis and as concerns which states may or may not be part of other smaller trading associations, is testimony to the difficulty of reconciling the ideal of open markets with the reality of national, governmental protection of favored industries.

Finally, official development *aid* is part of a system set up by eighteen of the richest nations (in a special Development Assistance Committee of the OECD) to give away capital (in the form of grants or concessionary [low-interest, long-term] loans) to some states so poor that, if they did not receive such funds, they would barely be able to function within the larger system— that is, they would not be able to buy the products, repay the loans, or provide the infrastructure for the investing, expanding capital of the core.

For most of the world, the liberal–capitalist system has been the operative system for many years. Parties attempting to change or reform it so that it produces greater wealth and comfort for more people (as opposed to the way it has typically functioned in states outside the core) will be termed leftist. Parties which champion the continued normal functioning of the system, or even its expansion beyond the control of nation-state governments, will be designated rightist.

One final aspect of the economic ideology of capitalism which must be addressed before moving on to this study's primary focus of comparative political systems is the importance of *growth*. Economic growth is the life-blood of the capitalist system. Without growth there is no generation of excess capital which can be invested back into economic enterprise to maintain the system (Thirlwall, 1995). Growth is also part of the ideology of development: the belief that by playing according to the rules, the less developed countries of the periphery will eventually grow to the level of modernization of the states of the core, an assumption which is not necessarily true but which is essential to the stability of the system (Bailey, Burtless, and Litan, 1993; Hunt 1989; Nossiter, 1987).

From this perspective, then, it is important to know which states are improving their relative lot within the system. Because statistics on economic growth vary considerably from year to year, the World Bank annually reports a multiyear figure. **Table 1b.iv** presents these data for 1980–1993, a display which reveals that the mature capitalist states of the European core grow relatively slowly but steadily (between 1.3 and 3.1% per year, if the former communist states in transition are excluded), whereas Asian states grew the fastest (about 6% per year on average) in the most recent decade. Other states in the periphery had rates both higher and lower than the steady European norm. The point is that these figures show that the risks of capitalism vary more widely the further one moves beyond the European (and north American) core.

These macro- and state-level statistics, however, do not say much about the standard of living for individuals within specific countries, a situation which is affected by the type of governments found in individual states and the policies they adopt. Some such quality-of-life measures will be presented in the final chapter of this book, after the study of the various forms of political systems, the central focus of this work, is covered in Chapters 2 through 6.

Table 1b.iv
GDP Growth, Average Annual Percentage, 1980–1993

Europe	Islamic	Africa	Asia	West. Hemisph.
			China 9.6	
			S.Korea 9.1	
			Thailand 8.2	
			Singapore 6.9	
			Vietnam 6.8 ('90-4)Δ	
			Malaysia 6.2	
			Pakistan 6.0	
			Indonesia 5.8	
	Turkey 4.6		India 5.2	
			Nepal 5.0	
	Egypt 4.3		Cambodia 5.0 ('94)Δ	Chile 5.1
	Israel 4.1	Uganda 3.8	Bangladesh 4.2	
		Kenya 3.8	Japan 4.0	
		Burkina F. 3.7	Sri Lanka 4.0	Colombia 3.7
Ireland 3.8	Tunisia 3.7	Guinea 3.7		
	Morocco 3.7	Tanzania 3.6		Costa Rica 3.6
Spain 3.1		Ghana 3.5		
Portugal 3.0				
		Senegal 2.8		Dom.Rep.2.8
UK 2.7		Nigeria 2.7		USA 2.7
Germany 2.6	Iran 2.6	Zimbabwe 2.7		Canada 2.6
Netherlands 2.3	Somalia 2.4^			Ecuador 2.4
Italy 2.2			Taiwan-n.a.	Jamaica 2.3
France 2.1	Uzbekistan 2.2		Afghan.-n.a.	Brazil 2.1
Belgium 2.1	Algeria 2.1	Ethiopia 1.8		Venezuela 2.1
Denmark 2.0	Syria 1.8^	Zaire 1.6°		
Sweden 1.7			Phil. I. 1.4	Guatemala 1.7
				El Salvador 1.6
	Jordan 1.2	Rwanda 1.1		Mexico 1.6
Greece 1.3	Libya-n.a.	Mozambique 1.0(war)		Panama 1.3
Bulgaria 0.9	Yemen-n.a.	S.Africa 0.9 (sanctions)		Bolivia 1.1
Yugo. 0.8^	Iraq-n.a.	Madagascar 0.9		
Poland 0.7		Zambia 0.9		Argentina 0.8
Czech. 0.6^	Saudi A. 0.4	Angola-n.a.	Myanmar 0.8	
Ukraine 0.5		Liberia-n.a.		
	Sudan 0.3°	Ivory Coast 0.1		
		Cameroon 0.0		

--NO growth--

Europe	Islamic	Africa	Asia	West. Hemisph.
Hungary -0.1	Kazakh. -0.6			Peru -0.5(war)
Russia -0.5	Tajik. -0.8			Haiti -0.7^
Romania -2.5	Azerb. -2.2			Nicarag. -1.8(war)
	Georgia -6.1(war)		N.Korea -7.6('92)Δ	Cuba -40('89-93)Δ
n=20	n=20,w/ 3 n.a.	n=20, w/2 n.a.	n=20, w/ 2 n.a.	n=20 (100)

Source: World Bank, *World Development Report (WDR)1995,* Table 2; ^ WDR 94,93,92 thru 92,91,90
  (Yugo., Czech.,Syria,Som.,Haiti); °UNDP *Human Development Report 1994* for 1980-91(Sudan,Zaire);
  and ΔEconomist or NYTimes 1993-94 (NK,VN,Cambodia,Cuba) for years indicated.

Notes: "mature" capitalist states of Europe grow relatively slowly (<2%/yr.); east Asian "tigers" grew fastest in
  1980s; Latin America's debt kept it sluggish.
    Growth "ideology" = belief that growth will bring economic well-being, without government efforts at
  direction/redistribution of surpluses.
    n.a. = data not available for Iraq, Libya, Yemen, Liberia, Angola, Taiwan, Afghanistan.

REFERENCES

Adams, N. A. (1993) *Worlds Apart: The North/South Divide and the International System.* London: Zed Books.

Ameringer, C. D. (ed.) (1992) *Political Parties of the Americas: Canada, Latin America, the West Indies.* Westport, CT: Greenwood Press.

Arrighi, G. and J. Drangel (1986) "The Stratification of the World Economy: An Exploration of the Semiperipheral Zone." Paper Presented at International Studies Association Annual Convention, Anaheim, CA: 1–64.

Baily, M., G. Burtless, and R. Litan. (1993) *Growth with Equity: Economic Policymaking for the Next Century.* Washington, DC: Brookings Institution.

Banks, A. S. (annual) *Political Handbook of the World.* New York: McGraw-Hill.

Barnet, R. J. and J. Cavanagh (1994) *Global Dreams: Imperial Corporations and the New World Order.* New York: Simon and Schuster.

Bebler, A. and J. Seroka (eds.) (1990) *Contemporary Political Systems: Classifications and Typologies.* Boulder, CO: Lynne Rienner.

Brown, L. R. (1981) *Building a Sustainable Society.* New York: W. W. Norton.

Bunce, V. (1990) "The Struggle for Liberal Democracy in Eastern Europe," *World Policy Journal* 7(3, Summer): 399.

Cantori, L. J. and A. H. Ziegler (eds.) (1988) *Comparative Politics in the Post-Behaviorist Era.* Boulder, CO: Lynne Rienner.

Chilcote, R. H. (1994) *Theories of Comparative Politics: The Search for a Paradigm Reconsidered.* Boulder, CO: Westview Press.

Clements Encyclopedia of World Governments (annual) Dallas, TX: Political Research Inc.

Culpeper, R. (ed.) (1995) *The Multilateral Development Banks*, vols. 1–5. Boulder, CO: Lynne Rienner.

Dahl, R. (1971) *Polyarchy: Participation and Opposition.* New Haven: Yale University Press.

——— (1979) "Procedural Democracy," in *Philosophy, Politics and Society*, edited by P. Laslett and J. Fishkin. Oxford: Basil Blackwell, pp. 97–113.

Day, A. J. and H. W. Degenhardt (1988) *Political Parties of the World.* New York: Keesings.

Delury, G. (1987) *World Encyclopedia of Political Systems and Parties.* New York Facts on File.

Europa Yearbook (annual) 2 vols. London: Europa Publications.

Farrell, D. M., I. Holliday, and K. Janda (eds.) (quarterly) *Party Politics: An International Journal for the Study of Political Parties and Political Organizations.* London: Sage.

Freedom House (1994) *Freedom in the World: Political Rights and Civil Liberties, 1993–1994.* New York: Freedom House.

Freeman, J. R. (1989) *Democracy and Markets: The Politics of Mixed Economies.* Ithaca, NY: Cornell University Press.

Fukui, H. (ed.) (1985) *Political Parties of Asia and the Pacific.* Westport, CT: Greenwood Press.

Hanley, D. (1994) *The Christian Democratic Parties: A Comparative Perspective.* London: Pinter.

Harris, N. (1987) *The End of the Third World: Newly Industrialized Countries and the Decline of an Ideology.* New York: Penguin Books.

Heilbroner, R. (1989) "The Triumph of Capitalism," *The New Yorker* 23 January, 98–109.

Hunt, D. (1989) *Economic Theories of Development: An Analysis of Competing Paradigms.* Lanham, MD: Barnes and Noble.

Jenkins, R. (1987) *Trans-National Corporations and Uneven Development: The Internationalization of Capital and the Third World.* New York: Methuen.

Kane, H. and L. R. Brown (1995) *Full House: Assessing the Earth's Population Carrying Capacity.* New York: W. W. Norton.

Kennedy, P. (1993) *Preparing for the 21st Century.* New York: Vintage Books.

Lipset, S. M. (1990) "The Centrality of Political Culture," *Journal of Democracy* 1(4): 80–83.

McHale, V. (ed.) (1983) *Political Parties of Europe.* Westport, CT: Greenwood Press.

Monshipouri, M. (1995) *Democratization, Liberalization and Human Rights in the Third World.* Boulder, CO: Lynne Rienner.

Moore, B. (1966) *The Social Origins of Dictatorship and Democracy.* Boston: Beacon Press.

Moran, T. H. (ed.) (1985) *Multinational Corporations: Political Economy of Foreign Direct Investment.* Lexington, MA: Lexington Books.

North–South Roundtable (1995) *The UN and Bretton Woods Institutions: Challenges for the Twenty-First Century.* London: Macmillan

Nossiter, B. D. (1987) *The Global Struggle for More: Third World Conflicts with Rich Nations.* New York: Harper and Row.

O'Connor, M. (1994) *Is Capitalism Sustainable? Political Economy and the Politics of Ecology.* New York: Guilford Press.

Organization for Economic Cooperation and Development (OECD) (annual) *Development Cooperation Report.* Washington, DC: OECD.

Panebianco, A. (1988) *Political Parties: Organization and Power.* Cambridge: Cambridge University Press.

Putnam, R. D. and N. Bayne (1984) *Hanging Together: The Seven-Power Summits.* Cambridge, MA: Harvard University Press.

Seligson, M. A. and J. T. Passé-Smith (eds.) (1993) *Development and Underdevelopment: The Political Economy of Inequality.* Boulder, CO: Lynne Rienner.

Shaw, E. and D. Bell (1994) *Conflict and Cohesion in West European Social Democratic Parties.* London: Pinter.

Susser, B. (1995) *Political Ideology in the Modern World.* Needham Heights, MA: Allyn and Bacon.

Thirlwall, A. P. (1995) *Growth and Development, with Special Reference to Developing Economies.* Boulder, CO: Lynne Rienner.

U.N. Development Program (UNDP) (annual) *Human Development Report.* New York: Oxford University Press.

U.S. Arms Control and Disarmament Agency (ACDA) (1995) *World Military Expenditures and Arms Transfers (WMEAT) 1993–94.* Washington, DC: U.S. Government Printing Office.

U.S. Central Intelligence Agency (annual) *World Factbook.* Washington, DC: U.S. Government Printing Office.

U.S. Department of State (various) *Countries of the World and Their Leaders: Background Notes.* Detroit: Gale.

Weiner, M. and S. Huntington (eds.) (1994) *Understanding Political Development.* Prospect Heights, IL: Waveland Press.

Williamson, J. and M. Miller (1987) *Targets and Indicators: A Blueprint for the International Coordination of Economic Policy.* Washington, DC: Institute of International Economics.

World Bank (1995) *World Development Report (WDR), 1995.* New York: Oxford University Press.

2

Power Sharing in Ten Political Systems

Before considering each of the ten types of political sytems, this chapter will cover certain common elements of the way power is shared in almost every state, regardless of its governmental structure. These include the following:

1. The way power is divided within the executive apparatus of government; that is, between the person representing the state and the person running the government. Also, the significance of the head of the party (in one-party polities), and of the leader of the military (in militarized political systems).
2. The role of the representative assembly.
3. Other divisions of power (either specified in the constitution or recognized by de facto political arrangements) within the government, in lower levels of governing administration, and among groups representing particular interests.
4. Evidence of the state's dependence upon other forces (external, historic, geographic) not previously mentioned.
5. Electoral systems for legitimating the government.

2a EXECUTIVE BRANCH HEADS

Within the top level of the executive branch of government, power is often divided among four significant institutions: the head of state, the prime minister of the government, the leader of the main political party, and the chief of the armed forces.

The head of state represents the country and possesses control of its most treasured symbols (the flag, the anthem, etc.); he or she generally holds office for an extended period of time, and is considered to be "above the battle" of partisan skirmishes for power. The title most commonly given to the person holding this position is "president," but "king," "chancellor," or "governor general" are among the others used in the 100 states chosen for further study in this book.

The head (or first minister) of government makes day-to-day policy, which often can be controversial, and therefore is supposed to be more readily accountable to the citizenry. As a consequence, he or she generally has a shorter term of office, and often can be removed in the middle of the term if confidence is lost, either by some representative assembly of the people or by the head of state. The title most commonly held by this person is "prime minister" (Rose, 1988).

In some political systems, there is an "executive head of state" who performs both the state ceremonial functions and is the actual head of government as well. But if these positions are divided between two persons—as is the case in 56 of the 100 states selected for further study in this work—then the relationship between the head of state and the prime minister of government is the first one which must be assessed in any analysis of power sharing.

Table 2a graphically distinguishes between those states which have divided the positions of head of state and head of government, and those where these positions are held by a single person. As one moves down the Comparative Government Spread Sheet from the multiparty to the one-party to the militarized party to the military/monarchical regimes (MPR to 1PP to MILP* to MIL°), it can be seen that the percentage of states where these two roles are divided drops from 80 percent to 68 percent to 48 percent to 31 percent. Conversely, where these two roles are concentrated the percentages rise from 20 percent to 32 percent to 52 percent to 69 percent as one moves down the CGSS to the less participative systems.

Two other institutions are important in one-party polities and militarized regimes. In one-party states, where the government is considered an instrument of the party's rule, neither the head of the government nor the head of state is the most significant position. Rather, the head of the party (variously called the "secretary general," "chairman," or "[party] president") is the most powerful political actor. This person may also serve as head of state or government, but it is from the party position that the greatest strength is drawn. (For more information, see Chapter 3, sections 3c, 3d, and 3e.)

In military systems, the armed forces are a more important institution than either the head of state, the first minister of government, or any party (if the latter is tolerated at all). The head of the military sometimes arrogates to himself some or all of these titles; but it is equally common that he remains behind the scenes installing pliant puppets to serve in these roles. (For more information, see Chapter 6, sections 6a, 6b, 6c, and 6d.)

For analytic purposes in this study, the number of people (one, two, three, or four) holding these main positions will be taken as evidence as to whether power is being shared at the highest levels of government. It will be deemed a sign of maturity in the political system if these few positions are separated and not held by a single individual.

Table 2a
Head of State/Head of Government Relationship

Europe	Islamic Zone	Africa	Asia		West.Hemisph.

States where Head of State and Head of Govt. are divided (n=56)

mpr & ~mpr

Europe	Islamic Zone	Africa	Asia	West.Hemisph.	
UK,Ireld.,Belg.,Neth.			Australia	Canada	
Sweden, Denmark					
France,Germany				Jamaica	
~Spain,~Port.,~Italy					
~Greece,~Bulgaria			~Japan		
~Pol.,~Hung.,~Czech.					80%
16			2	2	(20/25)

1pp

Ukraine	Uzbekistan	Madagascar	Malaysia,Singpore		
Russia	Iran	Tanzania	Vietnam,Taiwan		
Romania,Yugo.	Tunisia,Egypt	Zimbabwe	China,N.Korea		68%
4	4	3	6		(17/25)

*mpr & *1pd

	*Israel		*India,*Pak.,*Nepal		
	*Turkey		*Thailand,*Phil.I.		
		*S.Africa	*Sri Lanka,*S.Korea		48%
	2	1	7		(10/21)

mil/mon

	Syria,Jordan		Afghanistan		
	Morocco		Myanmar		
	Algeria,Libya	Uganda	Cambodia		31%
	5	1	3		(9/29)
(20)	(11)	(5)	(18)	(2)	(56/100)

States where Head of State = Head of Govt. (n=44)

mpr & ~mpr

Europe	Islamic Zone	Africa	Asia	West.Hemisph.	
				USA, Costa Rica	
				~Dom.Rep.,~Venez.	
				~Ecuador	20%
				5	(5/25)

1pp

		Iv.Cst.,Senega,Kenya		Mexico	
	Kazakhstan	Cameroon, Malawi		Cuba	32%
	1	5		2	(8/25)

*mpr & *1pd

			*Bangladesh	*Arg.,*Brazil,*Chile	
				*Bol.,*Colombia	
				*Panama,*Nicaragua	
			*Indonesia	*ElSalv.,*Guatemala	52%
			2	9	(11/21)

mil/mon

	Georgia,Iraq	Liberia, BF,Nigeria		Peru	
	Yemen,Saudi A.	Guinea,Ghana			
	Sudan,Somalia	Zaire,Rwanda,Ethiopia			
	Tajik.,Azerb.	Angola,Mozambique		Haiti	69%
	8	10		2	(20/29)
(0)	(9)	(15)	(2)	(18)	(44/100)

TOT: 20	20	20	20	20	(100)

There are some explanations beyond polity type which account for how these top positions in the executive branch might be allotted. These relate to region and culture and can be inferred from **Table 2a**. In the Western Hemisphere, 18 of 20 states, including all the Latin American countries, plus the United States and Haiti (both of whose systems have some French influence), have the two top posts consolidated (Linz and Valenzuela, 1994; Pierce, 1994); only Canada and Jamaica, with their northern European heritage, have the positions divided. In Africa, 15 of the 20 countries concentrate the heads of state and government, whereas in Europe, all 20 states have them divided, as do 18 of 20 in Asia. A more mixed pattern appears in the Islamic zone (11 divided, 9 concentrated).

2b REPRESENTATIVE ASSEMBLIES

A directly elected representative assembly (also called a parliament, congress, legislature, etc.) is a second institution which might share power in a government. The number of these which are truly independent and serving such a function is only about half of those which exist in the world (Olson, 1994); the rest are, rather, rubber-stamp bodies created by and serving a legitimating purpose for either a ruling dominant party or a military regime. Some states have no representative assemblies at all (Sullivan, 1991: 330; Copeland and Patterson, 1994; Norton, 1995). Depending on the strength of the assembly, the resulting government will be one of the following three types.

In *parliamentary* systems (usually multiparty republics, with weaker variations in other polity types), the leading ministers of the government (i.e., the cabinet, including its prime minister) must be nominated by the legislature and come from within its membership. The executive is thus, in some respects, a creature of a relatively strong representative branch. In most political systems, however, power is concentrated in the executive branch, either in a president directly elected by the people, or in a president or prime minister, perhaps formally ratified by the representative assembly, but actually chosen by the dominant party or the military (Lijphart, 1992; Shugart and Carey, 1992).

There are a few *mixed* parliamentary/presidential systems where a directly elected president is chosen separately from the assembly and sometimes vies for power with the prime minister, who comes out of the relatively strong representative body (e.g., France, Portugal, and four others in Chapter 3, section 3a). In *presidential* systems, the head of state, whether directly elected or chosen by a weak assembly, may appoint a prime minister who serves as head of the government at the pleasure of the president (e.g., Ghana and many African states), or the president may reserve this role for himself (e.g., Argentina and most Latin American states).

Regardless of whether the assembly is strong or weak, **Table 2b.i** lists the number of representatives in each assembly for this study's 100 states. It also draws attention to a few other matters characteristic of this institution of alleged mass-political participation, whose purpose is often, surprisingly, to *dilute* the representation of the popular will. Working up from the bottom of Table 2b.i, these features would include the following.

Eight states have no functioning assembly, as of 1995. One of these countries (Saudi Arabia) has never had such an institution: Its totally appointive "counsultative council" is not considered to be a representative assembly according to this book's definition; it has only advisory, and no decisional, powers. The other seven countries—Algeria, Nigeria, Myanmar, and so on—have had experience with a representative decision-making body, but it has been suspended by the current ruling military junta. Such expressions of the peoples' will, however weak or symbolic, are usually among the first political institutions to be eliminated when a military regime takes control of government.

Three countries (Libya, Sudan, and China) have representative assemblies which are indirectly elected by lower levels of government or by the ruling party. Other states may also have a small number of members of the representative assembly either indirectly elected or appointed (usually by the head of state or head of government), sometimes to give representation to minority ethnic or political groups, sometimes to increase the power of the ruling party.

Among the 89 remaining representative assemblies, the number of representatives ranges from 57 in Costa Rica to 945 in Italy's bicameral body. These numbers could be divided into the population to see how many citizens are representated by each member of the assembly, and states ranked accordingly.

With respect to second houses of assembly, **Table 2b.ii** shows that most (or 54) of the 100 states have unicameral assemblies. In the 35 states which have two chambers of representation, the larger Lower House (LH) has most or all of its members directly elected by the people, whereas a more significant percentage of members of the smaller Upper House (UH) is often appointed, or indirectly elected, in a way which ensures representation of certain interest groups in society. Even if the Upper House is entirely directly elected, each member represents a larger constituency than would be the case in the Lower House, or sometimes represents federal or other geographic subdivisions. In 6 of the 35 states with Upper Houses, the members are predominantly appointed.

2c CONSTITUTIONAL AND OTHER POWER DIVISIONS

Other dimensions of power sharing within political systems involve constitutional or more informal arrangements which provide for the participation in government of important societal groups. Several of these mechanisms will be discussed in the four parts of this section.

i Constitutions, Courts, and States of Emergency

The constitution is a written document which sets down the basic power relationships between the main actors in a government, especially its execu-

Table 2b.i
Numbers Elected to Representative Assemblies

Europe	Islamic Zone	Africa	Asia	West. Hemisph.	
Italy 945			India 792		
France 898			Japan 752	Brazil 594	
Germany 740		Zaire 310-780		Cuba 589	
Russia 628			N.Korea 655-87		
UK 651	Turkey 550	Ethiopia 548		Mexico 592-624	
Poland 560		S.Africa 490	Indonesia 500	US 535	
Spain 558->607	Egypt 444				
Romania 484			Vietnam 395	Argentina 321	
Ukraine 450			Thailand 391		
	Morocco 333				
Hungary 386			Bangladesh 330		
	Yemen 301			Canada 295	
Sweden 349			Pakistan 304		
	Iran 270	Mozambique 250	S.Korea 299	Colombia 263-4	
	Syria 250	Tanzania 244			
Greece 300	Iraq 250		Phil.I. 274-5		
Czech.Rep.281	Uzbekistan 250	Angola 223	Nepal 265	Venezuela 250	
	Georgia 250	Uganda 200			
Bulgaria 240		Kenya 200			
Portugal 230		Ghana 200	Sri Lanka 225		
			Australia 224		
Ireland 226	Tajikistan 181	Cameroon 180		Chile 158-166	
Netherlands 225	Tunisia 163	Ivory Coast 175		Bolivia 157	
Belgium 221		Zimbabwe 150	Malaysia 192	Dom.Rep.150	
Denmark 179		Zambia 150	Taiwan 164	Peru 120	
Yugoslavia 178	Azerbaijan 125	Madagascar 137		Haiti 110	
	Israel 120	Senegal 120		Nicaragua 90	
		Guinea 114	Cambodia 120	El Salvador 84	
		Burkina Faso 107		Guatemala 80	
	Jordan 80		Singapore 81	Ecuador 72-77	
				Panama 67	
	Kazakhstan 67			Jamaica 60	
				Costa Rica 57	
n=20	n=15	n=17	n=17	n=20	(89)

- -

	Libya 618-631†		China ~3000†		(3†)
	Sudan 300†				

† = mainly indirectly elected

- -

None=0	None=3	None=3	None=2	None=0	(8)
	Saudi A.(never)	Liberia(80-90)	Myanmar (489)		
	Somalia(177)	Rwanda (70)	Afghanistan(426)		
	Algeria(430)	Nigeria (670)			
20	20	20	20	20	(100)

Notes: Totals do not include Upper Houses whose members are predominantly appointed
(e.g., UK, Jordan, Thailand, Malaysia, Jamaica, Canada); they are included if appointed number is minimal.
Parentheses indicate number in last assembly before abolition.

Table 2b.ii
Number of Houses of Assembly

Europe	Islamic Zone	Africa	Asia	West. Hemisph.

Unicameral Assembly, directly elected, n=54

Europe	Islamic Zone	Africa	Asia	West. Hemisph.
Sweden	Israel,Syria	Burkina Faso,Guinea	Bangladesh	Ecuador
Denmark	Turkey	Senegal,Iv.Coast	Sri Lanka	Peru
Ukraine	Iran,Iraq	Ghana, Cameroon	IndonesiaΔ	El Salvador
Bulgaria	Ga.,Azerb.	Zaire,Angola	TaiwanΔ	Nicaragua
Portugal	Tajik.,Uzbek.	Kenya,Uganda	NKor.,SKor.	Panama
Greece	Kazakhstan	Tanzania,Zambia	VN,Cambodia	Guatemala
Hungary	Morocco,Yemen	Mozmbq.,Zimbabwe	Singapore	Costa Rica
	Egypt,Tunisia	Madagascar,Ethiopia		Cuba
7	14	16	9	8 (54)

Δ = 2nd houses serve primarily as presidential electoral colleges (Taiwan, Indonesia). (See 2e.)

Bicameral Assembly, mostly elected (incl. indirectly elected=†), n=29

Europe	Islamic Zone	Africa	Asia	West. Hemisph.
Italy 630+315			India 542+250	Brazil 513+81†
France 577+321†			Japan 500+252	Mexico 500+92(-128)†
Russia 450+178			Pakistan 217+87	US 435+100
Germany 672+68				Argentina 252+69
Spain 350+257(208+49)		S.Africa 400+90		
Poland 460+100			Phil.I. 250+24	
Romania 341+143			Nepal 205+60	Colombia 160+100
Czech.Rep. 200+81			Australia 148+76	Venezuela 201+49
Ireland 166+60				Chile 120+38
Netherlands 150+75†				Bolivia 130+27
Belgium 150+71				Dom.Rep. 120+30
Yugoslavia 138+40				Haiti 83+27
12		1	6	10 (29)

Bicameral Assembly, predominantly appointed Upper House, n=6

Europe	Islamic Zone	Africa	Asia	West. Hemisph.
UK (~1150)	Jordan (40)		Malaysia (58-69)	Canada (104)
			Thailand (270)	Jamaica (21)
1	1		2	2 (6)

- -

NOT Primarily Directly Elected (†), n=3

Europe	Islamic Zone	Africa	Asia	West. Hemisph.
	Libya,Sudan		China ~3000>135	
	2		1	(3)

> = China has "inner core" of assy. with higher (often "standing") duties.

(See also: pre-1993 Russia, and ministates Norway, and pre-1992 Mongolia).

- -

No currently (12/95) elected representative assembly, n=8

Europe	Islamic Zone	Africa	Asia	West. Hemisph.
	Saudi Arabia	Nigeria	Myanmar	
	Somalia	Liberia		
	Algeria	Rwanda	Afghanistan	
	3	3	2	(8)
TOT: 20	20	20	20	20 (100)

tive and representative branches (Goldwin, 1990). The constitution is some-times interpreted and enforced by a third, or judicial, branch of government whose independence is often compromised by a powerful executive in many states.

The existence of an independent judiciary enforcing a rule of law is signifi-cant in defining the relationship between the executive apparatus of the state (the bureaucracy) and its citizenry. This relationship is in turn determined by the degree of subservience or dominance between the courts (particularly the highest court in the land) and the executive branch of government. This equa-tion is influenced by such factors as how many actors within the political system have control over the appointment and dismissal of judges, the term of office of judicial appointees, and whether the courts have judicial review powers (i.e., can the courts declare actions of the government to be illegal or unconstitutional?).

With respect to the appointment of judges to the national court, the best way to ensure judicial independence is to have more than one political actor involved, such as the head of government recommending names for approval by a representative assembly, with final appointment by the head of state. In many countries, only one or two of the above participants are involved; in one-party states, the input of the ruling party may be the only significant factor. (For variations of practice across different cultural traditions, see But-ler, [annual]; Franklin and Baun, 1994; Khadduri, 1984; Verner, 1984.)

Concerning term of office, judges, to be independent, should not serve terms concurrent with those of their appointers. Most countries ensure that judges have fixed terms longer than those of the executive or legislative branch of the government that names them (i.e., generally in the range of five to ten years; often until some fixed age like seventy or seventy-five; sometimes for life). Finally, many high courts have powers of review over civil and criminal matters adjudicated in lower courts, and over political matters decided at lower levels of government. Very few courts, however, have such judicial review power with respect to acts of the national executive or legislative branches of the government (Fletcher, 1987; Cappellitti, 1971).

Regardless of the normal relationship between the courts and the ruling administration, the powers of the judicial branch, and indeed the constitution itself, can be suspended if the government declares a state of emergency (Chowdhury, 1989; Finn, 1991). Among the 100 states in the Comparative Government Spread Sheet, virtually all of the military regimes have at some point abolished or suspended the constitution and ruled using martial law, which transfers the entire judicial process to military courts, making it easier to imprison anyone disagreeing with the military seizure of power. Such states of suspended law are also frequently invoked by civilian governments when they are challenged by insurgencies or riots, and sometimes even when they are faced with more peaceful general strikes or mass political demon-strations. In civilian regimes in general, however, such states of emergency are limited with respect to time and place.

Charles Humana (1992), in his classic study of human rights based upon state compliance with forty different instruments of international law, ranks states on the basis of the independence of their judiciaries. Using the methodology employed by Sullivan (1991: 240, 292), Humana's states can be ranked on a scale of 1 through 4, with 1 being the most independent court system. The results of this scoring are produced in **Table 2c.i.**

ii Cabinets, Councils, Conferences, and the Like

Additional insight into how power is shared in a government can be gained by analyzing the role of the prime minister's cabinet, as well as that played by any important councils, committees, commissions, conferences, and conventions.

The cabinet consists of the persons chosen by the head of government to administer the various agencies and departments of the executive branch. The size of the cabinet can vary from a few persons, in cases where the prime minister wants to centralize power, to several dozen, in cases where the head of government uses the cabinet to reward political supporters from diverse constituencies. Sometimes rivals or leaders of contending factions within the ruling coalition use their Cabinet Ministries (particularly departments with large budgets or a military–security mission, like Defense or Interior) to build alternative bases of power and patronage (Rose, 1987).

As mentioned earlier, in parliamentary systems of government, all Cabinet Ministers must also be elected members of the representative assembly (i.e., they are politicians who are aided in their new posts with deputies drawn from society's technocratic elite or from the bureaucratic career civil service). In other systems, prime ministers may appoint Cabinet Ministers from any strata of society and indeed often use this power to reward or co-opt important interest groups in the country.

Councils—also often called commissions or committees—are groups of persons in, or on the fringes of, government who sometimes assume unexpected importance depending on the ad hoc circumstances of particular regimes and countries. In one-party states, the party's politburo (political bureau) and central committee are more important than the representative assembly whose members they propose to the electorate for endorsement (see Chapter 3, section c). In military regimes which have not built any other institutional structure, a military council (which often goes by a name such as the "committee of national salvation") initially serves as the junta's cabinet, and often remains in an oversight capacity during the transition back to civilian rule (see Chapter 6c and 6d). First-generation revolutionaries sometimes play a similar role (e.g., Iran has three councils of revolution defenders). Monarchies often try to create the appearance of representativeness with the appointment of "advisory" councils. In all polities, inner sanctums of the larger cabinet exist, such as the "National Security Council" of those ministers dealing with war and peace issues.

Table 2c.i
Independence of Judiciary Systems/Courts

Europe	Islamic Zone	Africa	Asia	West. Hemisph.
		1 (n=23)		
UK, Ireland,France				US, Canada
Belgium, Nethrlds.	Israel	Senegal	Australia	Costa Rica
Denmark, Sweden		Zimbabwe		Argentina
Spain, Portugal				Brazil
Italy, Greece				
Germany				
Hungary,Bulgaria				
14	1	2	1	5
		2 (n=35)		
Czechoslovakia	Turkey	Ivory Coast	India,Bangladesh	Chile, Peru
Poland	Egypt		Sri Lanka,Nepal	Bolivia,Ecuador
Romania	Saudi A.	Mozambique	Thailand	Venezuela
USSR	Algeria	S. Africa	Singapore	Jamaica
				Nicarg.,Panama
	Jordan	Ethiopia^^	Japan	El Salvador
			S. Korea	Guatemala
	Morocco	Zambia	Philippines	Dom.Rep.
4	6	5	9	11
		3 (n=19)		
Yugoslavia	Iraq	Ghana, Nigeria	Afghanistan	Colombia
	Yemen	Cameroon	Pakistan	Mexico
	Tunisia	Rwanda, Uganda	Indonesia	
	Kazakhstan^	Kenya, Tanzania	Malaysia	
		Angola		
1	4	8	4	2
		4 (n=15)		
	Iran		Myanmar	Cuba
	Syria	Zaire	Vietnam	
	Libya,Sudan		Cambodia	
	Azerbaij.^,Somalia^		China	
	Tajik.^,Uzbekistan^		N.Korea	
0	8	1	5	1
n=19	n=19	n=16	n=19	n=19 (92)
n.a.=Ukraine	n.a.=Georgia	n.a.=Guinea,Liberia	n.a.=Taiwan	n.a.=Haiti
		Burkina F.,Madag.		

Sources: Humana, 1992, Table 27, for n=104 states, including 18 states not in CGSS's n=100; ^Freedom
House, 1994, for n=5 (ex-Soviet Islamic, Somalia); and ^^*Economist,* July 30, 1994, n=1 (Ethiopia).
Note: n.a. = data not available for n=8 states.

Finally, the device of a national all-party conference, or convention, has been used by many countries, particularly in Africa in recent years, to open up tightly constricted political systems. The Conference on Democracy in South Africa (CONDESA) brought together 26 parties between 1991 and 1994 to plan the transition away from apartheid; similar bodies performed comparable roles, with varying degrees of success, in Zaire, Ethiopia, and Madagascar (see Chapters 3d and 6c).

iii Decentralized Federal and Autonomous Units

No matter how small, the 187 states identified in the Introduction are *sovereign,* that is, they admit to no higher legal authority over themselves in any matters, regardless of political reality. About one-third of the 100 states in the Comparative Government Spread Sheet, however, have provided for decentralization of power which transfers some degree of authority over political matters to small units within the larger jurisdiction. The reason for only an approximate number of states identified with such subunits relates to the various ways in which power is shared between the national, or central, government and its lower levels of jurisdiction, and the fact that there is some ambiguity as to exactly what is meant by terms such as "federal" and "autonomous," used to describe these subunits of government (Ornstein and Coursen, 1992). **Table 2c.iii** lists states in three types of such lower levels of government after defining relevant terms in Part a.

Federal or *federated* subunits are those which have most rights of government permitted to them, except those few (generally relating to the army, currency, international trade, and foreign policy) reserved for the center. Most important, such subunits can elect their own governors and representative assemblies, can tax their citizenry, and can run their own schools and police forces. They also often have specific input into the composition of the national government, sometimes with respect to the selection of the head of state (as in the U.S. electoral college), more commonly in the Upper House of the representative assembly. Part b of **Table 2c.iii** identifies seventeen states with federated subunits of varying degrees of strength (e.g., Russia, India, United States) and weakness (e.g., Belgium, Venezuela).

Autonomous subunits have only those rights of government which are explicitly permitted to them by the center. They generally relate to language, religion, schools, and cultural matters, and are usually granted to territorial jurisdictions where people are of a different ethnicity from the majority in the larger society (Coakley, 1993; Duchacek, 1987). There are 15 states with autonomous sub-units of some significance displayed in Part c of **Table 2c.iii**, a list which could be expanded if the definition of "significance" were expanded, and if more de facto as well as de jure situations were included (see Iraq, Tajikistan).

Table 2c.iii
Significantly Decentralized States

(a) - Most Important Decentralization Definitions

sovereign entities - admit of no higher legal authority in any matters.

federal entities - most rights permitted to them, except those reserved for the center (army, currency, trade, foreign policy, etc.)

autonomous entities - have only rights explicitly permitted to them by center (generally relating to language, religion, schools, cultural matters, etc.)

colony - the direct rule or control by people in one political jurisdiction over *another* nation or people, generally geographically separated. (See Chapter 6f.)

Europe	Islamic Zone	Africa	Asia	West.Hemisph.
(b) - Federated Subunits, n=17				
√Russia (89:21+66+2)		Nigeria (30)	India (26+6u)	US (50+1)
Germany (16)				Mexico(31+1)
			Malaysia (13:4+9r)	Brazil (26+1)
			Australia (6)	Colombia(27)
Belgium(3)				Argentina(22+1+1)
				Venezuela(20+2+1)
Yugoslavia (2)		Tanzania (2)	Pakistan (4)	Canada (10+2)
n=4		n=2	n=4	n=7 (17)
(c) - States with Important Autonomous Subunits, n=15				
√Russia (21)	Georgia (2)	Ethiopia('94:9:7+2)		
Italy (20)	Uzbekistan (1))		China (5)	
Spain (17)	Azerbaijan (1)		Bangladesh (3)	
Portugal (2)	Tajikistan(pre-'92:1)		Sri Lanka (2)	
Ukraine (1)	Iraq('70-4,'91ff:1))		Philippines (1)	
n=5	n=5	n=1	n=4	(15)

(d) - colonies and "possessions," especially of former empires, n=47

UK=14 - incl.: Hong Kong (scheduled return: 1997), Channel I., I. of Man, Bermuda, Gibraltar, Caymans, Virgins, Montserrat, Turks & Caicos, Anguilla, St. Helena, Falkland I., British Indian Ocean Territories (Diego Garcia), & Pitcairn I.

France=9 - including: Reunion, Guadeloupe, Martinique, Polynesia, New Caledonia, French Guiana, Mahore/Mayotte, Wallis & Fortuna, St.Pierre & Miquelon.

US=8 - incl.: Puerto Rico, Guam, Virgins, N.Marianas, Am.Samoa, Midway I., Wake I., Johnston Atoll.

Australia=3 - Coco I., Xmas I., Norfolk I.	N.Zealand=3 - Cook I., Niue, Tokelau.
Denmark=2: Greenland, Faeroes	Spain=2: Ceuta, Melilla .
Neth.=2: Antilles(Aruba,Bonaire,Curacao), Aruba .	Norway = 1: Svarlbaard
Port.=1: Macao (sked. return: 1999)	Finland=1: Aaland I.
Chile=1: Easter I.	

Notes:

+ = special districts (e.g., Washington, D.C.; union territories in India; royal states in Malaysia; etc.).

√ = Russia in both lists, with 21 former Soviet ethnic republics (16) & oblasts (5) now autonomous, and 68 other geographic regions (including Moscow and St. Petersburg cities) having federal status.

See also Table 4c for names of identifiable ethnic groups in subunits.

Finally, many countries have *colonies* or *possessions*—a phenomenon discussed at greater length in Chapter 6f—which today have a greater degree of self-government than in the past. A complete list of forty-seven such entities is found in Part d of **Table 2c.iii**.

iv Interest Groups

The power of interest groups in government is covered in many other sections of this work (e.g., ethnic and religious groups in Chapter 4, the military in Chapter 5), but the concept deserves some additional elaboration here, before the discussion of power sharing is completed (Thomas, 1993).

Important economic groups include workers and peasants, corporate businesses and trade unions (Brown, 1990; Davis, 1989; Frenkel, 1993). Particularly in states heavily dependent upon one or two natural resources or crops, the transnational corporations which produce and market the product often have a special significance in the political arena (Moran, 1985; Turner, 1991). Sometimes the permanent government bureaucracy itself is a signficant actor, wielding power as elected politicians come and go. Japan—especially its Finance Ministry and Ministry of Industry, Trade, and Investment—is particularly notable in this regard (Koh, 1989; Palmer, Leila, and Yassin, 1988).

The concept of a niche in government for aristocratic nobles or wealthy landholders was the historic justification for many of the Upper Houses of assembly (e.g., England's House of Lords; Malaysia's Senate, where eighteen of the sixty-nine members come from the assemblies of nine states with hereditary rulers). Thailand reserves many seats in its Upper House for the military. In Jordan, Canada, Jamaica, and Nepal, the appointed Upper Houses include a mixture of important economic actors and politicians. Finally, the power of a family of a charismatic leader still commanding political loyalty years after it has lost its official position (e.g., the Bhuttos in Pakistan, the Nehru–Gandhi family in India, Rockefellers and Kennedys in the United States) might be noted.

Although ethnic groups will be discussed at greater length in Chapter 4, some mention might be made here of a few examples of explicit ethnic representation in the representative assembly (see Chapter 2b) and in federated or autonomous entities of government (see 2c.iii). With respect to representation, Singapore requires its thirteen legislative constituencies to be represented by three-member teams, one of whom has to be non-Chinese. Pakistan and Egypt used to set aside seats in their assemblies for women; Pakistan still has separate electoral rolls for ten non-Muslim seats, and Egypt reserves places for "workers and peasants." Jordan saves eighteen seats out of forty in its Upper House for Bedouins, Christians, and Circassians.

Of the seventeen federal states noted in the previous section, eight are explicitly and substantially subdivided along ethnic lines: Russia, Belgium, Yugoslavia, Nigeria, Tanzania, India, Malaysia, and Pakistan. (This is not the case in Germany, Australia, or in the seven states in the Western Hemisphere, with the lone exception of one of Canada's ten provinces [Quebec].) Of the fifteen states with autonomous subunits, all have subdivisions based upon ethnicity, some of great political significance (e.g., Russia's Tatarstan, Spain's Basque region, Ukraine's Crimea, Iraq's Kurdistan [1970–1974 de jure; via outside duress since 1991], China's Tibet, and Sri Lanka's Jaffna [Tamil] peninsula).

Finally, religion, in addition to being an aspect of ethnicity, is a deep-seated part of the culture in many states, which may or may not become politically relevant depending upon the actions of both the political and the religious elites (Juergensmeyer, 1993; Moen and Gustafson, 1991; Williams, 1989).

For some examples of non-ethnic interest groups, see line 2c.iv in the *Excerpts* from the power-sharing data bank for nineteen states at the end of this chapter.

2d OTHER DEPENDENCIES

There are other factors, not directly connected to immediate political institutions, which affect the way power is shared in any polity. These would include international dependencies (e.g., military, economic) and the weight of a country's history and geography.

Militarily, many states are dependent upon outside powers for their security. The degree of dependence can range from membership in a protective alliance, to the establishment of a military aid and trade relationship, to the actual hosting of another country's troops on one's soil.

A state's membership in a military alliance could involve nothing more than one state's "promise to consider" coming to another's defense in case of an overt attack. Other alliance memberships entail a network of trade in military hardware (planes, tanks, armor, etc.), which often brings with it an economic aid component of credits to finance the purchase of the arms, as well as the sending of military trainers to explain the proper use of the equipment purchased (Sullivan, 1991: 72–73; Klare, 1984; Louscher and Salamone, 1987; Pierre, 1995). Finally, each of the previously mentioned functions might bring with it the permanent stationing of troops of the more powerful partner in an alliance in the territory of the less powerful member.

An extreme example of military dependency would be the NATO and Warsaw Pact Cold War alliances, which established permanent bureaucratic machinery dominated by the two super powers, and the "hosting" of hundreds of thousands of troops of the two dominant partners on the territories of the smaller alliance members. But a degree of exclusivity to the point of dependence regarding aid, trade, and basing rights can also characterize other more ad hoc military relationships between stronger and weaker parties (Catrina, 1988; Harkavy, 1989).

Economically, dependence is created when a smaller country develops a near exclusive trading or investment relationship with a more powerful "partner." As with ties in the military sector, extremely poor countries often become dependent upon economic aid from the larger party (or its multilateral lending organizations—see Chapter 1b) in order to finance the trade purchases or the infrastructure to lure investments. Even large countries like Mexico and Canada have more than half of their trade dependent upon a single country (the United States); the situation is more precarious for some of the former African colonies of France which, in addition to having only one main trading partner, also produce only one main product to be purchased by this partner (Cunliffe and Laver, 1985; Cardoso and Faletto, 1979; Emmanuel, 1972).

The establishment of stronger and weaker parties in these military and economic arrangements often traces itself back to some enduring historic and geographic realities.

Table I.2a indicated in capital letters the dominant state (or states) in each region. According to this framework, there were 20 states in the world with hegemonic positions in their respective regions—the United Kingdom, France, Italy, Germany, Russia, Turkey, Iran, Saudi Arabia, Israel, Egypt, Nigeria, Zaire, Ethiopia, South Africa, India, China, Japan, Brazil, Mexico, and the United States—including six regions (northern Europe, central Europe, west Asia, Arabian peninsula, central-east Africa, central America) where dominance is shared, or contested, between two countries. Although some of these countries are fairly insignificant by many absolute measures of power (e.g., Israel, Zaire, Ethiopia), within their regions they carry a disproportionate influence. Other states (e.g., United States, United Kingdom, France, Russia) carry a weight beyond the confines of a single region, or even a single zone (Camilleri and Falk, 1992). One of the main reasons for this is the history of European colonization over the past 125 years.

Table 2d is a schematic display of the decolonization process which has created some 121 new states since the end of World War II. Of these states, 50 were former colonies of Great Britain and 26 of France (actually 50.5 and 26.5, respectively; Vanuatu, the former New Hebrides, was jointly colonized by the United Kingdom and France), and these two colonial powers continue to retain significant economic and cultural (e.g., through the *lingua franca*) power in these countries today. This situation also obtains for the lesser historic colonial powers like the United States (vis-à-vis the Philippines), Portugal (vis-à-vis Angola), Russia (vis-à-vis Georgia, Azerbaijin, etc.), Japan (vis-à-vis Korea), and others.

Table 2d.i gives some selected examples from the Data Bank associated with this book of military, economic, regional, and neo-colonial dependencies still affecting countries (and the way power is shared in these countries) to this day. More can be found in line d of the *Excerpts* from the Power Sharing Data Bank for nineteen states at the end of this chapter.

Table 2d
New States

Islamic Zone	African	Asian	West.Hemisph./Eur.
ex- (22-Egypt)	57-Ghana	47-India	62-Jamaica
B 32-Iraq (M)	60-Nigeria	47-Pakistan(E&W)	62-Trinidad
R 46-Jordan (M)	61-Sierra Leone	48-Myanmar (Burma)	66-Guyana
I 48-Israel(M)	61-Tanzania(M)	48-Sri Lanka (Ceylon)	66-Barbados
T 56-Sudan (w/Egypt)	62-Uganda	(49-e.China)	73-Bahamas
I 60-Somalia(w/Italy)+	63-Kenya	57-Malay(si)a	74-Grenada
S 60-Cyprus	64-Zambia,Malawi	65-Singapore	78-Dominica
H 61-Kuwait	65-Gambia	65-Maldives	79-St. Lucia
67-(S.)YemenΔ	66-Lesotho,Botswana	70-Fiji	79-St. Vincent
71-Bahrain,Qatar	68-Swaziland	71-Bangladesh(E.Pak.)	81-Antigua,Belize
(n= 71-Oman,UAE	76-Seychelles	78-Solomons	83-St.Chris/Nevis
50.5)	80-Zimbabwe	84-Brunei	64-Malta

-- 80-Vanuatu --

Islamic Zone	African	Asian	West.Hemisph./Eur.
ex- 43-Lebanon (M)	58-Guinea		
F 44-Syria(M)	60-Cameroon(M),Togo(M)	54-Laos	
R	60-Gabon,Senegal	54-Cambodia	
E 56-Morocco(&W.Sah.)+	60-Benin(Dahomey)	54-Vietnam(N&S)	
N 56-Tunisia	60-Burkina F.(UVolta)		
C 60-Mauritania(&W.Sah.)+	60-Mali,Madagascar		
H 60-Chad	60-Niger,Ivory Coast		
62-Algeria	60-C.Af.R., Congo		
(n= 77-Djibouti	68-Mauritius		
26.5)	75-Comoros		

	African	Asian	West.Hemisph./Eur.
14 ex- 91-Ga.,Armenia,Azerb.			91-Latvia,Lith.
RUS/ 91-Kaz.,Kyrg.,Uzb.			91-Estn.,Belar.
USSR 91-Tajik.,Turk.			91-Ukraine,Moldv.
4 ex-YUGO:			90-Slov.,Croat.
4 ex-PORT.	74-Guinea Bissau		91-Bosn.,Maced.
4 ex-USA:	75-Angola, Moz.,76-CVerde		
4 ex-USA:		46-Philippine I.	
		86-Marsh.,Micron.(T);94-Palau(T)	
3 ex-JAPAN:		48-N.Korea & S. Korea	
		49-Taiwan & (ne China)	

	African	Asian	West.Hemisph./Eur.
ex:BELG.	60-Zaire, 62-Rw.,Bur.(M)		
SPAIN (76-W.Sahara)+	68-Eq.Guinea,75-STP		
ITALY 51-Libya; 60-Somalia (w/UK)+			
NETH.		49-Indonesia	75-Suriname
NZ/AUSTRL:		62-W.Samoa(T);75-Papua NG(T)	
DNMK.			44-Iceland
GER./S.AF.	90-Namibia(M)		
CZECH:			93-Slovakia
ETHIOP. 93-Eritrea			

Subtot:	30	39	25	13	13	(121)
(NEVER	Iran,Turkey,(Egypt)	Ethiopia	(China),Jap.,Thaild.,	22 in WH		
recently	Saudi A.,(N.)YemenΔ	s-Liberia-1848	Afg.,Nep.,Bhut.,Mong.		29 in EUR.	
COLONIZED)		s-S.Africa-1910	s-Australia,N.Zealand			
	5	3	9	22	29	(67)
TOT.	35 w/ Δ=2 Yemens	42	34	35	42	(188)

Notes: #=yr. of indep.; M=Mandate; T=Trusteeship; s=settler state, pre-1945; ( )=never *fully* colonized;
+ = ex-Spanish Sahara absorbed by two state, Somalia emerged from two states.

Table 2d.i
Notable International "Dependencies"

Ireland - EU subsidies; UK economy; US emigrants. Dependent on UK for N.Ireland solution.
Italy - heavy US influence since WWII occupation. Still 13,000 troops.
Germany - EEC/EU, NATO, G7 multilateral memberships to divert post-WWII fears of neighbors.
Russia - $28bil. aid from G7, promised 6/93; via: World Bank & IMF ($10b. tot.), European Regional Bank, &
  especially from US,Germany,Japan. Also, $16bil. in stretched out debt service.
ex-USSR republics now dependent on Russia and Commonwealth of Independent States (n=12). 12/93
  Tashkent meeting established mutual tax policies, joint military headquarters for "technical cooperation",
  stationing of Russian troops still in Belarus, Armenia, Georgia, Kazakhstan, Kyrgystan, Tajikstan.

Georgia - dependent on Russia since 1801 liberation from Persia; 1993 mutual defense treaty allows 10,000
  Rusian troops to stay indefinitely in bases (land,sea,air) including key spots like Poti, on Black Sea.
Tajikistan - 25,000 Russian troops protecting vs. Afghan.& Tajik rebels there. '94 Russ. aid = 70% CGE, 30%
  more than when part of USSR. 12/93 conversion to new Russian rouble after $100m. loan.
Israel - US $3 bil./yr. aid since 1979 Camp David Agreement; $10b. '93-97 loan guarantee delay led to
  government change in '92. $56 b. in US aid since '48; + diplomatic/military protection. US aid, loans, gifts
  = 12% GNP(=$60b.). Leading trade (X+M=$2.8 bil.) partners: 1. US, 2. Germany.
Egypt = US $2.3bil./yr. aid since 1979 Camp David Agreement; $35 b. in US aid,1975-93, incl. $19b. econ.,
  $16 b. military. Gets 10% of all OECD DAC aid = ~$6 b./yr. Got $2.3b./yr. from Persian Gulf states after
  sending troops to1991 Iraq-Kuwait war. US forgave its $9b. bilateral debt for help during this war.
Jordan - historic $1m./yr. US CIA retainer for King. $500 m./yr. fm. Gulf Arabs until '91 war tilt toward Iraq.
Sudan - since 12/91, Iran sends free oil, Revolutionary Guard trainers (n=1500), sells arms.

Ivory Coast - n=500 French troops; 40% exports needed to service debt, paid by France in '92.
Zaire - historically dependent on Belgium,US,World Bank & IMF; all boycotting in $-transfers since '91.
Uganda - 60% Cent.Govt.Expenditures from Western aid keeps country to economic right, 3/93.
Kenya - Western aid cut-off (~$1 bil./yr., #1 & 2 = Japan and UK) led to multi-party elections in 12/92,
  acceptance of IMF austerity package, 2/93.
Angola - UN peacekeeping; US-Portugal-S.Africa oversight. Oil = 95% exports; 75% of its exports to US (its
  #1 trading partner), incl. 65% its oil. 60% oil export-$ from Cabinda enclave. #2 export=diamonds.

Nepal - landlocked dependency on India, home to politically important Koirala family when in exile.
Taiwan - diplomatic relations with only 29 states (6/95), up from low of 21 in 1979. Ties to China despite non-
  recognition, esp. in economy: $14 bil. in trade, 20,000 business with $20 bil. invested (1993).
Cambodia - UN peacekeeping; Japan economic ties; China, Vietnam, Thailand strategic dependence.
Korea - historically dominated by either: 1. China; 2. Japan; 3. Russia; 4. successors thereto (US).
N.Korea - $1.1b./yr. in remittances (of $26 b. GNP) from 300,000 Koreans in Japan. 6/95 nuclear reactor deal
  with US-Japan-S.Korea consortium will increase dependence on them.
Phil. I. - still strong dependence on colonial power US (50% foreign investment, 40% its exports) despite
  departure of its 17,000 troops in 1992.

El Salvador - UN peacekeeping; US military & economic aid, especially in 1980s ($300m./yr.=$30b. total).
Panama - historic dependence on 1903 neo-colonial creator/midwife USA. Most recently 1989-94 govt. via
  US invasion. 10,000 troops, now "renting" in returned Canal zone; "national" currency is US dollar.
Nicaragua - US aid: $535m. in 1st 2 Chamorro years '90ff, one of highest per cap.; + $284 forgiven debt; '92-
  93 aid (~$100m./yr.) often delayed for President's not getting rid of Sandisita DM (Ortega) fast enough.
Mexico - US economic influence, esp. after 1/94 North American Free Trade Agreement. More than 2/3
  trade (X+M) with US. 1/95 $40 billion bail-out of peso by US.
Dom.Rep. - US mil. intervention & show of force (respectively) in 1965 and 1978 government changes.
Canada - US economic influence. ~2/3 trade (X+M) with US, including 75-80% exports (=20% GDP).

2e ELECTIONS AND ELECTORAL SYSTEMS

The final aspect of governance to be discussed in this chapter relates to elections, exercises in political participation often proclaimed as the ultimate in power sharing between the governed and their rulers. In fact, it will be argued here that elections are generally evidence not of popular participation in the choice of leaders, but rather of acquiescence in selections made by other, more signficant actors in the political process. Especially in one-party states, military regimes, and monarchies, the electoral process serves the legitimating function, whereas the true choice of leaders occurs within the party, the military, or the royal family. Even in multiparty states, the election is often the last act of a drama in which the final choices have been structured by more signficant personalities (party leaders, wealthy supporters of individual candidates) earlier in the process (Lewis-Beck, 1988; Booth and Seligson, 1989; Bartolini and Maaiar, 1990; Sullivan, 1991: 321–323).

To understand this thesis, one must study the modes and forms of elections held across the 100 states chosen for study (Jennings and Mann, 1994; Taagepera and Shugart, 1989). **Table 2e** is presented to help in this analysis. It shows (section A) that of the 100 states, 35 do not have direct elections for the head of state or government at all, but only for a representative assembly, and that 12 governments have had no recent legitimizing electoral exercise at all (section D) as of 1995. The remaining 53 countries have had elections for both a representative assembly and an executive head of state): 34 of these (section B) being elected at different times for different terms of office (a device for increasing the power and independence of each institution at the expense of the other) and 19 of these (section C) being elected at roughly the same time for the same term of office (a situation which generally enhances the power of the executive branch).

The assembly-only electoral route to executive selection—the most common situation, in 35 of the 100 states—results in the indirect selection of a country's leaders. The most common example of the indirect election of the head of government occurs in the parliamentary multiparty republics (the most "democratic" form of government in the popular mind), where the only election that is held is for the representative assembly (and this may not be a national referendum at all, but rather a series of local contests), which then chooses the head of government from among its members. According to **Table 2e**, this is the situation in 20 multiparty republics (including the weak and militarized variations), as well as in 15 other one-party and military regimes where elections are generally more tightly restricted than in the mprs.

Direct elections, in which the head of state or government is chosen by unfiltered universal adult suffrage, occur in the 53 countries of the electoral Categories B and C on **Table 2e**. But of these, only 24 are in multiparty republics (and, of these, 7 are weak ~mprs and 13 are militarized *mprs, each

Table 2e
Electoral Systems by Three Main Types

Europe	Islamic Zone	Africa	Asia	West.Hemisph.

A. Assembly only (incl. parl. Leg.>PM type) (n=35)
mpr,~mpr,*mpr (n=20)

Europe	Islamic Zone	Africa	Asia	West.Hemisph.
UK,Sweden,Denmark			Australia	Jamaica
Belg.,Nethrlds.,Germany				Canada
~Spain,~Greece				
~Italy,~Czech.Rep.			~Japan, *Nepal	
	*Israel		*India, *Pakistan	
	*Turkey		*Thailand	

1pdom,1p-oth.,*1pd (n=6)

Europe	Islamic Zone	Africa	Asia	West.Hemisph.
Yugoslavia		*S.Africa	Malaysia	Cuba
			Vietnam, N.Korea	

mil^,mil°,mon(n=9)

Europe	Islamic Zone	Africa	Asia	West.Hemisph.
	^Iq.,°Ga.,^Yem.	^Uganda	Indonesia (Δ)	
	^°Jord.,^°Mor.	^Ethiopia	°Cambodia	

B. Separately elected Pres. & Assembly, for different terms of office(n=34)
mpr,~mpr,*mpr(n=15)
(incl. 5 or 6 Europ. "mixed" mprs by defn.; assy somewhat strong than in "C")

Europe	Islamic Zone	Africa	Asia	West.Hemisph.
Ireland,France			*Bangladesh	USA
~Portugal				~Ecuador
~Hungary			*S.Korea	*Chile,*Argentina
~Bulg.,~Pol.			*Phil.I.	*ElSalv.,*Brazil

1pdom,1p-oth.,*1pd (n=12)

Europe	Islamic Zone	Africa	Asia	West.Hemisph.
Russia	Egypt,Iran	Zimbabwe	Singapore	Mexico
Ukraine	Uzbek,Kazakh.	Cameroon,Madagascar	Taiwan(Δ)	

mil^,mil°,mon(n=7)

Europe	Islamic Zone	Africa	Asia	West.Hemisph.
	^Syria,°Azerb.°Tajik.	^Ghana,^Guinea		^Haiti
		^Burkina Faso		

C. Separately elected Pres. & Assembly (~same year & term) (n=19)
mpr,~mpr,*mpr(n=9)

Europe	Islamic Zone	Africa	Asia	West.Hemisph.
				CRica,~DomRep.,~Ven.
				*Bolivia,*Colmb.*Peru
				*Guat.,*Nicrg.,*Panama

1pdom,1p-oth.,*1pd(n=8)

Europe	Islamic Zone	Africa	Asia	West.Hemisph.
Romania	Tunisia	Senegal,Iv.Coast		
		Kenya,Tanz.,Zambia	*Sri Lanka	

mil^,mil°,mon(n=2)

Europe	Islamic Zone	Africa	Asia	West.Hemisph.
		°Angola,^Mozambique		

- -

D. No Recent/Never Any(√)/Direct Elections (i=indirect only)(n=12)
1. Assy. only states (n=7)

Europe	Islamic Zone	Africa	Asia	West.Hemisph.
	^Libya-i		China-i	
	°Sudan-i	°Liberia	°Myanmar	
	^°Saudi A.√		°Afghan.	

2. Pres & Assy. States (n=5)

Europe	Islamic Zone	Africa	Asia	West.Hemisph.
		^Nigeria		
	°Algeria	°Zaire (1987)		
	°Somalia	°Rwanda		

Summary of types: 36+33+19=88 (active, direct elections) +12 (not functioning or indirect) = 100.

Note: Δ = Indonesia has second house of assembly which serves primarily as a presidential electoral college; Taiwan had a similar arrangement before 1996 (see 2b.ii).

with its own problems with respect to "representativeness" and "participation"—see Chapters 1, 3, and 6). The remaining 29 are either one-party states (12 Type B + 8 Type C = 20) or military regimes (7 Type B + 2 Type C = 9) where the election often serves only the legitimizing function of popular acquiescing in the choice of the single dominant party or the military junta (Hermet, Rouquie, and Rose, 1978; Ginsberg and Stone, 1991).

Whether elections are direct or indirect for the executive or for the representative branch, there are certain practices which can undermine their legitimacy as a tool for registering the expression of popular will. Many candidates of ruling regimes have no opponents, or their resources are so vast that any opposition is only token or symbolic. Also, elections can be stolen or rigged by those in charge of the electoral machinery, usually the governing regime. Chapter 3d, on one-party polities, provides a list of such tactics, but they can also be employed in mprs if elections are not administered by authorities independent of the government. Finally, there is the matter of turnout: who votes. Most states have elaborate systems of voter registration and of purging voting rolls of people who die or do not vote, or of refusing to register people who do not sign up by some date, perhaps long before the election day. The opportunity for abuse of such systems is obvious.

Even if actual election day procedures are fair, the electoral system can be structured in such a way as to help one or another of the contesting parties (Brennan and Lomasky, 1993; Lijphart, 1994). For example, elections to the representative assembly can be run in one of two ways. Under the system of *proportional representation* (PR), votes are cast not for an individual but for a political party; the party draws up a list of candidates equal to the number of seats to be filled (generally nationwide in small countries like Ireland, Denmark, and Greece; in large states, sometimes for a subregion, like Germany's federal lands, Japan's prefectures, or Russia's republics). The party wins a number of seats proportionate to the percentage of votes it receives in the designated district; the actual holders of those seats would be those individuals listed at the top of the party list down as far as the place on the list where the percentage won would mandate a cutoff. This system favors political parties and their leaders over more independent (or possibly just wealthier or more notorious) candidates.

Proportional representation is the most common form of election to the representative assembly. It is particularly prevalent in Scandanavian, central European, Mediterranean, and Iberian (and hence Latin American) states. Often a "threshold" of from 2 to 5 percent is stipulated before a party is awarded any seats. States with a lower percentage (e.g., Israel before 1992, Poland in 1989 to 1993) run the risk of having their assemblies overrun with many small parties.

The *first-past-the-post* (FPP), or *single-member-district* (SMD), system employed in the United States and many other countries with Anglo-Saxon traditions is based upon geographic representation by a single person. It favors candidates with a local reputation (or the money to buy one quickly), small regional parties, or large national parties with strong grassroots organizations (as opposed to national parties whose strength is their ideology). Within this system, one candidate out of several may win with a simple plurality of votes (as in the United States and United Kingdom); or there could be a requirement of a 50 percent majority, with a run-off election between the top two candidates if no candidate received 50 percent in the first round of a multicandidate contest (as in France and many Latin countries). Run-off elections favor large parties; the possibility of plurality victories favors small or single-issue parties and insurgent candidates.

Several states (e.g., Germany, Bulgaria, Japan, South Africa) have assemblies resulting from a combination of PR and FPP systems. Other countries (e.g., France, Greece in recent years) have switched back and forth between one and the other (PR and FPP), depending on which system the government in charge of the election thought favored its chances for victory.

Finally, in addition to the Lower House electoral college for selection of head of government in parliamentary systems, many heads of state are chosen by slightly larger colleges of the Lower House plus the Upper House (e.g., Italy, South Africa) plus, in some cases (e.g., Germany, India, Pakistan), by some representatives from lower levels of government as well.

There are two interesting cases worthy of note (designated by Δ in **Table 2e**) concerning unique bodies chosen specifically for the purpose of electing the head of state. In Indonesia, the president is chosen by the "Peoples Consultative Assembly," consisting of the 500-member House of Representatives, plus 500 others indirectly elected by provincial assemblies, political parties, and the military (which has 230 of the 500 seats—see *Excerpts*). Until recently, Taiwan had a similar arrangement. The "National Assembly" (as distinguished from the Legislative Yuan) elected the president but did little else during its six-year term. This situation was not too significant because the composition of both these bodies was determined by the dominant Kuomingtang Party. In keeping with the move to more competition in recent years, this system is scheduled to change to a directly elected president in 1996.

The United States has a peculiar system in which presidential electors represent the fifty states based on a formula reflecting population (i.e., one electoral vote for each member of the Lower House plus one electoral vote for each of its two members of the Upper House). The electors invariably follow the will of the majority popular vote in each state, but the system gives added importance in presidential campaigns to large states (though actual added weight on a per capita basis to smaller states).

2f FORMAT AND DISPLAY OF DATA BANK EXCERPTS

This chapter concludes with four pages of *Excerpts* from the Data Bank associated with the research for this book. Nineteen states drawn from a representative sample of zones and polity types are displayed following the *For-mat* for 2abcde—Power Sharing Data Bank, whose structure parallels the main sections of this chapter.

This combination of *Formats* and ***Excerpts*** is the first of eleven to be found here and in Chapters 3, 4, 5, and 6. The ***Excerpts*** in this chapter are generally

Format for 2abcde Power Sharing Data Bank

Name of state - polity type

2a - names of Head of State, Head of Govt., & (if relevant) Head of Party, Army; with summary of their relationship (<, >, and = used to describe <u>actual</u> (not formal) power relationships; i.e., Queen<PM, exec. Pres.>PM, etc.
Official titles (including Interim & Acting), and dates of accession & relegitimation (i.e., election); also: how each chosen (on what basis does Pres. appt. PM), term of office for Pres. (does term for PM depend most on Pres. or on Assy.), etc. from 2b, 2e, etc.

b - representative assembly:
i. total number of members: lower + upper houses (LH+UH);
ii. how chosen: # elected (dir.v.indir.(by whom)); SMD/FPP v. Prop.Rep.(% threshold); # appointed (by whom; on what basis). Terms of office for all.
N.B. total # often varies due to ex-officios, appointees, etc., especially in UH; # directly elected usually fixed, but often increases as population rises.

c - significant constitutional (or other) balancing arrangements re 2a & 2b, and as concerns other important power centers such as:
i. constitution - date, number; contitutional assys. & courts?; State of Emergency (SOE) allowed to suspend?; number of parties stipulated (especially in 1pps)?; role for military reserved (especially in *^°s)?
ii. cabinet (if notable for its size, or policy orientation, [e.g., # with military title], councils (military, revolutionary, advisory [to monarchs], etc.; committees; conferences, etc.
iii. # administrative subunits & whether or not decentralized "federal" states or "autonomous" regions, provinces, republics; for n=~30 countries only. Also note: any "problematic" regional (> ethnic) provinces (whether or not federal or autonomous);
iv. interest groups (economic; also, ethnic, religious, military [related to Chptrs. 4 ,5,6]; plus: charismatic personalities, political families, etc.).

d - other dependencies
i. international: military (aid, trade relationship); economic(aid, trade,investment), etc.
ii. geographic/historical (including colonial).

e - electoral systems (if not covered earlier)
i. Type A (assy.), B (assy. & Pres., different terms), or C (assy. & Pres., same terms)
ii. direct or indirect, PR or FPP/SMD; where significant and not covered in 2a or 2b
iii. other unique electoral colleges or election rules.

of more permanent features in each political system, whereas the *Excerpts* in future chapters are more reflective of current realities (e.g., election results, military power distributions, etc.).

In all cases, the *Format* generally follows the organization of the relevant chapter, and the *Excerpts* from the Data Bank are chosen to give a representative mix of states and regions to exemplify the main themes covered in this chapter. Because the purpose of these displays is to give only a sample of the data available for comparing countries along a particular dimension, and because of space constrictions, not all sub-category items in the *Format* will necessarily appear among the data in the *Excerpt* for each state as it is displayed in this publication.

For power sharing categories 2abcde, the states in the *Excerpts* are presented in geographic-region order, and include the following (by zone):

Region	State(s)
northern Europe	Netherlands
southern Europe	Italy
central Europe	Poland
west Asia	Kazakhstan
Arabian peninsula	Jordan
north Africa	Tunisia
west Africa	Nigeria
central-east Africa	Zaire, Rwanda, Ethiopia
southern Africa	South Africa
south Asia	India
east (mainland) Asia	Thailand, Taiwan
offshore (ocean) Asia	Indonesia
south America	Argentina
central America	Panama
Caribbean	Jamaica, Cuba

The states in the *Excerpts* that are cross-referenced by polity type and selected in proportion to the number in each polity type include the following:

Polity Type	State(s)
multiparty republic (mpr, 2 of 13)	Netherlands, Jamaica
weak multiparty republic (~mpr, 1 of 8)	Italy
ex-communist (ex-com, 3 of 14)	Poland, Kazakhstan, Cuba
one-party dominant (1pdom, 2 of 8)	South Africa, Taiwan
one-party other (1p-oth, 1 of 7)	Tunisia
militarized multiparty (*mpr, 4 of 20)	India, Thailand, Argentina, Panama
moderating military (mil^, 3 of 14)	Zaire, Ethiopia, Indonesia
entrenched military (mil°, 2 of 13)	Nigeria Rwanda
monarchy (mon°, 1 of 3)	Jordan

Excerpts from Power Sharing Data Bank

EUROPE

Netherlands - mpr: parl.

2a. Queen Beatrix (1980; hereditary accession) <
   PM Willem Kok (5/94), appointed by Head of State from majority in assembly.
b. representative assembly, n=225: LH n=150 + UH n=75; all dir. el., 4 yr.terms. Prop.Rep. 1% threshold.
c.i. 1814 constitution;   ii. Cabinet n=13
d. dependent since 1945 on BeNeLux customs union, forerunner of ECSC,EEC,EC, EU (Europ.Union).

Italy - ~mpr: parl.

2a. Pres. Oscar Luigi Scalfaro (5/92) < PM Lamberto Dini (1/95). Pres. indirectly elected by full rep. assy.
   (n=945)+ representatives from regions (n=~70), 7 yr. term; appoints PM fm. assembly majority.
b. assy. n= 945: LH n=630 (dir. el., 5 yr. terms) + UH n= ~315 (5 yr. term, indir. el. by regions, [7 ea. x 20
   autonomous regions = 140, + 3 fm. each regional council x 58 = 174; + 5-7 appointed for life by
   Pres.]). LH & UH have equal power. See recent 2e changes.
c.i. 1948 constitut., revised 4/93 (see 2e).   ii. Cabinet members need not be members of parliament.
 iii. n=20 autonomous regns.(5 w/ "special status" incl. Milan, Lomb ardy, & German-speaking Alto Adige).
 iv. Mafia a significant political force in Sicily, Sardinia, parts of mainland south. Vatican still important
   despite 1990s ending of 1928 Lateran Treaty which gave it special status.
d. dependence on US since 1942 occupation, CIA election financing of non-Communist parties (1948-
   71), declining in favor of EU ties; though still n=12,000 US("NATO") troops.
e. rep. assy. previously elected by strict (≤1%) Prop.Rep. resulting in many small parties, coalition (and
   short-term) govts. 1993 law changed basis for both LH & UH to 75% FPP/SMD, 25% Prop.Rep. with
   4% threshold, requiring parties to form coalitions to win FPP/SMD seats.

Poland - ex-com-----> ~mpr(∂): mixed, pres./parl.

2a. Pres. Lech Walesa (12/90) ?=? PM Josef Oleksy (2/95). Pres. directly elected, 5 yr. term (2 maximum),
   appoints PM from majority choice of assy. Any other president other than anti-communist
   dissident/hero Walesa would probably be less significant than PM.
b. assy. n=560: LH n=460 (dir. el., 4 yr. term, Prop.Rep. in 37 districts, 5% threshold) + UH n=100 (2
   seats ea. x 49 provs. + 2 seats for Warsaw and Krakow, 4 yr. term).
c.i. constitution of 1952, amended in 1989 at end of 1pcom system.   ii. Cabinet n=26
  iv. Trade union Solidarity (leader, Walesa) important in effecting change from communism. Catholic
   Church (and Polish Pope) has some political influence.
d. Economic depedence during post-Communist transition on OECD aid, IMF/World Bank loans.

ISLAMIC ZONE

Kazakhstan - ex-com----->1pdom

2a. Pres. N. Nazarbayev ('84; 4/90 by CP assembly; 12/91 by direct election, 5-yr. term; 4/95 referendum
   extends term 4 yrs. to 12/2000) > PM A. Kazhegeldin (10/94)
b. assy. n=358, part-time in 1990 1p-com system; reduced to 177 full-time in 3/94; then to 67 in 8/95
   constitutional revisions which extended president's term and increased his powers.
c.iii. ex-Soviet republic declared sovereignty 12/90, independence 12/91; renounced USSR treaty,
   joined Commonwealth of Independent States (CIS), 12/91.
d. still heavily dependent on Russian military through CIS "collective security" treaty of 1995.

Jordan - mon

2a. King Hussein (8/52) > PM Field Marshall Zaid bin Shakr (1/95). King's PM changes with policies.
b. rep. assembly, n=120; incl.: National Consultative Council (House of Deputies), n=80; el.,4 yrs.; +
   Senate n=40, appointed by King, 8-yr. terms. Weak; dissolved (1967-84 and 7/88-11/89) by King.
c.i.1952 constitution.   ii) Cabinet n=26.
 iii. renounced claim to West Bank, 7/88; perhaps federation/confed. some day with new Palestinian Authy.
 iv.*Palestinians* are majority ethnic group (see 4b-Cat.3=minority rule), but no special treatment; Seats in
   rep. assy (10 in LH, 18 in UH) reserved for minority Bedouins, Christians, & Circassians.
e. electoral districts drawn to favor rural villages (over cities which are mainly *Palestinian*).

Tunisia - 1p-other
2a. Pres. Zine al abideine Ben Ali (11/87; 4/89; 3/94) > PM Hamed Karoui (8/89; 3/94). 5-yr. terms, 2-terms maximum. Age limit of 70 (after experience with senility-removed independence era leader Habib Bourguiba (1956-87).
  b. rep. assy. n=163: 144 FPP/SMD + 19 Prop.Rep.; dir. el., 5 yr. terms, concurrent with president.
  c.i. 6/59 constitut. amended 7/88 to allow other than independence-era Destourian Socialist Party if no appeals to "religion, language, race or (?)regime".
   iv. Labor unions (esp. General Union of Tunisian Workers) and outlawed fundamentalist Islamic Tendency Movement (MTI) are major opposition to government.
   e. PR seats created in 1993 for non-dominant parties who lose in FPP/SMD districts. Winning party gets 50% of seats even if not 50% of votes. Govt. subsidies to parties (half before, half after election) winning 3% assy. vote, 5% pres. vote. (See 3de text on 1pdom tactics.)

AFRICA

Nigeria - mil°
2a. Pres. Gen. Shani Abacha (11/93) is Head of State and Government. Military coup voided presidential election of 6/93 whose winner (Chief M. Abiola, of Soc.Dem.P.) was never allowed to take office by Transition Council of previous 1985ff. mil. govt. of Gen. I. Babangida.
  b. rep. assy. n=661: 577LH + 84UH elected (4 yr. terms) in 7/92, first in nine years since Gen. M. Buhari coup of 12/83; abolished by coup of 11/93.
  c.i. 10/92 constitution for transition to civilian rule preempted by coup of 11/93.
   iii. 31 decentralized states (incl. Lagos and new capital Abuja). Earlier constitutions had 22 subdivisions (1987), 19 (1976), 12 (1967), and 5 (1963); all were unsuccessful efforts at sharing power among two main religions, three main ethnic groups (see 4abcd).
   iv. Military has been main actor to control population politically split between Moslems (50%, esp. in north among Hausa-Fulani=30% population), and Christians (40%, in south; divided between Protestant Yoruba, 18% pop., in southwest, and Catholic Ibos 22% pop., in southeast.). 1993 winning presidential candidate Abiola was a (rare) Yoruba Moslem and wealthy (election voided).

Zaire - mil^
2a. Pres.=Field Marshall Jos. D. Mobuto Sese Seko('65 coup; '67 el. by MPR party; '70,'77, '84 el. by direct vote for 7 yr. terms; 7/91 election postponed) > PM Kengo wa Dondo (5/94 appointed by Pres., 7/94 accepted by rival PM E. Tshisekedi [who had been elected by National Conference, 8/92]).
  b. Natl. Leg. Council, n=310, directly elected, 5-yr. term, last in 9/87. Extended, then rivalled by (1992), then merged with (1994) all-party National Conference. (then merged with (1994) all-party National Conference.)
  c.i. 2/78 constitut. specified 1 party (Mobuto's MPR); modified 6/90 for multi-party elections (never held).
   ii. Cabinet n=30. 8/92ff National Conference attempting transition to multiparty elections, their own PM, etc., but President Mobuto thwarting its efforts, 1992ff (see 6c Data Bank).
   iii. No federalism; historic 5b secessionist problems in southeast Shaba province (Katanga).
   iv. Pres. Mobuto, a northern Ngbandi/Mangbutu, favors Katangans & Lunda in southern Shaba, more than did rival PM Tshisekedi, a Kasai from the center. See 4b-Category 3 "minority rule" Data Bank.

Rwanda - mil°
2a. Pres. P. Bizimungu (7/94) < PM Faustin Twagiramungu (6/94), two Hutus
        both < VP & DM Gen. Paul Kagame, Cmdr.-in-Chief of Tutsi-dominated RPF Army, (7/94).
  b. No assembly since Rwanda Patriotic Front (RPF) violent ouster of Hutu-dominated govt. in 1994.
  c. Professed desire to follow terms of earlier 8/93 accord for Hutu-Tutsi power sharing.
  d. Tutsi-RPF Govt. has long-standing military ties with Uganda (English speaking); vs. overthrown Hutus who were dependent on France, now in exile in Zaire (French speakers).

Ethiopia - mil^
2a. Pres. Meles Zenawi (7/91; chosen by Natl. Conf. reps. of winning armed groups at end of civil war); was elected PM (5/95) by new directly elected national representative assembly (see 2b).
  b. assy., n=548, directly elected from new regions (see 2c.iii); terms not specified.
  c. i. constitutional assy. elected 6/94 to approve Natl.Conf. draft transition to new govt., including:
    iii. n=9 new regions: 8 ethnic (Tigre, Afar, Somali, Oromo, Amhara, Sidamo, Shankella, Guarage) + capital (Addis Ababa). Southern Oromos are largely boycotting, rebelling (see 4b, 5b Data Banks).
    iv. *Tigreans* dominate EPRDF government over Oromos, Amharans, etc. See 4b,5b(Oromo) & 6c.

South Africa - 1pdom

2a. Pres. Nelson Mandela (5/94), executive Head of State, indirectly elected by transitional (5-yr.) "power-sharing" parliament & Cabinet, with two VPs: ex-Pres. F.W.deKlerk (ANP), ?next-Pres.T.Mbeki (ANC).

b. assy. n=490: LH=400, all dir. el. by Prop.Rep., 200 on national level, 200 on province level; + UH=90, indir.el. by 9 provincial assemblies (x 10 ea.). MPs lose seats if they bolt party.

c.i. 11/18/93 post-apartheid (4th) constitution includes: list of fundamental rights, limits on St.of Emerg., & a Constitutional Court, n=11 (named by Pres., from lists prepared by impartial commission).

ii. Cabinet, n=27, with proportionate representation (of parties with 5% el. threshold) for first five years.

iii. n=9 provinces, with own police, schools, right to tax, select UH; but NOT autonomous as desired by Inkatha in KwaZulu-Natal. Others: NorthWest, N.Transvaal, Pretoria, E.Transvaal, Orange, N.Cape, E. Cape, W. Cape (majority coloureds). Have replaced1951-90 apartheid tribal homelands (Bantustans).

iv. pre-'93 Army and 5b ANC guerillas being merged; whites will still dominate civil service and bureaucracy (job security, pensions, etc. during 5-yr. transition.)

ASIA

India - *mpr: parl.

2a. Pres. Shankar Dayal Sharma (7/92) < PM P.V. Narasimha Rao (6/91).

Pres. elected by both houses of Parliament plus 26 state assemblies, 5 yr. term.   Leg>PM, 5 yrs.

b. Parl.=792: 542 Lok Sabha (House of People,LH), 540 directly elected, 2 (English) appointed, 5 yrs. + 250 Rajya Sabha (Council of States,UH); 232 indir.el. by state assys., 18 apptd., 6 yrs., 1/3 ev. 2 yrs.

c. i. Constitution of: 1950.   ii. Large "patronage" Cabinet of: 25(Banks)-40(CIA)

iii. 26 federal states, language-based, of which 3+ in almost constant state of rebellion (5b): Moslems in Kashmir, Sikhs in Punjab, and several northeast tribes (animist, Christian). Also: n=6 centrally administered "Union territories" (Andaman I., Chandrigarh, Pondicherry, etc.) w/ 20 seats in assy.

iv. Nehru-Gandhi (Indira, Rajiv) family ruled for 38 of first 43 yrs.   Ethnic probs. w/ 12% *Moslem* population (>100m.).   Scheduled castes and tribes have reserved assembly seats (see 4abc Data Bank).

d. interdependence/competition with Pakistan over divided state of Kashmir (see 5b).

Thailand - *mpr

2a. King Bhumibol Adulyadej (6/46) < PM Barnharn Silpa-archa (7/95).

b. assy. n=661: 391 LH dir.el., 4 yrs. + 270 UH appointed by King on recommendation of PM & military, 6 yr. terms. UH cannot be more than 3/4 size of LH.

c.i. 12/91 constitution is 15th since 1932 end of absolute monarchy (avg. length, < 4 yrs.).

ii. ~15 in Cabinet, of which ~3 military.   iii. 72 provinces, centralized.

iv. military rule for 39 of lst 49 years, and 15 to 20 coup attempts since military replaced monarchy as major political actor in 1932. King appoints PM (often a retired General) after elections and "consultations" with the military. Many appointments to Senate are also military officers. Military are in many parties which are often weak and formed solely to back particular officers' political ambitions and/or business interests.

e. Lower House election districts jerrymandered to favor more conservative rural areas over Bangkok.

Taiwan - 1pdom

2a. Pres. Lee Teng-hui (1/88, 3/90) > PM Lien Chan (2/93). Pres. indirectly elected by (2e) Natl. Assy. electoral college, 6-yr. term (to change to directly elected in 1996); PM fm. (2b) rep.assy.

b. assy.(Leg.Yuan) n=164: 125 dir. el., 3 yr. terms, FPP in multi-mbr. districts; + 39 apptd. Majority of assy. dir. el. for first time in 12/93. Previously majority were members with "permanent" seats won in mainland China election of 1948; these members finally pensioned off in 1993 reform.

c.i. 1946 constitution, with 1992 revisions, still claims to cover all of China. State of Emergency/martial law from 1949-87 was used to perpetuate rule of dominant KMT (mainlander) party.

iv. 87% Taiwanese islanders gain first seats in assy. in 1980s, presidency in 1988; but 10-12% mainlanders, or their descendants, still prominent in dominant party (most important actor).

d. Security Treaty with US ended in 1979; colony of Japan, 1904-45. These two powers still vie with China for influence over Taiwan.

e. Natl. Assy. = Electoral college for president and, after last 12/91 election (6-yr. term), to revise constitution to provide for future direct elections; n=~400, with minority of mainland holdovers.

Indonesia - mil^
2a. Pres. Suharto is Hd. of State & Govt., elected by Assy.,5 yr. terms ('66;'68;'73;'78;'83;'88,'93).
b. Assy n=500 House of Reps. (400 el.,100 apptd.), 5 yr. terms. (weak; no Leg. initiative).
c.i. '85 law requires all groups to endorse five tenets of *Pancasila* ideology (1. one God; 2. national unity; 3. humanitarianism; 4. consensus democracy; 5. social justice) which virtually outlaws sectarian (i.e., Islamic Fundmentalist) politics.
  iii. 13,000 islands, 900 populated, 50% pop. on one (Java),but very centralized, almost colonial in rule, esp. over ethnic Timorese, Papuans, Aceh in n.w. Sumatra (see 4b/5b).
  iv. military powerful since 1965 coup. '88 law enshrined its role (*dwifungsi*) in politics (incl. 230 Assy. seats). Dominant Golkar Party of '65 coup leaders continues to dominate. Pres. appointees=60% Peop. Constultative Assy. (see 2e). 4/93 VP Sutrisno, likely next Pres., sympathetic to more military influence.
e. Peop.Consultative Assy=1000 mbrs: 2b House of Reps. + 500 Others (indirectly elected from provinces, parties, military, & govt. appointees) to elect Pres. only (i.e., electoral college).

WESTERN HEMISPHERE

Argentina - *mpr: pres.
2a. Pres. Carlos Menem (7/89; 5/95) is Hd. State & Govt., directly elected to second (4 yr.) term in accordance with 11/93 Olivos Pact w/ opposition party to allow for pres. re-election (starting in 1995) in exchange for shorter (than original 6-yr.) pres. term, increased powers to rep. assy. (incl. new dir. el. UH), and creation of Coordinating Minister of Cabinet (=~PM) answerable to assy.
b. Assy. n=321: LH n=252, dir. el., 4 yr. terms, 1/2 el. every 2 yrs.; + UH n=69, 3 ea. dir. el. fm. 23 provinces, 9 yr. terms, 1/3 el. every 3 yrs., including 1 fm. ea. province guaranteed to opposition.
c.i. 4/94 constitut. assy. ratified most of Olivos Pact which modified 1983 post-Falklands War constitution.
  iii. 23 autonomous provinces with separately elected governors & power in Upper House.
  iv. military still important political actor despite end of coup-rule in 1983. (See 5c.i,ii,iii data.)
e. Former presidential electoral college which gave power to states, replaced in 1994 by new rule requiring 2 rounds of dir.el., unless leader in Rd.1 has 45% vote (which Menem got in 1995), or 40% vote + 10% lead.

Panama - *mpr
2a. Pres. Ernesto Perez Balladares (5/94) is Head of State and Govt.; directly elected, 5 yr. term.
b. Natl. Leg. Council, n=67, directly elected, 5 yr. terms; Proportional Representatioń, 2% threshold.
c.i. 1972 constitution (4th since 1903 violent independence secession from Colombia).
d. US historic power since its role in 1903 secession from Colombia; 10,000 troops permanently there (in 10 bases w/ 6500 jobs generating $500 mil. = 10% GNP annually; also, 2000 US civilians, 20,000 dependents). US troops invaded in 12/89 to install Endara, alleged winner of 5/89 election.

Jamaica - mpr: parl., SM (3/91)
2a. Head of State: QEII/Gov.Gen.Howard Cooke (8/91) < PM Percival Patterson (3/92, 3/93). Governor General appointed, serves at Queen's pleasure; names PM who commands majority of LH.
b. Parliament n= 81: LH=House of Reps. (n=60, el. dir., FPP/SMD, 5 yrs.); + UH=Senate (n=21, appointed by Gov.Gen.(13) & PM (8), also for 5 yr. terms).
c.i. 1962 independence constitution. 5/91ff constitution review considering change to republican status (i.e., end tie to UK, QEII/Gov.Gen. Head of State).
  ii. Cabinet n=18; Privy Council n=6 (high court in UK). iii.13 parishes, centralized.
  iv. Trade unions are strong, and have close ties with one party (PNP; see 3a).

Cuba - ex-com----->1p-other
2a. Head of State,Govt. & Party: Pres. and lst Secy. CCP: Fidel Castro (1/59; '76;'81;'86)
b. National Assembly of Peoples Power (n=589); 5 yr.terms; directly elected for 1st time in 2/93, though: n=169 nominated by municipal assys. directly elected in 12/92; + n=420 directly elected fm. single list.
c.i. '76 constitution, appved. by 98% in referendum: freq.,regular elections at local levels w/ >90% turnout.
  ii. Cabinet n=26, of which 6 military. Also: block Committees for Defense of Revolution
  iv. charismatic '59 revolution leader Castro dominates; his brother Raul is Armed Forces Minister. 1.5 million Cuban Americans in Miami influential via $400 mil./yr. in remittances.

REFERENCES

Bartolini, S. and P. Maaiar (1990) *Identity, Competition, and Electoral Availability: The Stabilisation of European Electorates, 1885–1985.* New York: Cambridge University Press.

Brennan, G. and L. Lomasky (1993) *Democracy and Decision: The Pure Theory of Electoral Preferences.* New York: Cambridge University Press.

Booth, J. A. and M. A. Seligson (eds.) (1989) *Elections and Democracy in Central America.* Chapel Hill: University of North Carolina Press.

Brown, N. J. (1990) *Peasant Politics in Modern Egypt: The Struggle against the State.* New Haven, CT: Yale University Press.

Butler, W. E. (ed.) (annual) *Yearbook on Socialist Legal Systems.* Ardsley-on-Hudson, New York: Transnational.

Camilleri, J. A. and J. Falk (1992) *The End of Sovereignty: The Politics of a Shrinking and Fragmenting World.* Brookfield, VT: Edward Elgar.

Cappellitti, M. (1971) *Judicial Review in the Contemporary World.* Indianapolis: Bobbs, Merrill.

Cardoso, F. H. and E. Faletto (1979) *Dependency and Development in Latin America.* Berkeley: University of California Press.

Catrina, C. (1988) *Arms Transfers and Dependence.* New York: Taylor and Francis, for the United Nations Institute for Disarmament Research.

Chowdhury, S. R. (1989) *The Rule of Law in a State of Emergency.* New York: St. Martin's Press.

Coakley, J. (ed.) (1993) *The Territorial Management of Ethnic Conflict.* Portland, OR: Frank Cass.

Copeland, G. W. and S. C. Patterson (eds.) (1994) *Parliaments in the Modern World: Changing Institutions.* Ann Arbor: University of Michigan Press.

Cunliffe, A. and M. Laver (1985) "African Aid Links and UN Voting: A Research Note," *International Interactions* 12: 95–107.

Davis, C. L. (1989) *Working-Class Mobilization and Political Control: Venezuela and Mexico.* Lexington: University Press of Kentucky.

Duchacek, I. D. (1987) *Comparative Federalism: The Territorial Dimension of Politics.* Lanham, MD: University Press of America.

Emmanuel, A. (1972) *Unequal Exchange: A Study of the Imperialism of Trade.* New York: Monthly Review Press.

Finn, J. E. (1991) *Constitutions in Crisis: Political Violence and the Rule of Law.* New York: Oxford University Press.

Fletcher, G. P. (1987) *Comparative Jurisprudence.* Dobbs Ferry, NY: The Oceana Group, Condyne Cassettes.

Franklin, D. P. and M. Baun (eds.) (1994) *Political Culture and Constitutionalism: A Comparative Approach.* Armonk, NY: M. E. Sharpe.

Freedom House (annual) *Freedom in the World: Political Rights and Civil Liberties.* New York: Freedom House.

Frenkel, S. (ed.) (1993) *Organized Labor in the Asia-Pacific Region: A Comparative Study of Trade Unionism.* Ithaca, NY: ILR Press.

Ginsberg, B. and A. Stone (eds.) (1991) *Do Elections Matter?* Armonk, NY: M. E. Sharpe.

Goldwin, R. A. (1990) "We the Peoples: A Checklist for New Constitution Writers," *The American Enterprise* (May/June): 70–75.

Harkavy, R. E. (1989) *Bases Abroad: The Global Foreign Military Presence.* New York: Oxford University Press.

Hermet, G., A. Rouquie, and R. Rose (eds.) (1978) *Elections without Choice.* London: Macmillan.

Humana, C. (1992) *World Human Rights Guide.* New York: Oxford University Press.

Jennings, M. K. and T. E. Mann (eds.) (1994) *Elections at Home and Abroad.* Ann Arbor: University of Michigan Press.

Juergensmeyer, M. (1993) *The New Cold War? Religious Nationalism Confronts the Secular State.* Berkeley: University of California Press.

Khadduri, M. (1984) *The Islamic Concept of Justice.* Baltimore: Johns Hopkins University Press.

Klare, M. (1984) *American Arms Supermarket.* Austin: University of Texas Press.

Koh, B. C. (1989) *Japan's Administrative Elite.* Berkeley: University of California Press.

Lewis-Beck, M. S. (1988) *Economics and Elections: The Major Western Democracies.* Ann Arbor: University of Michigan Press.

Lijphart, A. (Ed.) (1992) *Parliamentary versus Presidential Government.* New York: Oxford University Press.

Lijphart, A. (1994) *Electoral Systems and Party Systems: A Study of 27 Democracies, 1945–90.* New York: Oxford University Press.

Linz, J. J. and A. Valenzuela (eds.) (1994) *The Failure of Presidential Democracy.* Baltimore: Johns Hopkins University Press.

Louscher, D. J. and M. D. Salamone (eds.) (1987) *Marketing Security Assistance: Perspectives on Arms Sales.* Lexington, MA: D. C. Heath.

Moen, M. C. and L. S. Gustafson (eds.) (1991) *The Religious Challenge to the State.* Philadelphia: Temple University Press.

Moran, T. H. (Ed.) (1985) *Multinational Corporations: Political Economy of Foreign Direct Investment.* Lexington, MA: Lexington Books.

Norton, P. (ed.) (1995) *Legislatures and Legislators.* Brookfield, VT: Dartmouth.

Olson, D. M. (1994) *Democratic Legislative Institutions: A Comparative View.* Armonk, NY: M. E. Sharpe.

Ornstein, N. and K. Coursen (1992) "As the World Turns Democratic, Federalism Finds Favor," *The American Enterprise* (Jan/Feb): 20–24.

Palmer, M., A. Leila, and E. Yassin (1988) *The Egyptian Bureaucracy.* Syracuse, NY: Syracuse University Press.

Pierce, R. (1994) *Choosing the Chief: Presidential Elections in France and the United States.* Ann Arbor: University of Michigan Press.

Pierre, A. (ed.) (1995) *Cascade of Arms: Controlling Conventional Weapons Proliferation in the 1990s.* Washington, DC: Brookings Institution.

Rose, R. (1987) *Ministers and Ministries: A Functional Analysis.* New York: Oxford University Press.

Rose, R. (1988) "Presidents and Prime Ministers," *Society,* 25(3): 61–67.

Shugart, M. S. and J. M. Carey (1992) *Presidents and Assemblies: Constitutional Design and Electoral Dynamics.* New York: Cambridge University Press.

Sullivan, M. J., III (1991) *Measuring Global Values: The Ranking of 162 Countries.* Westport, CT: Greenwood Press.

Taagepera, R. and M. S. Shugart (1989) *Seats and Votes: The Effects and Determinants of Electoral Systems.* New Haven, CT: Yale University Press.

Thomas, C. (1993) *First World Interest Groups: A Comparative Perspective.* Westport, CT: Greenwood Press.

Turner, L. (1991) *Democracy at Work: Changing World Markets and the Future of Labor Unions.* Ithaca, NY: Cornell University Press.

Verner, J. G. (1984) "The Independence of Supreme Courts in Latin America: A Review of the Literature," *Journal of Latin American Studies* 16: 463–506.

Williams, P. J. (1989) *The Catholic Church and Politics in Nicaragua and Costa Rica.* Pittsburgh: University of Pittsburgh Press.

3

Civilian Political Systems

Chapter 1's Comparative Government Spread Shead proposed five political systems in which civilian actors and the rule of law predominated. There are four main categories—the multiparty republic (mpr); the weak multiparty republic (~mpr); the one-party dominant system (1pdom); and the one-party "other" system (1p-oth)—and one additional category of ex-coms, or "communist states in transition," made necessary by the collapse of communism in the Soviet Union and eastern Europe (and de facto in China and east Asia as well). The one characteristic all these polities have in common is that the political process is essentially in civilian hands. As is the case throughout the entire CGSS, arguments could be made for different placements of certain countries; the main point of this study is to employ the definitions of the various governing systems, and to test indicators for measuring whether states conform to the categories in which they have been put.

Throughout the analysis of civilian political systems in this chapter, consideration will be given to the alleged global "trend toward democracy" since the collapse of communism in eastern Europe in 1989 (Huntington, 1991; Liu, 1993; Diamond and Plattner, 1993; Pridham, 1994). One of the premises of this study is that even at the height of the Cold War, the idea that the world was dominated by only two political systems—multiparty democracies and one-party communist dictatorships—was a gross oversimplification. There were only about 35 well-functioning democracies among the 140-odd states of the alleged "free-world West," and there were, at most, 15 states faithfully adhering to the principles of Marx and Lenin in the "communist East" (Sullivan, 1991: 317–325). Most (i.e., about 90) of the the world's polities were something else (i.e., one of the CGSS's other eight types) then, and they are still today. So the end of the Cold War has not had that much of an effect on the framework of analysis first developed for the study of 162 states in this author's *Measuring Global Values* (1991).

It should also be mentioned that this study of measurable political institutions does not even use the word "democracy" in describing the most open, participative governmental form (the multiparty republic), because it does not analyze at great length certain elements of democracy, such as minority rights, the rule of law, and civil liberties (Budge and McKay, 1994; Horowitz, 1990; Inkeles, 1991; Legters, Burke, and Diquattro, 1994). Such prerequisites of the democratic condition are discussed elsewhere in this book (e.g., minority rights in Chapter 4c; the rule of law in Chapters 2c.i and 5b, and civil liberties in Chapter 7a), but are not among the dimensions against which our ten political types will be explicitly measured.

3ab MULTIPARTY SYSTEMS (mpr,~mpr,*mpr)

According to the Comparative Government Spread Sheet, there are three forms of multiparty systems: the (regular) multiparty republic (mpr), the weak multiparty republic (~mpr), and (on CGSS, page 2) the militarized multiparty republic (*mpr). Before discussing each of these polity types at length, some general remarks about the archetype, and the *Format* to be employed for its analysis, will be made.

Regardless of which of the three types of mprs is being studied, certain basic bits of information must be confronted in order to analyze the way the system is functioning at any particular time. These are summarized in the *Format* for 3ab—mpr, ~mpr, *mpr Data Banks, and include the following four points.

The first (paragraph i in the *Format*) indicates whether the mpr system is parliamentary, presidential, or mixed (words defined in Chapter 2b). If the system is parliamentary, then it must be determined whether the members of parliament coming together to form the government are from a single party's simple majority in the representative assembly, or from a coalition of parties. If they come from a single party, they will be designated as a *simple majority* (SM) government. If it takes more than one party to generate the 50 percent of the votes needed to command the support of the parliament, then it will be called a multiparty *coalition* (CO) government.

One final variation—which historically accounts for 30 percent of all parliamentary governments (Stromm, 1990)—must be mentioned: the *minority* (MIN) government, which does not command the support of the majority of parliament but does not have a majority of members opposed to it either. Minority governments might be made up of a single party, or of several parties, without majority support. They are sustained in power by some "silent partners" among the other parties which do not join to form the government (and hence do not control any Cabinet Ministries) but which abstain on any votes of no confidence to terminate the rule of the government (i.e., cause the government to "fall").

Format for 3ab Multiparty (mpr,~mpr,*mpr) Data Banks

---

i.) **State** + note if **PARL.(14 + *7)**, **PRES.(5 + *12)**, or **MIXED(7 + *1)** system;
& if parl., whether simple majority **(SM)**, coalition **(CO)**, or minority **(MIN)** government;
& if mixed, the form that predominates (parl. or pres. type).
Plus: **# of parties** (major, with seats; &/or total on ballot in last election).
Also: n = # of parties with seats in the significant (generally, lower) house;
+ = if larger total # of parties, or # parties on ballot, is known;
* = # seats needed to govern (usually LH/2); in a few cases *both* houses, (LH+UH)/2.

ii.) - <u>Party strengths</u> in latest (and, if appropriate, any earlier) elections; in ideological
order (i.e., left-thru-right; see below reprint from Table 1b.i), abbreviated in left-hand
margin before name of party.
= number of seats in significant house, won by party, (in 21 parl. & 7 mixed systems);
% = % popular votes for party's Pres. candidate, (in 7 mixed & 17 Pres. systems).
* = annotation to numbers for governing coalition partners;
^ = annotation for sustainers of minority governments.
For each major party, give: name of leader, date party established (if available).

iii.) <u>Remarks</u> relevant to the distribution of power such as:
% required for representation in Prop. Rep., to avoid runoff in SMD, systems;
turnout (t.o.);   term of office (after last date, if not obvious fm. earlier results);
history of: CO or SM rule; 1-party(~) or (*)military dominance.

iv.)(where appropriate): why **~mpr** "weak" (∂, ≈, or *; see 3b *format* for n=12 ~mprs); or,
why ***mpr** "militarized" (war, coup, other; see 6a *format* for n=20 *mprs).

In presidential systems, such bargaining between parties in the assembly is not as important, because the winner of the presidential election is the most significant actor in determining the composition of the government. In mixed systems, the strength of the directly elected president, and that of the assembly-generated prime minister, as well as the relationship (both institutional and personal) between them, must be taken into account (see Chapter 2, *Format* for 2abcde—Power Sharing, line a).

The next step (paragraph ii in the *Format* for 3ab) in analyzing the way mpr systems function is to display the results of the most recent election for each party, with reference to the percentage of the vote won, and the number of seats attained in the parliament. Under strict proportional representation, the percentage of votes would correspond to the percentage of seats, a situation obviously not achieved in FPP/SMD electoral systems, and only approximated in PR electoral systems with a threshold of more than 1 percent (see Chapter 2e). For directly elected presidents, the percentage of the vote for each major candidate also should be indicated.

Parties coming together to form the government are annotated with an asterisk (*) next to the number of seats won (Sjolin, 1993). Silent sustainer-parties of minority governments are annotated with a caret (^). To aid in understanding the ideological composition of a government, parties are displayed in the Data Bank and in its *Excerpts* here in a left-through-right order, as these terms were defined in Chapter 1b (see Table 1b.i)

Finally (paragraphs iii and iv of the *Format* for 3ab), any additional remarks relating to electoral practices (turnout, percentage of vote required for representation in PR systems, percent needed to avoid run-offs in FPP systems, etc.), term of office, or history of coalitional, single-party, or military-dominated rule might be noted. It is these last two factors which will provide substantiation as to why a multiparty republic might be designated "weak" (~) or "militarized" (*). (For further explanation of these terms and abbreviations, see section 3b.)

Table 3ab.i presents the mpr polity types based upon the manner in which the head of state is chosen for each of the 45 multiparty political systems—13 mprs, 12 ~mprs, and 20 *mprs. It reveals that the most common form of mpr is the parliamentary, with 21 states, followed by 18 countries having strong presidential systems and 6 being mixed. Of the 21 parliamentary types, 8 have constitutional monarchs as the head of state, 3 have governors general appointed by a constitutional monarch, and 10 have indirectly elected civilian heads of state.

With respect to heads of government in the 21 parliamentary systems (**Table 3ab.ii**), as of mid–1995, thirteen preside over coalitions, seven are sustained by the simple-majority support of a single party, and there is one one-party minority regime; (minority coalitions are counted among the coalition governments). Of the 6 mixed systems, 4 are from weak ~mprs, and 3 have coalition governments, 3 are simple majority. Of the 18 presidential systems, 13 are from militarized *mprs, and the terms minority and majority (which relate to the assembly) are not as significant as the party of the president. (Summaries can be confirmed by reference to specific states in Tables 3a.ii and 3b.ii in the relevant subsections.)

From this survey, it seems that the most common form of multiparty republic is the parliamentary mpr with a coalition government in which more than one party is represented. For this reason, the number, names, and strengths of parties will be the key variable in the analysis of multiparty systems which follows and which includes many states which do not mirror the prototype but which are commonly asociated with the term "multiparty democracy," like the United States, the United Kingdom, and France. Their particular variations from the norm will be explained in their respective *Excerpts* from the Data Bank at the end of subsection 3a.

With this background for all three multiparty types, it is now appropriate to give greater attention to the two civilian versions, mprs and ~mprs; study of the militarized *mprs will be deferred to Chapter 6.

Table 3ab.i
Selection of Head of State (n = 45 mprs: 13 mpr, 12 ~mpr, 20 *mpr; with indication of how head of government data are encoded in 3ab and 6a Data Banks)

Parliamentary: (n=21: 9+5~+*7; 2e Elec.Type A: Leg>PM)
Head of State for Life (contitutional monarchs), n=8:
UK, Netherlands, Belgium, Sweden, Denmark; ~Spain; ~Japan; *Nepal
-------Hd.Govt. fm. # seats in Leg. (5+2~+1*)

Head of State (Governor General) appointed by Head of Commonwealth, n=3:
Australia; Jamaica, Canada.
-------Hd.Govt. fm. # seats in Leg. (3+0~+0*)

Head of State (indirectly) elected (by rep. assy. or some other electoral college), n=10:
Germany, ~Greece, ~Italy, ~Czech.
*Also: Turkey, Israel, India, Pakistan, Bangladesh, Thailand
--------Hd.Govt. fm. # seats in Leg. (1+3~+6*)

Mixed (n=6: 2+4~; Elec.Type B: Leg>PM and dir.el.Pres., different terms)
Head of State directly elected, but is NOT Hd. of Govt. which comes out of Leg..
France, Ireland; ~Poland, ~Bulgaria, ~Hungary, ~Portugal.
(in approximate order of Pres. strength, within mpr type)
-------% vote Pres. and # seats Leg. both in 3ab Data Bank

Presidential (n=18: 2+3~+*13; Elec.Type B,C: Assy. & dir. el. Pres.)
Directly elected Head of State who is also Hd. of Govt:
~Venezuela, ~Ecuador, ~Dominican Republic, Costa Rica, USA.
*Also: Sri Lanka, S.Korea, Philippine I.; *Madagascar.
+ 9 Latin Am.: Arg., Brazil, Chile, Bol., Col.; Panama, Nic., Guat., & El Salvador.
-------%vote Pres. more impt. than #Leg. seats in 3a Data Bank

Head of State and the Head of Government *both* directly elected: NONE√

Total n=45:   (45:21+7+17)

Note: √But Israel scheduled to move to this system in 1996.

Table 3ab.ii
Selection of Head of Government in 45 mprs, as of December 1995

(For details, see Tables 3a.ii, 3b.ii, and 6ab.i)
parliamentary, n=21: 9+5~+*7
coalition, n=13; 1p minority, n=1; simple majority, n=7;
mixed, n=6: 2+4~
coalition, n=3; simple majority=3.
presidential, n=18: 2+3~+*13
terms coalition, minority, majority, etc. are not applicable.

Note: In 6 mixed and 18 presidential systems, the Data Bank includes results of both the parliamentary and the presidential elections.

3a Multiparty Republics

Multiparty republics are countries with essentially civilian political structures, with a (generally divided) executive (see 2a) sharing power with an independent representative assembly (see 2b) with law-making power (i.e., a legislature), an independent judiciary to enforce this rule of law (see 2c.i), and legitimation from regularly scheduled elections in which opposition parties have a realistic chance of coming to power (see 2e).

Table 3a reproduces the 13 mprs from the CGSS, a display which shows the preponderance of European states (8, with 3 of the remaining 5 descended from the British system). The United States has elements of both the British and the French (the strong president) systems.

The 13 mprs are next divided into four subtypes in **Table 3a.i**. The most common form, in 5 states, is the parliamentary mpr employing proportional representation, assembly only elections. This system is most typical of (Protestant) north-central Europe—Sweden, Netherlands, Denmark, and Germany—where there is great historical suspicion of concentrated authority; it is also found in Belgium (which has ethnic divisions which must be carefully reflected). Four of these countries have kings as ceremonial heads of state, and one (Germany) has an indirectly elected, relatively weak president.

The second significant mpr subtype—the parliamentary mpr with first-past-the-post/single-member-district, assembly only, elections—is found in the United Kingdom and three of its former colonies: Australia, Canada, and Jamaica.

Nine of the 13 mprs are thus distinctly parliamentary systems. The United States (along with Costa Rica) is in a minority among mprs in having a strong presidential system. France and Ireland have mixed systems with independently elected presidents. France's relatively strong president shares power with a prime minister, whose appointment must be approved by a majority in the assembly; twice since 1958, when this system was established, it has resulted in "cohabitation" in government between two parties. Ireland's relatively weak president cannot even comment on political matters; its mixed system is heavily tilted toward the parliamentary side.

All 13 states in this category have been mprs since the late 1940s, and all except Germany for many years before that. Since the most significant feature of the mpr polity type is the variety of political parties defining the system, **Table 3a.ii** summarizes the number of parties comprising each government as of late 1995. It reveals 5 parliamentary coalition governments (one of which is a minority coalition) in Denmark, Belgium, Germany, Netherlands, and Sweden, and 4 ruled by a single party with a simple majority (United Kingdom, Australia, Jamaica, and Canada), a division which reflects precisely the electoral systems in the two groups of states. In the United States and Costa Rica, the party in charge of the presidency is most significant, but they each have a vigorous assembly in which the opposition is strong. In the

Table 3a
Multiparty Republics (mprs)

Europe	Islamic Zone	Africa	Asia	West.Hemisph.
		3a. mpr=multiparty republics (n=13)		
UK, Ireland			Australia	Canada
Belgium,Nethrlds.				Jamaica
Denmark,Sweden				USA
Germany, France				Costa Rica
TOT: 8			1	4 (13)

Table 3a.i
mprs by Subtype

parl., PR, assy. only els. (n=5): Sweden, Netherlands, Denmark, Germany, Belgium
parl.,FPP/SMD, assy. only elections (n=4).: UK, Australia, Canada, Jamaica
presidential (n=2): United States, Costa Rica;   mixed (n=2): Ireland, France

Table 3a.ii
Number of Parties Forming Governments in 11 of 13 mprs, as of December 1995
(includes 9 parliamentary and 2 mixed systems)

Europe	Asia	West. Hemisph.	
?LEAST STABLE/MOST RESPONSIVE			
parliamentary CO govts. (n=5)			
4 parties: ^Denmark 9/94,Belgium 5/95			(2)
3 parties: Germany 10/94,Nethrlds.5/94			(2)
1p minority^: ^Sweden 9/94			(1)
parliamentary SM govts. (n=4)			
UK 4/92	Australia 3/93	Jamaica 3/93, Canada 10/93	(4)
mixed govts. (n=2)			
3 parties,CO: Ireland 12/94			(1)
1p SM: France 3/93			(1)
not applicable: strong Pres. govt. (n=2)			
		USA 1/93 ,Costa Rica 2/94	(2)
TOTS: 8	1	4	(13)
		MOST STABLE/LEAST RESPONSIVE?	

Note: ^ = minority govt. (n=2, Sweden, Denmark). Parties don't need majority to rule, just no majority *against* their rule (i.e., some non-governing parties abstain on votes of confidence).

two mixed systems, the three-party parliamentary-based coalition has the most power in Ireland, whereas, in France, a Conservative president shares power with a de facto simple-majority (the several right-of-center parties ran as a team) Conservative prime minister.

A factor to balance against the high degree of fluidity in party participation in governments in parliamentary, mpr-coalition states is frequent changes in administration before legislative terms are completed caused by these coalition governments losing votes of confidence in the assembly. There is some debate over whether governments' reconstituting themselves (without necessarily calling for new elections) is evidence of instability or a reflection of popular will (Damgaard, 1992; Vanhanen, 1990; Lijphart, 1984; Powell, 1982); the annotations relating to stability and responsiveness at the top left and bottom right of **Table 3a.ii** are intended to note this tension.

All 13 mprs have a number of strong political parties. Whether they are in or out of government at any given moment, most have considerable longevity as part of each state's political system. According to **Table 3a.iii** (which gives abbreviated names for the main enduring parties in each state), the average number of major parties is 4.2, and at the present time they share an average of 96.5 percent of the seats in the 13 mpr parliaments. The total number of parties required to fill all assembly seats is, on average, 6.4. In the weak and militarized mprs to be discussed later, there are typically fewer main parties (3.5 and 3.4, respectively) comprising a smaller percentage of the representative assemblies on average (87.6%, 86.3%), with a larger total number of parties needed to account for the rest of the assembly (7.6 and 10.5, respectively).

Excerpts from the Data Bank associated with this study, generally employing the *Format* from Table 3ab in the previous section (but not necessarily denoting each subhead explicitly), are presented next for 3 parliamentary mprs (2 of the 5 coalitional [Denmark and Germany], 1 of the 4 simple majority [United Kingdom]), for 1 (of the 2) presidential mprs (United States), and for 1 (of the 2) mixed systems (France). Data in the *Excerpts* in this chapter are less enduring than those for the structures in Chapter 2 and are subject to amendment as governments and power change.

Table 3a.iii
Number of Parties in Representative Assemblies in 13 mprs, as of December 1995

Number (& Abbreviated Names) of *Main* Political Parties	% of Assy. Seats Held by Main Parties		Total # of Parties with Assy. Seats	
Belgium 10 (EF,EW,PSB,BSP,CVP,PSC,PVV,PLP,VU,VB)	Sweden	170/170=100%	Belgium	13
Denmark 8 (PP,CPP,LDP,CDP,CPP,RSLP,SDP,SPP)	Denmark	175/175=100%	France	11+
Sweden 7 (LP,SDP,CP,LP,MP,CDP,NDP)	Jamaica	60/60=100%	Nethrlds.	9
France 5+ (CP,SP,UDF,RPR,NF)	USA	434/435=99.8%	UK	9
Canada 5 (PCP,LP,NDP,NRP,BQ)	Canada	294/295=99.7%	Denmark	8
Netherlands 4 (PP,CDP,D66,LP)	Australia	146/148=98.6%	Sweden	7
Germany 4 (CDU,CSU,FDP,SPD)	Belgium	205/212=96.7%	Germany	6
Ireland 3 (FF,FG,LP)	France	557/577=96.5%	Canada	6
UK 2 (CP, LP)	Germany	631/656=96.2%	Ireland	5+
Australia 2 (Lib.,Lab.)	Costa Rica	54/57=94.7%	Costa R.	3+
Jamaica 2 (PNP,LP)	UK	607/651=93.2%	Australia	2+
Costa Rica 2 (NLP,SCUP)	Netherlds.	137/150=91.3%	Jamaica	2
USA 2 (DP, RP)	Ireland	146/166=88.0%	USA	2
Average: 4.2 main parties with 96.5% seats			Avg: 6.4+ parties	

Excerpts from Multiparty Republics Data Bank

Denmark - parl, CO - 4p^ (9/94)

n=10+ 175/2=88 to *	5/88	12/90	1/93	9/94
f-l: Unity List (ex-communists)	0	0		6 (3.2%v)
l: Socialist Peop. P. (anti-NATO,EU; ldr. Nielsen)	24	15 (8.3%v)		13 (7.3)
c-l: Soc.Dem.Party(anti-nuke; PM Rasmussen); #1 in % votes	55	69 (37.4)	*	62* (34.6)
c: Rad.Soc. Libl P. (rgt.on econ, left on foreign; Jelved)	10*	7^(3.5)	*	8* (4.6)
c-r: Center Democratic P.	9^	9^(5.1)	*	5* (2.8)
c-r: Christian Peoples P.	4	4^(2.3)	*	0 (1.8)
r-c: Liberal Dem. P. (ldr. Ellemann-Jensen)	22*	29* (15.0)		42 (23.3)
r: Conservative Peop. P. (ex-PM Schluter, since '82)	35*	30* (16.0)		27 (15.0)
f-r: Progress P. (anti-: tax,immigrants,EU; Kjaersgaard)	16^	12^(6.4)		11 (6.4)
	175	175		175
+Regional Reps: Greenland P. (2), Faeroes (2)	4	4	2*	4(1*)
(* = # in governing coalition:	67*	59*	91*	76*)

Govt. changed in 1/93 without an election as 3 c-r parties shifted support to SDP to get its support for EU
Maastricht Treaty for monetary union which was defeated in referendum 6/92, then passed 6/93.
With 2% threshold for a Prop.Rep. seat, Denmark has *never* had a simple majority govt.; rather *minority*
govts. where ^ = caucus to form, but don't share in, govt. (no majority to rule, just no majority against rule).

Germany - parl, CO - 3p (10/94)

n=6 w/ seats; §656/2=329 to*	12/90 (t.o.:77.8%)	10/94
f-l: PDS=Dem.Soc.P.(fd.'46; ex-E.Ger. CP; ldr. L. Bisky)	17 (2.4%v:0w.,10e.)Δ	30 (4.4%v)
mbrs: 130,000 ('94), incl. 20,000 unreconstructed; #1 in east		
l: Greens=Ecology P.(fd.'79; ldr.J.Fischer; 1/93 merge w/...	0 (3.9: 5,0)	49 (7.3)
l: Alliance '90(east N.Forum reformers+e.Greens); 37,000 mbrs.	8 (1.2:0,10)	n.a.
c-l: SPD=Soc.Dem.P. (fd.1870s; ldr: LaFontaine	239 (33.5:37,24)	252 (36.4)
c: FDP=Free Dem. P.(ldr. W.Gerhardt,FM Kinkel)	79* (11.0:11,13)	47* (6.9)
c-r: CDU=Christian Democ.Un. (fd.'45; Chancellor Kohl)	268* (36.7:36,43)	244* (34.2)
r: CSU=Xtn. Social Union (fd.'46, Bavaria; Fin.Min.Waigel;)	51* (7.1: 9,0)	50* (7.3)
f-r: Republican P. (neo-Nazi, Schonhuber; ~25,000 mbrs.)	0 (2.1: 2,1)	0 (1.9)
Total:	662 (98.1%)	672 (98.4%)
	*=398 w/6§	*=341 w/ 10§

Voting system combines 1/2 SMD/FPP & 1/2 PR. Each voter has 2 votes: 1st vote for a specific cand.,
2nd vote for a party list drawn up for each state, and number seats party receives is determined by its total
nationwide share of the 2nd vote (Kohl has always been elected from the list). Very stable system; only one
Chanc.has lost post after natl. el (Kiesinger), others all changed by parliamentary bargaining.
§=When a party wins more direct mandates than it w/b entitled to under Prop.Rep, it gets "surplus seats".
In '90, CDU got 6 such, raising tot. # in LH to 662 (& 331 needed to govern*). In '94, CDU got 8 extra seats,
and other parties got 8, raising tot. # in LH to 672 (& 337 needed to govern *; Kohl got 338, of 341 *MPs).
ΔFor 12/90 el. only: Fedl.Constitut.Court ruled 5% cutoff for Prop.Rep. did not have to be met nationally
for former e. German parties, but only within ex-east Germany, allowing PDS to get in LH w/o 5% threshold.
UPPER HOUSE, n=68 indirectly elected by 16 state govts. as they are elected. Results as of 10/94:

SPD delegations:	26 seats, 7 states (Saar,NR-W,LSax,Hmbg,S-H,Brdbg.,Berlin)
SPD-minor party (FDP and/or Green) delegs.:	15 seats, from 4 states (Bremen,Hesse,Rh-Pal.,Sax.Anh.)
SPD/CDU Grand Coalition delegations:	17 seats, fm. 3 states (Meck-WP,Thurg.,Bad-Wurt.)
CDU/CSU delegations:	10 seats, fm. 2 states (Bavaria, Saxony)

PRESIDENT: indirectly elected by LH n=660 + 660 from state assemblies; need majority to win in 1st 2
rounds, plurality thereafter. Results, 5/94: CDP's R. Hergzog over SDP's Rau by 696-605 on 3rd ballot.
Other votes in earlier rounds: FDP's Hamm-Brucher 126 on 2nd (to Herzog on 3rd); Reich (E.Ger.) 62 on
1st; and Repub. P.'s Herzel 12 on 1st.
Other parties: f-r: Ger.Peop.Union (G. Frey), ~25,000 mbrs., combined with Repubs. in 8/94; Citizens P.
Outlawed (Nazi) parties: German Alternative, Free Ger.Workers P., National Front et al. (n=10 total, 2/95).

United Kingdom - parl, SM

		'79	6/83	6/87	4/92
n=2 main parties,9 w/ seats	651/2=326 to *				
l:Labor P. (fd.:1900; Kinnock; Smith; Blair; 280,000 mbrs.)		268	209	229	271
c:Liberal P.('79) + Soc.Dem.P.('82) = Alliance ('83,87)		11	27	22	n.a.
......merged ('90) into Lib.Dem.P.(Ashdowne; 100,000 mbrs.)		n.a.	n.a.	n.a.	20
r:Conservative P. (Thatcher,'79,83,87; Major,'90,92; 500,000 mbrs.)		339*	397*	375*	336*
r:Regional Parties (#s fm.'79, '83,'87,'92 elections):		17	21	24	24 (9^)

N.Ireland (gen'ly 13:4 = Prot:RC, of 17 seats despite only 9:6 pop.ratio):
  OUP=Offic.Unionist P. (Molyneux,moderates 3X more pop.; 11,9,9^);
  Dem.Un.P.(Paisley; 3,3,3,3),Un.Ulst.Pop.Un.P.(Kilfeder;1,1,1,1);
  Soc.Dem.&Lab.P.(fd.,70:mod.RC,Hume;1,3,4,4) finally talked 5/93 to:
    Sinn Fein (front for mil. IRA, legal,'74, Adams;1,1,0,0; but 33%v.),
    Alliance P. (ldr. Alderdine; non-sectarian 60:40=Prot:RC 0,0,0,0).
  Scottish Natl. P.: Salmond; 2,5,3,3; of n=72 Scotld. seats + see below
  Welsh Natl.P./Plaid Cymru: 2,3,4,4; of n=38 Wales seats; + see below

	TOTAL:	650	650	650	651

4/92ff: Cons. P. 11-vote margin of 336-315 made shaky by presence of ~40 "Euroskeptics". In 5/93
  Maastricht EC Treaty vote (which passed 292-112-247 abstaining), 41 voted no, 2 abstained. In 7/93 vote of
  confidence on PM, 23 voted no, but offset by 10 Ulster Unionists in OUP. Since then, opp. won 7 by-
  elections in 1993, reducing margin to 329-324. In 12/94, 9 Euroskeptics drummed out of party leaving
  Cons. 4 short of majority without Off.Unionist P. (^) support. They were restored by time of 7/95 vote on
  Major's party leadership which he won 218-89-22(abstentions, etc.) showing ~2/3 party still behind him.
Party vote for 6/94 European Union MPs: Labor 44%, Conservative 27%, other 29%.
Party vote for 5/95 els. to 346 local councils: Labor 48%, Conservative 25%, Libl.Dems. 23%, other 4%.
Voting system: Due to FPP, non-PR system, Conserv.P. with 42%v. twice, got 58%s in '87, 51%s in'92;
  whereas Labor, 31%vote, 35%seats in '87; 34% vote, 42% seats in '92; and
  Lib.Dems. (strong in local pockets, not nationally) had 23%vote, 3% seats in '87; 18%vote, 3% seats in '92.
Fm. Scotland in parl.(n=72; '87,'92): Labor (50,49) w/ ~55%v, Libl.Dems.(8,11), Cons.(9,11). + Scot. Natl. P.
  (3,3) w/ ~25% vote. (Fm. 2c.iii: In 3/79 referendum, Scotland devolution preferred, but not by 40% of total
  electorate (low turnout); SNP withdrew support fm. Lab.P. govt. for not pushing hard enough, & govt. fell.)
Fm. Wales i n parl .(n=38 total): Labor 27, Cons. 6, other 5, in '92. Wales devol. defeated in referendum, 1979.
Re N. Ireland, (17 seats): Sinn Fein gen'ly gets NO seats despite 33% RC vote in N.Ireland; ≤2%v. in Ireland.

USA - presidential

Recent presidential election results (n=2 main parties):

11/88 Pres.	11/92 Pres.
c-l: Democ.P.: Dukakis=46%v., 112 electoral	Clinton = 43%v., 370 electoral*
c-r: Repub.P.: Bush = 54% 425 electoral*	Bush = 38% 168 electoral
Bentsen = n.a. 1 electoral	Perot = 19%, 0 electoral
TOTALS: 100%v. ,538 w/D.C.(n=3)	100%v., 538 w/D.C.(n=3)

*Electoral college vote, favoring largest states and intended to create mandate, has agreed with popular vote
winner in all US elections for past 104 years; earlier exceptions: 1824 J.Q.Adams 1876 Hayes, 1888
B.Harrison.
  A strongly 2-party system; 3rd party presidential candidates seldom survive to next 4-year election cycle.

Recent bicameral assembly election results: 435/2=218 to control LH; 100/2=51 to control UH.

	11/90 assy.	11/92 assy.	11/94 assy.
c-l: Democ.P	267 LH + 56 UH	258 LH + 57 UH	204 LH + 47 UH
c-r: Repub.P.	167 LH + 44 UH	176 LH + 43 UH	230 LH + 53 UH
TOTALS:	434+ 100	434+ 100	434+ 100

Note: + = 1 independent (Socialist); otherwise, strongly 2-party; 3rd parties seldom win seats in Congress.
Opposition party control of Congress (1986-92; 1994ff) somewhat of a restraint on otherwise activist
  executive branch.

Excerpts from Multiparty Republics Data Bank *(continued)*

France - mixed: pres≥parl (> when same party ['88-93,'95ff]; = when co-habit ['86-88, '93-95])

Presidential elections:	'81 Rd.1	'81 Rd.2	'88 Rd.1	'88 Rd.2	'95 Rd.1	'95 Rd.2
I: CP=Marchais '81,Lajoinie '88	15.3	–	6.6	–	Hue 8.5%	
c-l: SP=Mitterand ('81,88)	25.9%	51.8%	34.2%	54.0%	Jospin 23.3	47.4%
c-r: UDF=Giscard '81,Barre '88	28.3	48.2	16.6	–	Balladur 18.6	
r: RPR=Chirac ('81,'88)	18.0	–	20.0	46.0	Chirac 20.8	52.6%
f-r: NF=Le Pen '88	–	–	14.4	–	Le Pen 15.0	
Others(Ecol.,Wrkrs.,Trots.)	13.5	–	9.2	–	n=4 @ 13.8	

Earlier Round #2 results: '74: Giscard 50.8, Mitterand 49.2; '69: Pompidou 58.2, Poher 41.8; '65: de Gaulle 55.2, Mitterand 44.8; '58 indir.: deGaulle.

Assy. elections (LH > PM)		3/86	6/88(Rd.1,2)	3/93
n=25, 5 main	577/2=289 needed to *	(3pCO)	1p min.	3p CO
f-l: CP=Communist Party (Marchais, Hue)		35	26^ (11,3%v.)	23 (9.2%v)
(%vote decline: '46=28%;'71=21%;'81=16%;'88=11%;'91=7%)				
l: Greens & Ecology Generation (n=2 parties)		n.a.	0	0 (7.0)
cl: SP=Socialist Party (Mitterand, Jospin) +Rad.Lft, U.of Lft, others		215	277*(35,45%)	70(20.3)
cr:UDF=Union Fr.Dem.(=Giscard/Leotard Repubs.+ Soc.Dem.Cntr.U.		127*	132(19,23%)	217* (44.2)√
rc: Other right: Soc.Dem.P., +: Radical P., CNIP, indeps.(Barre)		14*	12	23* (44.2)√
r: RPR=Rally for Republic(Gaullists, Chirac), incl.: Pasqua populists;		149*	129(18,21%)	247* (44.2)√
Balladur businesmen; ex-Un.Dems.fRepub.,Indep.Repubs.,RefrmstMvmt.				
fr: NF=National Front (Le Pen)		35	1 (10,1%)	0 (12.4)
Others (incl. Pacific & other territories)		2	2	0 (6.9)
TOTAL		*290/577	*277/577	*484/577

√ = combined vote of 3 right-parties for 3/93 ; 44% of votes yielded 84% seats; largest majority since 1815.

3/93 assy. vote: Rd. 1 results: UDF/RPR/other right, aligned in "Union for France" in all but 70 districts, won 39.5%v. (as in '88!) & 80 seats outright; Soc. P. only 18-20%v. (down fm. 34.7% in '88!), & NO seats outright. Others: #3=NF (12.4% vote); Commies (9.2%v.); Environnmntlst Alliance (Green P. + Ecol.Gen.) (7.6%); others on far right & left, 13.7%. Turnout: 69% (=low).

In Rd. 2: Soc. P. asked all on left to back non-right cands.; Communists agree; Greens didn't & lost their 2 chances. Chirac, leader of #1 RPR party, appoints Balladur as PM while biding time to run for Pres.

FPP/SMD + 2 Rounds favors large parties: right's 40% vote = 80% seats; Green's and Natl. Front's 20% vote (total) = 0 seats. Earlier....

3/86 - Prop. Representation system favored small parties; 5% minimum. NF got 35 seats. Changed in......

6/88 - FPP/SMD constituencies(favored large parties, esp. vs. Natl.Front [got 1 seat w/ same % vote]).

^ = Communists support of 6/88 minority Soc. P.govt.; caused >25 censure motions to fail (6/88-10/92).

Less Impt. UH=Senate - 1/3 *indirectly* elected every 3 yrs. for 9 yr. terms. Recent results:
9/86: CP 15; Soc.P. 64; indeps. & others 9; UDF etc. 154; RPR 77. TOT: 319
9/89: CP 16; Soc.P.66; indeps. & others 6; UDF, etc. 143; RPR 91. TOT: 321.
9/92: CP 17; Soc. P. 73; indeps. & others 3; UDF, etc. 132; RPR 96. TOT: 321

After 1995, right controlled 4/5 LH, 2/3 UH, 19/21 regional councils, 4/5 department councils (n=96), and most municipal councils.

3b Weak Multiparty Republics (~mpr)

Weak multiparty republics also have two or more parties participating in a civilian political system with elections in which more than one party has a credible chance of gaining power. (See **Table 3b**, which reproduces the 12 ~mprs from CGSS.) But these system are weak, or immature, due to one of three reasons, each of which is illustrated in the following discussion of the three subtypes of the 12 states described in **Table 3b.i**.

In the first case are two states, normally described as democratic but where, although elections are formally fair, one party has ruled for almost every year under analysis: Italy and its Christian Democratic Party (CDP) from 1948 to 1994, and Japan and its Liberal Democratic Party (LDP) from 1954 to 1993. This situation is the result of political systems originally imposed by World War II occupation forces and perpetuated during the Cold War era by U.S. military troops staying on under treaty arrangements. Each system was truncated in a different way. Italy had fifty-two governments in forty-six years (an average of one every ten months); all coalitions dominated by the CDP, which never won a majority of the vote in a system which was structured to keep the second largest party (the Communists) out of power (Kurth and Petras, 1993). Japan had nineteen governments in forty years, all led by the LDP with weak prime ministers and in the manner of a one-party-dominant system (Hayao, 1993; Pempel, 1992). It was only with end of the Cold War that the first governments without CDP or LDP were formed in Italy and Japan, respectively. These two ~mprs are coded ≈ in **Tables 3b.i** and **3b.ii**.

The second subtype of ~mprs includes 6 states which have been moved up to this category from the militarized multiparty systems of the CGSS, page 2 of Table 1a. These countries have not been militarized for fifteen to twenty years now, but are still a generation behind the (regular) mprs in civilian experience. They include the following: Greece, Spain, and Portugal in Mediterranean Europe (all of which ended their military dictatorships in the early 1970s), and Venezuela (1961), Dominican Republic (1965), and Ecuador (1979) in Latin America, whose transitions to civilian rule occurred in the years indicated. These states will be coded * in **Tables 3b.i** and **3b.ii**, reflecting their emergence from CGSS category *mpr (Higley and Gunther, 1992; Mainwaring, O'Donnell, and Valenzuela, 1992).

The final group of ~mpr states (coded ∂ in **Tables 3b.i** and **3b.ii**) has been moved up to this category from the one-party (specifically one-party communist) polities only in the last few years: Czech Republic, Hungary, Poland, and Bulgaria. It is unclear whether the transition to "democracy" has been successfully made in these countries. After non-communist parties won the first post-communist elections, power was returned to communists (renamed and ruling in coalition) in subsequent elections in Poland, Hungary, and Bulgaria. Thus, it would be prudent to wait a few more electoral cycles, preferably ones in which power changes hands again, before any of these countries are moved definitively up to the mpr category (Wightman, 1994; Zloch-Christy,

Table 3b
Weak Multiparty Republics (~mprs)

Europe	Islamic Zone	Africa	Asia	West.Hemisph.
	3b. ~mpr=_weak_ multiparty republics (n=12)			
Italy,Greece			Japan	Venezuela
Spain, Portugal				Ecuador
Czech.,Hungary				Dom.Rep.
Poland,Bulgaria				
TOT: 8			1	3 (12)

Table 3b.i
~mprs by Subtype

(≈) = WWII/Cold War 1pdom (n=2): Italy, Japan
(*) = ex-military (n=6): Greece, Spain, Portugal; Venezuela, Dom. Rep., Ecuador
(∂) = ex-1-party (esp. 1p-communist) (n=4): Czech Republic, Hungary, Poland, Bulgaria

Table 3b.ii
Number of Parties Forming Governments in 9 of 12 ~mprs, as of December 1995
(includes 5 parliamentary and 4 mixed systems)

Europe		Asia	West.Hemisph.	
LEAST STABLE/MOST RESPONSIVE				
parliamentary govts. (n=5)				
3 party CO: ∂Czech.1/93,				(1)
2 party CO:		≈Japan 7/94		(1)
1p minority^: *Spain^ 6/93				(1)
1p SM: *Greece 10/93				(1)
0p technocrat: ≈Italy 1/95				
mixed govts. (n=4)				
2p CO: ∂Poland 10/93, ∂Hungary 7/94,				(2)
1p SM: *Portugal 10/91, ∂Bulgaria 12/94				(2)
not applicable: strong Pres. govt. (n=3)				
			*Dom.Rep.,*Ven.,*Ecuad.	(3)
TOT: 8	0	0	1 3	(12)
			MOST STABLE/LEAST RESPONSIVE	

Note: ^ = minority govt.(n=1, Spain). Parties don't need majority to rule, just no majority _against_ their rule;
    i.e., some non-governing parties abstain on votes of confidence.

1994). (This phenomenon has not occurred in the Czech Republic, and is probably not likely to, since most politicians who were inclined in that direction were in the Slovak republic which broke off to form its own state in 1993.)

Regardless of the reason for the weak ~mpr designation, the distinguishing feature of these twelve governments today is the number of parties (government and opposition) participating in the political process. Following the _Format_ of the previous section, **Table 3b.ii** reveals (as of late 1995) 5 parliamentary governments (2 with coalitions, 1 simple majority, 1 minority, 1 nonparty technocrat), 4 mixed (with 2 CO and 2 SM), and 3 presidential (all in Latin America).

Table 3b.iii shows that, on average, the number of main parties of long standing is somewhat fewer than in the mprs (3.5 versus 4.2) and that they comprise a smaller percentage of assembly seats (87.6% versus 96.5%). The most significant feature in this regard is the total number of parties gaining assembly representation (7.6), with 5 of the 13 states each having 10 or more viable parties. It is a distinguishing characteristic of the more "mature" mprs, placing higher in the CGSS, that such minor parties eventually become subsumed into some of the larger major groupings.

The *Excerpts* for this section are for Japan (as an example of the ~mpr [≈]), and Greece and Venezuela (exemplars of the ~mpr[*]). The displays of the ~mpr(∂) type are deferred to section 3c, on ex-communist countries.

3c COMMUNIST STATES IN TRANSITION (ex-com)

The previous discussion of the 4 ex-communist eastern European states which appear to have adapted multiparty modes—and the difference between these states and the other European countries in that category, like Italy, Spain, and Greece—highlights the fact that states evolving from the one-party communist system might deserve to be analyzed separately in their own right.

Ex-Communist polities (ex-com) are former one-party communist states— that is, Leninist vanguard parties with a monopoly of political power over a Marxist government-controlled economy (see definitions in Chapters 1a and 1b)—now in transition. They may be evolving into one of the following:

weak multiparty republics (ex-com——>~mpr) (3cb), if the ex-Communist Party has lost power in a multiparty election, as in Czech Republic, Hungary, Poland, and Bulgaria; but because this trend is not guaranteed to continue, especially if ex-communists rename themselves and win power in subsequent elections (some-

Table 3b.iii
Number of Parties in Representative Assemblies in 12 mprs, as of December 1995

Number (& Abbreviated Names) of *Main* Political Parties	% of Assy. Seats Held by Main Parties		Total # of Parties with Assy. Seats	
Italy 8+ (FI=3,PA=5)	Dom.Rep.	118/120=98.3%	Italy	12+
Japan 6+ (LDP,JSP,Kaishin=3+,CGP)	Venezuela	?197/201=98.0%	Japan	12
Poland 4 (DLA,PPP,DU,LU)	Greece	281/300=93.6%	Spain	11
Ecuador 4 (PSCP,RUP,RP,DL)	Italy	579/630=91.9%	Hungary	10+
Venezuela 3 (COPEI,AD,RC)	Poland	418/460=90.9%	Ecuador	10+
Dom.Rep. 3 (SCRP,DRP,DLP)	Bulgaria	217/240=90.4%	Czech.	7+
Hungary 3 (SP,AFD,DF)	Portugal	202/230=87.8%	Poland	7
Czech. 3 (CDP,CDA,LB)	Spain	300/350=85.7%	Greece	5+
Greece 2+ (PASHOK, ND)	Japan	434/511=84.9%	Venezuela	5+
Spain 2+ (PP,SWP)	Hungary	316/386=81.7%	Portugal	5
Portugl 2 (PSD,SP)	Czech.	74/99=74.7%	Dom.Rep.	4
Bulgaria 2 (BSP,UDF)	Ecuador	53/72=73.6%	Bulgaria	3
Average: 3.5 parties with 87.6% seats.			Avg: 7.6+ parties	

Japan ~mpr(≈): parl.	SM	CO,7p.min	CO,3p	
n=12+ LH: 511/2=256 to *	2/90 el.	7/93 el.	7/94 re-align	UH,11/93
f-l:JCP=Jap.("Euro-") Communist P.	16 (8%v)	15	15	11
n=470,000 members; ldrs: Miyamoto,Wada				
l:(United) Soc.Dem.Fed./New Wave (Eda/Shibuye)	4	4*	0	
lc:JSP=Jap. Socialist (Dem.,7/91) P. (PM Murayama vs...	136 (24%)	70*	74*	74
...SG Kubo w/ faction of ~40); controls largest union				
cl:DSP=Democ.Socialist P. (JSP rightists)	14 (5%)	15*	15	12
ldrs. Nagasue, K.Ouchi; public sector unions				
c-l:New Harbinger P.(Sakigake), 7/93,Takemura	n.a.	13*	22*	
c-r:JNP=Jap. New Party, fd. '92, Hosokawa	n.a.	35*	40	
c-rr:Renewal(Renass.,NewBirth); 6/93exLDP Hata,Ozawa	n.a.(36,6/92)	55*	52	
√r-c:Kaishin(Innovation, 4/94,Ozawa bloc w/o JSP,Harb.,JNP + some LDP)		(~128)		
√√r-c:New Frontier P.,11/94,SG Ozawa,Chm.Kaifu + 9p. incl. Harb.,Renewal		(~178)		
(≈)r-c:LDP=Liberal Democratic P. SG Kono	275*(+11*=286)	223(-)	206*	107
(founded, 1955 with CIA funding & support for years after)	(46%v;54%s)			
rr-c: Clean Govt.P.(=Komeito; Buddhist; fd.'64)	45 (8%)	51*	52	24
8m.mbrs., city social work in Soka Gokkai relig. group				
ensures 80% t.o.; women; ldrs: Yano,Ishita				
Others, independents, vacancies	22(11*,LDP;7%)	30(15,+)	35	24
TOTAL:	512	511		252
* =	275*	243*	302*	n.a.

7/93: + = indeps. linked with LDP; - = LDPs before defections of 4 in 11/93 incl. T.Nishioka, 6 in 1/94, 5 in 4/94 fm Watanabe wing forming Libl.(Fam.Values) P. under S.Arai.

7/93 minority CO of 243 (+19 indeps. & LDP defectors = 262 total) ended 38-yr. LDP rule. But only lasted until 4/94 creationof Kaishin bloc(√) which caused 7/93 Govt. to fall, JSP to switch support to LDP & new (Soc.PM) Govt. in 7/94. 3 new center parties (JNP,Harbinger,Renewal) differed on WWII apology, global role, electoral reform, & opening of economy, even before Ozawa moved, 4/94, to create new r-c Kaishin (√) "bloc" with "progressive" defectors from LDP (incl. Kaifu, Nakasone, Watanabe; also Yokomichi's Council for Dem. Govt. on his left). Ozawa's LDP to Renewal to Kaishin to 11/94 New Frontier(√√) maneuvering perpetuates tradition of weak parties and shifting Govt. (see below ~mpr[≈]).

Electoral System: LH incl. 130 multi-seat (3,4,5) districts (means factions in LDP get 1st 3 seats, minority parties 4th and 5th). Also, drawn to favor rural areas (3:1) over cities; (in worst cases: 3.34:1 in LH; 6.5:1 in UH.) In UH, 60% SMD districts, 40% PR at large acc. to party % & ldrs.' whim. PM Kaifu 7/91 reform would have 300 SMDs, 171 Prop. Rep. (tot. 471), ea. voter picking 1 of each. Rejected/ousted by party bosses 9/91. 11/93 Govt. proposed, 7/94 Govt. continues more viable plan: LH of 500, w/ 300 dir. el. SMD (favors larger LDP), 200 PR in 11 multimember districts.

~mpr(≈) due to dominance of political system by one party (LDP) over several weaker ones since 1955; opposition has ruled only in short 7/93-4/94 period (though if united they would still have majority). System started in '55 with 2 main coalitions: LDP (encourdaged by US, financed by CIA) & JSP. "Hakuchusen", or near-parity politics, with "consultative" (nearly 1pdom) relation of LDP to other parties. 45% LDP seats virtually inherited to 2nd generation MPs in 1992.

(≈) Within LDP: 4 main factions (until 1993 break-up); their approx. #s in LH+UH pre-'7/93 el.):
1. Tanaka, '71 PM (pre-Lockheed). Then:Takeshita (PM pre-Recruit) + Kanemaru (godfather, creator of 4 PMs, toppler of 2, before out 8/92). n=~109 MPs til faction splits 12/92 when Obuchi & Kajiyama defeat Hata & Ozawa, by roughly 60-40. Losers defect to form "Reform (of $ politics) Forum 21" w/dozens of younger mbrs.(e.g.,Aichi,Hosokawa),35 LH seats; reducing #1 faction to #4. 6/93 they bolt with 34 MPs in no-confidence vote, topple govt., form Renewal P. 10 others(Takemura,Mihara) form Harbinger P.
2. Nakasone/Watanabe (=ex 1980sPM/1991 FM). n=67-87 MPs; disparaging remarks on US blacks,'90.
3. Miyazawa - n= ~88; allegedly more progressive; but 12/92 names LDP SG Kajiyama (vs.elec. reform).
4. Mitsuzuka & Mori (successors to Abe), n=~81-89..

Party leader (=Pres, not SG) (&PM, limited to two 2-yr. terms.) chosen by LDP MPs, plus representatives of 1.75m. party mbrs.(=496 voters). Great deference to seniority.

Unsure if ~mpr(∂) ended by "unnatural" 7/93 coalition which lasted only nine months. LDP still #1 with 37% plurality vote; three new center-right parties only got 20%. But Ozawa predicts 7/94 government of old-LDP-right/old-JSP-left coalition is inherently unstable and his NFP(√√) right-center coalition is wave of future (vs. left-center coalesced around JSP [which has always been #2 in vote %] in new 2-party system).

Greece - ~mpr(*): parl.

n=3+ 300/2=150 to *	CO 11/89	SM 4/90	SM 10/93(4yrs)
f-l: Green Party	0	1	0
l: KKE=Communist P.(legalized in '74;Florakis,Kyrkos)	n.a.	n.a.	9 (4.5%v)
l-c: Left coalition of KKE Communists, Jt.PASHOK/KKE, and others.	21 (11%v)	21 (9%v)	0 (2.9)
c-l: PASHOK-Pan-Hellenic Soc.Mvmt; Papandreou	128* (41)	125 (38.6)	171*(46.8)
c-r: NDP-New Democracy P.(Karamanlis,Mitsotakis,Evert)	148* (46)	150* (46.9)	110 (39.3)
r: Dem.Renewal (n=10 ex-NDP'87; Stefanopoulos)	0	1*	n.a.
r: Political Spring (n=12 NDP '93 defectors on Macedonia; Samaras)	n.a.	n.a.	10 (4.9)
Other, including ethnic Turks from Thrace	3(2%)	2	0
TOTAL:	300	300	300

Govt. has changed voting system within 6 months of election in 9 of 12 elections since 1951. In 6/89 PASHOK made system more strictly proportional so that expected winning NDP party would need 47%+ of vote to get 50% of seats (it failed). 11/89 grand coalition created a "reinforced" PR system with 56 districts (# seats ranging from 1 to 26) structured so that greatest number of seats would go to party with greatest number of votes. PR threshold raised to 3% (v. Thrace Moslems who were getting 2 seats w/ <2% vote).

3/95 Pres. el. - PM Papandreou acquiesced in choice of conservative Stefanopoulos as Pres. (elected to 5 yr. term by 60% [n=180] vote of assy.) to avoid new gen.election if no pres. cand. got 60% assy.vote.

~mpr(*) due to 1967-74 military dictatorship, and unstable US CIA-dominated regimes before that, going back to 1946-49 civil war. Today's two main parties trace roots to 1974 liberalization (though Papandreou's PASHOK descended from his father's US-harassed Socialist Party).

Venezuela - ~mpr(*): strong pres. > parl.   n=2+ parties

	88LH	88UH	88Pres.	93LH	93UH	93Pres.
12/88 and 12/93 elections		turnout: 82%			turnout: 62%	
l: RC=Radical Cause (fd. '82; Maniero, Velasquez)	3	0	n.a.	40	9	21.9%
lc: MAS=Movement to Socialism (fd.'71Petkoff)	18	3	3%	26*	4*	*
cl: AD=Democ. Action (fd.'39; Lusinchi,Perez,Fermin)	97*	23*	54%*	55	18	23.6%
c:Convergence, '93 17-party COalition of	-----n. a. -----			-------n.a. -------		
ex-Pres. Caldera + MAS +15 sm. left, 2 sm. rights				24*	3*	30.5%*
cr: COPEI=Soc.Xtn.P.(fd.'46;Fernandez,Alvarez Paz)	67	22	40%	54	15	22.7%v.
r:NGD=New Dem.Genrls.P.('79;Gen.A.Castro)	8	1	n.a.	*	*	*
Others: DRU,NO,CP,RM,NIM,UNA,etc.;+indeps.	8	0	4%	8?		1.2%
	201	49	100%	199-207?	49	100%

Strongly presidential thru 1988 when legislators had to be elected on pres. ticket on basis of Prop.Rep. lists controlled by party bosses. '93 reform: 1/2 MPs to be filled by candidates not on party-controlled slates.

Strong 2-centrist-party system (COPEI,AD) until 1993. In 1988 AD split between Pres. Lusinchi (who wanted O.Barretto as successor), & ex-Pres. C.A.Perez, who won nomination in party electoral college & general election. By 1993, both parties seen as autocratic, remote, corrupt; ex-Pres. Caldera, age 77, founder of COPEI, ran as independent on Convergence slate, allying with old left MAS (& 17 small, mostly left, parties) vs. new left RC and discredited centrist AD & COPEI.

~mpr(*) due to lingering manifestations of militarism from 4 coup-regimes during 1948-59, esp. in light of rising public discontent with ineffective and corrupt govts . Some examples:

2/4/92 coup attempt: leader Lt.Col. Hugo Chavez & his Bolivarian Revolution Movement; ~40 killed in try, 300 in riots after. 1800 arrested, of wh. 1750 released w/o trial. Forces Pres. Perez into natl.unity coalit. govt. w/ COPEI; collapses 6/92. Mil. unrest temporarily defused with: pay raise, command changes, housing loans, overseas scholarships,more mil.intelligence, Genl. apptd. Foreign Minister, etc.

11/92 coup attempt:ldr. AF Gen. F.Elfrain Visconti, + video fm. imprisoned Col. Chavez. 230 dead, 377 wounded; arrested; 1200-1300 miliary incl. 500 offs. & non-coms; 93+leader escape to Peru.

1/94: Col. Chavez pardoned by new Pres. Caldera. Chavez, 39, is most popular political figure in public opinion polls & esp. among about 80% of the 6000-man officer corps (of 75,000 man army).

6/94: "Economic" State of Emergency declared. Many constitut. guarantees suspended: arbitrary arrests, searches, travel bans; killings and torture by police tolerated.

Spring '95: 150 Chavez followers detained to deter protests in food price riots as SOE goes into 2nd year.

thing that has already occurred in three countries), these states were separated from the other ~mprs in section 3b, and will be discussed at greater length here.

one-party dominant states (ex-com———>1pdom) (3cd), if the ex-Communist Party (or its leading members with a changed party name) held power in a multiparty election which it ran and tried to control (e.g., Romania, Russia, Ukraine, Uzbekistan, and Kazakhstan).

other one-party (ex-com———>1p-oth) (3ce), if the Communist Party has still not relinquished its monopoly of power in the political arena, even if it has allowed "liberalization" in the economic sphere (e.g., China, Vietnam, North Korea, and Cuba). Also in this category is the special case of Yugoslavia. Most of that former republic is enmeshed in war, but the nominal successor-state in the rump areas of Serbia and Montenegro has a similar one-party modality; since the focus of this analysis is on the political process there, the decision is made to keep Yugoslavia on the first page of the CGSS because it is civilian, though the war allows it to be authoritarian in the manner of the other four ex-com states in this category.

entrenched military regimes (ex-com———>mil°) (3c/6d), where ex-communist countries are currently in the midst of civil wars (e.g., Georgia, Azerbaijan, Tajikistan, Afghanistan, and Cambodia). These will be covered in Chapter 6.

It has been noted that there were, at most, 15 states which might have been realistically labeled "communist" among the 160-odd countries which existed at the end of the Cold War in 1989. Even with the increase of 23 new states from the former USSR (15), Yugoslavia (6), and Czechoslovakia (2), the number of recognizable communist or former communist countries among the 100 chosen for scrutiny in this study is still less than 20 (see **Table 3c**). Although these polities could be mentioned in their respective sections (as were the ex-com———> ~mprs), it might be helpful to compare all of them at this point, in order to understand how these states attempted to make the transition from the one-party communist system and how they respectively succeeded or failed (Holmes, 1993; Pei, 1994; White, Gill, and Slider, 1993).

The 19 former communist states among the CGSS's 100 include 7 former constituent republics of the Soviet Union (Russia, Ukraine, Georgia, Azerbaijan, Kazakhstan, Uzbekistan, and Tajikistan), 5 eastern European states upon whom the one-party communist system was imposed by the USSR at the end of World War II (Czech Republic, Poland, Hungary, Bulgaria, and Romania), and 4 states whose post–1945 communist systems resulted from indigenous revolutionary struggles (Yugoslavia, China, Vietnam, and Cuba).

Three ex-communist states have rather murky origins with respect to their roots (indigenous versus external). North Korea was not an independent state but rather a Japanese colony before the Soviet Army liberated it in 1945, so it was more a matter of trading one externally imposed political system for another. The kingdom of Afghanistan had an indigenous revolution and coup (in 1973 and 1978, respectively), but required the intervention of Soviet troops in 1979 in order to maintain its new system. Cambodia had a nationalist communist (Khmer Rouge) revolution in 1975, but the Vietnamese Army replaced

Table 3c
Ex-Communist States in Transition (n = 19: 4 + 5 + 5 + 5)

Europe	Islamic Zone	Africa	Asia	West. Hemisphere
		3cb. **ex-com---->~mpr** (n=4)		
Czech.,Hungary				
Poland,Bulgaria				
Sbtot: 4				(4)
		3cd. **ex-com---->1pdom** (n=5)		
Romania				
Russia	Uzbekistan			
Ukraine	Kazakhstan			
Sbtot: 3	2			(5)
		3ce. **ex-com---->1p-oth** (n=5)		
Yugoslavia			China	Cuba
			Vietnam	
			N.Korea	
Sbtot: 1			3	1 (5)
		3c/6d. **ex-com---->mil°** (n=5)		
	Georgia		Cambodia	
	Azerbaijan			
	Tajikistan		Afghanistan	
Sbtot:	3		2	(5)
TOT: 8	5		5	1 (19)

----

ex-com states, by historic origins of communist rule, n=19+3^
ex-Soviet republics (n=7): Russia, Ukraine, Georgia, Azerbaij., Kazak., Uzbek.,Tajikistan.
east European WWII (n=5): Czech Rep., Hungary, Poland, Bulgaria, Romania.
indigenous revolutions (n=4): Yugoslavia, China, Vietnam, Cuba.
unclear(n=3): N.Korea, Afghanistan, Cambodia.
Note: ^Never 1p-communist, despite Reagan Doctrine claims (n=3): Angola, Ethiopia, Nicaragua.

it with another communist regime in 1979. (Three allegedly communist states, according to the 1985 "Reagan Doctrine"—Angola, Nicaragua, and Ethiopia—will not be discussed here, for they never had the degree of popular participation in the party or government control of the economy to deserve that designation (Sullivan, 1991: 366; Colburn, 1990; Somerville, 1986; Tiruneh, 1993).

The origins of communism in each of these 19 states is relevant to the enthusiasm or reluctance with which each abandoned the old system after 1989. Those which had the system imposed upon it (Czech Republic, Hungary, Poland, Bulgaria, and Romania) moved the fastest to embrace multiparty republican forms. Those which had genuinely indigenous roots (Yugoslavia, China, Vietnam, and Cuba) have been the most reluctant to let the system go. The Cambodian and Afghan communist regimes, though of local origin, were aided by external force; they have returned to violence today. North Korea is unclear in the wake of the 1994 death of its founder, Kim Il Sung.

The former USSR republics can be divided between those in which ex-communists are trying to engineer one-party dominant systems (Russia, Ukraine, Uzbekistan, and Kazakhstan) and those which have fallen into civil wars (Georgia, Azerbaijan, and Tajikistan) (Bremmer and Taras, 1993). Since they are all ethnically divided, the only pattern which emerges for differentiating between them is geography (i.e., distance from Moscow; the further away, the more likely war becomes [Dawisha and Parrott, 1994; Motyl, 1992]). Similarly, the 8 smaller ex-Soviet states not covered in this study can be divided into 6 aspiring to 1pdom status (Latvia, Lithuania, Estonia, Belarus, Turkmenistan, and Kyrgyzstan), and 2 with civil wars (Armenia and Moldova).

The evolution of the historic communist experiment in government can best be understood by analyzing the tactics of Mikhail Gorbachev, who attempted to reform (i.e., save and improve) the one-party communist system of the Soviet Union in the years 1985 to 1991 (Kaminski, 1992; Sakwa, 1990; Walker, 1993; White, 1990). The fact that Gorbachev was ultimately unsuccessful and that his "reforms" led to the end of Soviet hegemony and communism in eastern Europe as early as 1989, and to the dissolution of the USSR itself in 1991, does not gainsay the fact that he had a plan—*glasnost, perestroika,* and "democracy" (no equivalent word in Russian)—which strove to keep reform communists in power in a vain effort to save a system on the verge of economic collapse under the weight of its own contradictions and a "generation of stagnation." His idea involved allowing restricted elements of capitalism (external corporate investment, some private ownership) into the Marxist (i.e., government-controlled) economic sphere and, in the political arena, certain incremental adjustments designed to keep "reformers" in control of what would essentially be, in this book's terminology, a one-party dominant system.

These steps included the following: first, the transference of the monopoly of political power from the Leninist "vanguard" party to the representative assembly (Jowitt, 1992; Urban, 1990); second, the making of elections to that assembly somewhat more meaningful (e.g., allowing one-third of the Soviet Congress of Peoples Deputies to be freely elected in 1989); third, having the party's Secretary General elected State President by the new assembly, then later increasing this President's power (and legitimacy) by having him re-elected in a direct election (organized by the still-dominant communist party); fourth, tolerating factions within the central party and permitting other parties (particularly on the decentralized, republican levels of government within the USSR); fifth, legalizing other parties on the national level after appropriate arrangements had been made to keep the communist party (perhaps renamed) as the dominant party; and sixth, relinquishing the party's legal, stipulated monopoly role in society (Waller, 1994).

Gorbachev travelled to eastern Europe, east Asia, and Cuba to encourage the one-party communist states there to embrace similar reforms and to alert them that Soviet subsidies sustaining their economic systems were to be phased out. Each state, in turn, adapted versions of the Soviet model. In eastern Europe, the legalization of other parties and the infiltration of Western capital and ideas led to the collapse of most of the communist systems by 1989 (Berglund and Dellenbrant, 1994; Rothschild, 1993; Stokes, 1993). In east Asia—particularly China and Vietnam—a variant of the Soviet experience allowed for wide-scale opening of the system in the economic arena without any relinquishing of control in the political domain (Nathan, 1990; Rozman, 1992; Scalapino, 1992).

Excerpts from the Data Bank associated with this project will be presented next for at least 1 state from each of the three civilian types of ex-communist states (3cb, 3cd, 3ce); analysis of the militarized ex-coms now in civil wars will be deferred to Chapter 6. The *Formats* to be employed precede the *Excerpts* and are also in the sections where their respective archetypes (3b, 3d, 6d) are covered.

Excerpts follow for 2 ex-coms evolving into weak multiparty republics (3cb), Hungary and Bulgaria; Russia, the most important example of a former Soviet republic where ex-communists (Yeltsin, Gaidar, Rutskoi, Zhironovsky, etc.) are trying to dominate a system (3cd) cluttered with weak parties (McFaul, 1994); and one state still primarily communist in its political structure (3ce), China.

Format for 3c Ex-Com Data Banks

State - i. notable dates on transition from 1pcom rule:
    a. date of transfer of power fm. party to assembly;   b. date Party SG elected Pres. by new assy;
    c. date this Pres. legitimated by direct popular election;   d. names (dates founded) of other parties;
ii. result of first multiparty (see **3 b** format for n=4), or 1pdom (see **3 d** format for n=5), or 1p-other (see **3e** format for n=5) elections.
iii. names and number of armed supporters of contending parties (see formats for **6 d°** and **5 b** for n=5) in states in midst of civil war.

Format for 3ce 1P-Other: Ex-Com Data Bank

State - i. name of party (&/or front), & SG   ii. party membership, % population
iii. results of most recent election to assembly. *(Any executive referendums?)*
iv. degree of choice (vs. single list), including status of non-party members; % of spoiled ballots, etc.
v. *other 1pcom info.* : e.g. # in Politburo & Cent.Cmtee; other positions & duration of SG; date & direction of most recent party congress or conference.

Excerpts from Ex-Communist States Data Bank

Hungary - excom---->~mpr(∂): parl.

	CO, 3p	CO, 2p
386/2 = 193 to *	4/90 Rd.2	5/94 Rd.2
f-l: SWP=Socialist Workers P.(unreformed communists: Grosz)	0 (3.6%v)	0 (<4%v)
l-c: SP=Socialist P. (reform communists: 50,000 mbrs.; '94 PM Horn)	33 (11%)	209* (32.7%)
c-l: Alliance of Free Democrats (old dissidents; urban intellectuals;	94 (21%)	70* (19.8%)
incl. 1990ff Pres. Goncz; also Kuncze, Tolgyessy, Peto)		
c: FIDESZ=Alliance of Young Democrats (Fabor, Orban)	22 (6-9%)	20 (<4%)
c-r: Democratic Forum (1990 PM Antall; Boross)	164* (25%)	37 (11.6%)
r-c: Independent Smallholders (pre-'48 party; Torgyan; 100,000 mbrs.)	44*(12%)	26 (<4%)
r: Czurka + n=15 MPs split from Dem.Forum, 5/93	n.a.	0 (1.3%)
f-r: Christian Dem.P. (Keresztes, Giczi; pro-RC Church,fast privtz.)	21* (7%)	22 (<4%)
Independents	8 (11.4%)	
Independents & Other parties, including:		2 (32.5%)
Social Democratic P., Entrepreneurs P., Peoples P.		
Patriotic Election Coalition, Agrarian Federation		
	386 (100%)	386 (97.9%+)

Electoral system (176 SMD, 210 PR w/ 4% threshold) rewards strongest parties with extra seats. Parties with less than 4% of PR vote won ~70 SMD seats in '94, but their divisions help largest Socialist Party of ex- (i.e.,reform)-communists which tripled its vote but increased its seats by six times over 1990.

~mpr(∂) = Former 1pcom state,1946-89. To get broadest possible base for transition from 1pcom system, center-right coalition government in1990 tolerated center-left president from opposition (but second largest) party. By 1994, reform communists had re-grouped and moved toward center to win majority, and number of parties with significant % of vote nationwide had dropped from 6 to 3. Anti-communist indirectly elected by (reform-communist) assy. to weak state presidency, 5/90 and 6/95.

Bulgaria - excom--->~mpr(∂): mixed

	1p min.	1pmin.	S M
n=30+ parties	6/90 el.	10/91 el. + 12/92	12/94
: BSP=Bulg.Socialist P.(fd. 4/90; ex-Communists)	211* (47%v)	106 (33%v) ^	125* (43%v)
(Ldrs.: Lilov, exPM Lukonov, PM Videnov)			
r:UDF=Unionof Dem.Forces (ex-PM Berov;Pres.Zhelev)	144 (36%)	110*(35%) *	~68 (26.5%)
(union of n=~17 in '91, split in '94, incl: monarchists, fascists,			
radical dems [ex-PM Dimitrov,Panov]; IMFers-I.Kostov)			
eth: MRF=Mvmt.f.Right & Freedom (*Turks;* A.Dogan)	23 (6%)	24^(7%)	
BANU=Agrarian Union (farmers; Ldrs. Barev, Petkov)	16 (8%)	0 (3.9%)	? (3.5%)
Others	6 (3%)	0 (21.1%)	~47(27.0%)
	400/2=200 to *	240/2=120 to *	240

4% threshold needed for the 50% of seats decided by proportional representation; 4 yr. term. Parties not getting it in 1994 incl: BANU, UDF(Center), UDF(Liberal), King's Party, Business Bloc.

1/1,1/92 Pres. election (5-yr. term)

	Rd.1(73%t.o)	Rd.2 (75% turnout)
l: BSP:V.Valkanov/VP Vodenicharov	31%	46%
r: UDF: ex-CP (1960s) Zhelya Zhelev/VP Dimitrova	45%	54%
20 others incl. G.Ganchev Petrushev of Business Bloc	24%	n.a.
	100%	100%

~mpr(∂) = ex-1pcom state; close ~mpr v. 1pdom decision as ex-coms. have been in charge for all except 13 months since 1989 end of communism. Also, only 34 state enterprises privatized (vs. 2098 in ~mpr Poland, and even 92 in 1pdom Romania.) MRF party declined to enter 10/91 minority govt. of Dimitrov on advice of Turkey; party is not even officially recognized as constitution bans ethnic ones. 11/92: Govt. fell on no confid.vote as MRF switched (pretext: govt. talking arms sales to Macedonia). In 12/92 , UDF chose technocrat caretaker PM and reliance on ex-cornmunist BSP for support. 12/94 election completed transition back to (reform) communist rule. Ex-communist party dissident has weaker presidency. Earlier transition fm. communism: 4/90: assy. revokes CP monopoly; 6/90 1pdom Assy. (53% seats w/ 47% votes; gerrymandering to overcome Soc.P. weakness in Sofia, cities) picks reformist ex-CPs Pres. Zhelev & PM Lukanov, but forced (when about 39 defect) to indep. PM Popov in 12/90 w/ Cab. of 8SP, 3UDF, 3Ag.U. 12/90: constitut. amendment revoking CP monopoly. But pres. remains weak, cannot dissolve BSP-dominated assy., even after 1992 direct election.

Russia - ex-com---->1pdom due to domination of weak multiparty system by ex-com Pres. (esp.
after 10/93 storming/closing of assy.), adoption of president-dominated constitution in referendum of 12/93; and growth of ex-coms in assy. after 12/95. (Earlier, reforming ex-coms had won 3 elections over left and right forces in 3 yrs: 3/89 USSR assy.; 3/90 Russian assy.; 6/91 Rusian Presidency [Yeltsin].)

Pres. Yeltsin elections - 5/90 el. by 3/90 CP-dom. assy. by 535-467; 6/91 - dir. el. as ex-CP/non-partisan with 57% vote; over CP Ryzhkov 16%, LDP Zhirinovsky 7.8%, Gen. A. Makashov 4%, et al. 75% turnout.

8/91 - 12/91: CP putsch vs. Sov.Pres.Gorbachev led to power shift away from Gorbachev to Russian Pres. Yeltsin and end of USSR. Summary of Russian assy. forces, 1992: c-l (for fastest change, PM Gaidar , Mvmt. Dem. Reforms, Dem.Russia), n=300, ~20% assy.; c-r: Civic Union (Volsky), Free Russia (VP Rutskoi), Dem.P. (Travkin), n=400 (~40%). r: Natl. Salvation Front (Konstantinov, Isakov), n=343 (33%).

12/92 vote for new PM (Pres. to choose fm. top 3): Skokov 637; Chernomyrdin 621 (named), Gaidar 400 (for vs. 492 against; ousted). New PM a non-party technocrat; vote defers exec. v. assy. struggle to .....

4/93 referendum: YES on Pres. Yeltsin 57%, his econ. policy 53%, for pres. election 49%, for parl. election 67%. (With 67% turnout, %s are: 38%, 34%, 31%, 43%), w/ Yeltsin winning 66/89 regions, 2/3 military.

9/93 - Pres. calls for new elections for 2-yr. assy. After assy. revolt put down, SOE suspends constitution, assy., parties. 13 parties approved for 12/93 election; 43 for 12/95 election. Turnouts over 60% in each.

Assy. Election Results (w/ 5% threshold for PR seats):

	12/93				12/95			
	% vote	PR	+ SMD	= Total	% vote	PR	+ SMD	= Total
f-l: Working Russ.(4.5%)/Peopl.Power(1.6%)	n.a.	n.a.	n.a.	n.a.	6.1%tot.	0	10	10
l: AP=Agrarian P. (Lapshin)	7.9%	21	34	55	3.8%	0	20	20
l: CP=Communist P. Bloc (Zyuganov)	12.4%	32	13	45	22.3%	99	58	157
l-c:Women of Russ. (Fedulova)	8.1%	21	2	23	4.6%	0	3	3
c-l: S.Fyodorov Party	founded in 1995				4.0%	0	1	1
c-l: Dem.P.(Travkin)/Mvmt.DemRef.(Sobchak)	9.6%	14	4	18	<2% ea.	0	0	0
c: SMD "independents"	n.a.	n.a.	45	45	n.a.	n.a.	77	77
c: "New Regional Policy" (n=9 SMD parties)	n.a.	n.a.	65	65	n.a.	n.a.	n.a.	0
c-r:YABLOKO (Yavlinsky ,Amb.Lukin)	7.8%	20	6	26	6.9%	31	14	45
c-r: Russia's Dem.Choice (Gaidar, Kozyrev)	15.4%	40	36	76	3.9%	0	9	9
c-r: P.of Unity & Accord (Shakrai)	6.8%	18	12	30	< 2%	0	0	0
c-r: Our Home is Russia (PM Chernomyrdin)	founded in 1995				10.1%	45	10	55
r-c: n=6 incl. Civic Union (Volsky)	18.8%	0	3	3	<2% ea.	0	0	0
r-c: Cong.o'Russ.Cmnties (Skokov,Gen.Lebed)	founded in 1995				4.3%	0	5	5
r: LDP=Libl.Dem.P. (Zhirinovsky)	22.8%	59	5	64	11.2%	50	1	51
Others without PR seats/None of Above	6.6%	0	0	0	≤19%	0	17	17
TOTALS	100%	225	225	450	~100%	225	225	450

In two assy. elections since 1991 end of SU, support for parties has moved from the center first to the right, then to the left. Shifting middle (n=~160) held balance of power in 1993-95 assy. between ~130 pro-Yeltsin "centrist reformers", and ~160 "red-browns" (left-right alliance of AP, CP, LDP). Less important Upper House, n=178 elected from 89 regions (x 2 ea./FPP), was more pro-Pres. Yeltsin/reformist.

In 12/95 election, better organized ex-coms move toward 1-party dominant goal as left ex-CPs rose from 20% vote and 100 seats, to 32% vote and 187 (i.e., 42% of) seats; right dropped from 23% vote and 64 seats to 11% vote and 51 seats. Unorganized center went from 57% vote and 286 seats, to 57% vote and 212 seats. 39 small parties split 49.5% PR vote among them, receiving no PR seats.

6/96 presidential election (probably between left and right survivors of Round 1 voting) will determine ultimate arbiter of power in president-dominanted system.

China - ex-com---->1p-other

i. Chinese Communist Party (CCP+Front): SG(6/89), Pres.(3/93), & Chm. Party Central Military Commission (3/93) Jiang Zemin > PM Li Peng; both < Deng Xiao Peng, retired Chm.,Cent.Mil.Cmsn.(1978-89).

ii. party members still (1995) ~4.4% pop. (53 mil./1.2 billion), despite economic liberalism.

iii. 3/93 assy., n=~3000 (elects SG as Pres; re-els. PM but with 10% (~330) spoiled ballots; then dismissed leaving rest of year's work to ~135-person standing committee. Reconvenes annually (n=2811 in 3/95).

iv. assy. indirectly el. for 5 yrs., by local assys,parties,ethnic groups & military units from approved CCP lists.

v. 10/92 14th Party Cong. (n=~2000 reps, selected fm. list w/ 5% "additional" cands. incl. 70% apptd. fm. lower levels (up from 50% in '87)), elects Central Cmtee of 170+110 alternates, Politburo of 17+1 alt., which dominates all sectors of govt. and army. Shared power during time of transition fm. Mao/Deng generation, esp. in Standing Cmtee. of Politburo (n=7). Army is strong militarily (#1 in world in size), economically (~15,000 companies under its control), and politically (23% Politburo, saved govt. during 6/89 Tien An Minh Square uprising).

3de ONE-PARTY POLITIES (1PP)

The Comparative Government Spread Sheet proposes two types of one-party political systems: one-party dominant and one-party other. In *one-party polities*, opposition political parties are either not allowed or are so severely restricted that they have no real chance of coming to power even though they may participate in an electoral exercise. In such polities, most meaningful political participation takes place within the structure of the ruling party; therefore, the character and size of this party, and the regularity and openness of its legitimizing electoral experiences, need to be assessed if one wishes to analyze the political system (Randall, 1988; Danopoulos, 1992).

Table 3de elaborates upon the CGSS for 1PPs by separating out the ex-communist states from the others in the 1pdom and 1p-oth categories. The display indicates that the 25 one-party polities are spread out across all five zones, with Africa and Asia having the most (8 and 6, respectively) and Latin America the least (2) (Fortes and Evans, 1987; Friedman, 1994; Pinkney, 1994).

Table 3de
One-Party Polities (n = 25: 13 + 12)

Europe	Islamic Zone	Africa	Asia	West. Hemisph.
		3cd. ex-com---->1pdom (n=5)		
Romania				
Russia	Kazakhstan			
Ukraine	Uzbekistan			
Sbtot: 3	2			(5)
		3d. 1p-dominant (n=8)		
		Senegal,Cameroon	Malaysia	
		Kenya,Zambia		Mexico
		South Africa	Taiwan	
Sbtot:		5	2	1 (8)
		3e. 1p-other (n=7)		
	Egypt	Ivory Coast		
	Tunisia	Tanzania	Singapore	
	Iran	Zimbabwe		
Sbtot:	3	3	1	(7)
		3ce. ex-com---->1p-oth (n=5)		
Yugoslavia			China	Cuba
			N.Korea	
			Vietnam	
Sbtot: 1			3	1 (5)
TOT: 4	5	8	6	2 (25)

Presidential Power in 1-Party Polities, n=25

Pres. without PM (n=5): Iran, Zimbabwe, Kenya, South Africa, Mexico.
Pres. > PM (n=13): Romania, Russia, Ukraine, Uzbekistan, Kazakhstan, Egypt, Tunisia, Senegal, Ivory Coast, Cameroon, Tanzania, Zambia, Taiwan.
Pres. < (Leg. > PM) (n=2): Malaysia, Singapore.
Pres. < decent. repub. Pres.(n=1): Yugo.   Pres. $\leq$ SG(n=4): China, N.Kor., VNam, Cuba.

Strongly presidential systems predominate, with 5 states having no prime ministers sharing executive power and 13 having weak prime ministers named by the president (Pres.>PM). Only Malaysia and Singapore have even the trappings of parliamentary systems (Leg.>PM). Yugoslavia has its own idiosyncratic system where a presidential decentralized subunit (the Serb Republic) dominates the larger parliamentary federation; and 4 states still have the communist system where the secretary general of the party is the most significant political actor. The *Formats* for the Data Bank entries for the one-party polities, which will be discussed next in their two main manifestations, are found preceding the *Excerpts* at the end of this chapter.

3d One-Party Dominant (1pdom)

One-party dominant systems are most like the mprs covered earlier in this chapter in the regularity of their elections and the ability of opposition parties to win some seats in the representative assembly; however, unlike the mprs (or even the weak ~mprs), other parties never win even a share of power in the administrative branch of government. This is because the 1pdom system is structured (i.e., rigged) so that only the one dominant party has a credible chance of gaining executive power in an election.

In this category, in addition to the 5 ex-com states trying to hang on to power by adopting 1pdom tactics (see section 3c), there are several successors to the historic mass nationalist–independence (or revolutionary) movements which have evolved into umbrella parties and have continued to rule. The classic model for single-party ruling longevity is Mexico, whose Institutional Revolutionary Party (PRI) traces its roots back some eighty years to the 1911 to 1919 revolution. Its constant co-opting of the opposition and tampering with electoral modalities has provided the blueprint for other dominant parties which attempt to perpetuate themselves by agreeing to share some perquisites of power in "reforms," most notably the ex-USSR (see previous section) and South Africa (to be discussed). Among other states where this has been done (in approximate order of their success in prolonging the power of the original party without resorting to undue use of military muscle) are Malaysia and Taiwan in Asia, and Senegal, Kenya, and Cameroon in Africa.

A second type of 1pdom polity, however, is provided by the historic transition in South Africa in 1991 to 1994. South Africa was effectively a classic one-party dominant state after 1948, when the Afrikaner Nationalist Party (ANP) ousted the ruling English-speaking party and then used its apartheid ideology to hold on to a near monopoly of power (in the white community) for the next forty-three years. Even in ceding some power after 1991, it built a power-sharing alliance with Nelson Mandela's African National Congress (ANC), from which it will retain significant influence through 1999. However, the size, scope, and internal history of the ANC is such that if it takes total control in 1999, as expected, South Africa will have effectively moved from one 1pdom government to another, with only the identity of the party changed. A comparable changing of the guard occurred in Zambia, where in 1991 a 1pdom state (under Kenneth Kaunda's United National Independence Party) yielded in its second generation to a similar domination by a different coalition (Frederick Chiluba's Movement for Multiparty Democracy). These two countries are designated √ on **Table 3d**.

While it might be argued that South Africa and Zambia are examples of nascent multiparty polities, it seems that such wholesale shifting of power is more reminiscent of the national conference/negotiated power-sharing phenomenon which has occurred in other smaller African states (not among the top 100 states recognized in the CGSS) in the early 1990s. In Benin, Togo, and Congo, power was transferred from longtime one-party or military dictatorships to a successor generation. However, it remains to be proven that the one-party habits are not so strong that that the change of power does not merely mean their assumption by the former opposition amidst the discrediting of the previous dominant party. This phenomenon is discussed further in Chapters 6b and 6c with respect to Madagascar, Zaire, and Ethiopia.

Despite the control of the executive branch of government by the dominant party in these 8 1pdom states, the other parties serve more than a representational function. In allowing genuine opposition parties to run and win elections for seats in the representative assembly, the 1pdom polities reflect some form of

Table 3d
Power Sharing in One-Party Dominant Polities

i - Rankings of n= 8 (of 13) 1pdoms in most recent elections, 1990-1995			
By dominant party % of Presidential vote		By dominant party % of Assembly seats	
Cameroon	35-40%	Cameroon	88/180	49%
Kenya	37%	Kenya	112/200	56%
Mexico	48.9%	Mexico	359/592	60.6%%
Taiwan-Assy	(79%; indir.electors; dir.in '96?)	Taiwan-Leg.	109/161	68%
Senegal	58.4%	Senegal	84/120	70%
Malaysia	n.a. (Assy. > Pres.)	Malaysia	162/192	84.3%%
√Zambia	75%	√Zambia	12/150	83.3% (MMD CO)
√S. Africa	n.a. (Assy. > Pres.)	√S. Africa	334/400	83.5 % (ANP/ANC CO)

ii - 1pdoms, party, recent electoral history; in order of openness		
State	Party, Date Estab.	Last Election(Pres.,assy.), Dubious Tactics
Mexico	PRI, 1929	8/94; Media control; last 200 LH seats, 4 of 31 fedl.states, OK to opp.
Malaysia	UNMO, 1958	4/95; Broad Front (n=14) co-opts other parties; monopoly over media.
Taiwan	KMT, 1920s	12/91,12/92; Govt. TV monopoly, money a significant factor
Senegal	SP, 1960	2/93,5/93 - opp. Pres. cand. arrested. Fraud, Violence, Low turnout
Kenya	KANU,'63	Constitut. required 1-party only frm 1982 to 1991. Public queuing.
Cameroon	CPDM'88	Successor to 1960 CNUP indep. mvmt. Opposition boycotts.
√Zambia	MMD'91	Since fair election, new 1pd party has declared SOE, jailed opp.,etc.
√S.Africa	ANP/ANC'94	See Text re ANP/ANC as new dominant force; Inkatha has Natal prov.

Note: √ = new dominant coalitions; others are from original mass independence/revolutionary movements.

legitimation and provide a safety valve to relieve pressure against the regime (Camp, 1993; Copper, 1994; Diamond, 1994; Means, 1991; Widner, 1992).

As evidence of political participation in such systems, it is instructive to identify the functioning opposition parties and some measure of their strength. **Table 3d** does this for the 8 1pdom states which were not formerly communist. (The 5 ex-com——>1pdom covered in section 3c are not discussed again here, for these governments have not yet achieved this degree of control over the opposition in their systems and could well evolve into ~mprs at the end of their transition from communism, or could degenerate into military systems as 5 other ex-coms already have.)

Table 3d.i ranks these 8 states in order of the strength and presence of the opposition parties in these systems, which are otherwise highly structured to perpetuate the rule of the governing party (i.e., Cameroon and Kenya being least 1p-dominant and most like ~mpr, South Africa and Zambia being most 1p-dominant). In Mexico's highly calibrated system, in recent years the president has received a decreasingly smaller percentage of the vote; in the most recent election only 48.9 percent, the first time the establishment candidate ever fell below 50 percent. The opposition has been given increasingly more seats in a progressively expanding representative assembly, but not enough to threaten the rule of the PRI on the national level (see **Excerpt**). Malaysia and Taiwan do not allow for direct election of the president (the first is parliamentary, the second has a special electoral college, at least until 1996), and their historic ruling parties (UNMO, KMT) have been skillful at buying off and co-opting the opposition over the years, as has Senegal's Socialist Party, even after the death of its independence-era leader. In Kenya and Cameroon, the systems seem the most open if only the percentage of votes for president and seats in assembly for the opposition parties are considered; but in both cases, the electoral exercises were considered fraudulent and were largely boycotted by the main opposition and no run-off was provided for the most powerful presidential post, which was achieved with less than 40 percent of the vote.

The brief remarks relating to the age of the dominant party and some of the electoral structures sustaining it in **Table 3d.ii**, along with the **Excerpts** from the 1pdom data bank presented for three states—Senegal (for Kenya, Cameroon), Malaysia (for Taiwan), and Mexico—reveal a number of tactics used by dominant parties to maintain their control. The most blatant examples of rigging the system occur on election day: ballot box stuffing, repeat voting, bogus voters, outright vote-buying, and the like. But these maneuvers, which can be found even in mprs in areas where only one party has a presence, can be curbed by ensuring that election boards—from the precinct to the national level—are staffed either with independents or with representatives from the various parties.

The more sophisticated structuring of the system occurs "upstream," long before the actual election day. Requirements for getting candidates' and even parties' names on the ballot can be onerous, requiring the signatures of many petitioners weeks or months before the scheduled election. The state's resources (especially its control over the media) can be thrown behind the campaign of the governing party. Campaign spending limits work against challengers and in favor of well-known incumbents (i.e., the ruling party). Districts can be gerrymandered, that is, drawn in ways that favor interests already represented in the governing party (Pempel, 1990).

Finally, electoral rules can be structured so that the opposition parties' percentage of seats in the representative assembly is much less than their percentage of votes. Sometimes the leading party is awarded 50 percent of the seats even if it does not get 50 percent of the votes (e.g., in Mexico in 1990); multimember districts often ensure that the most seats are won by the largest party and keep the smaller parties fighting among themselves for the remaining seats. This is a more sophisticated variation of the rule that, in some states, blatantly prohibits minority parties from forming coalitions to contest elections. Similarly, saving a specific number of seats for the opposition is not a favor to them but often condemns them to vying with one another for these few places (e.g., Mexico, Singapore). In decentralized states (Mexico, Malaysia, South Africa), the opposition is often allowed control of lower-level jurisdictions in return for not protesting fraud or tampering at the national level.

3e Other One-Party Systems

The *one-party other* (1p-oth) category will be reserved for three situations of extremely limited civilian rule.

The first—designated *1p-other: constricted opposition* in the *Format* for 3e—resembles 1pdom, but the political space in which other parties are allowed to operate is so constricted that they achieve only minimal (if any) representation in the assembly and, of course, no opportunity to share power in the executive branch (Clapham, 1993). There are 6 such states, 5 of them in Africa (including Islamic north Africa), plus Singapore. They are identified in **Table 3e**, without the √. The distinguishing feature about most of them, as compared with the 1pdoms in the previous section, is that they have not made the transition from the first-generation mass independence (or revolutionary) party with as much flexibility or tolerance within their highly structured electoral systems. Indeed, some, which seemed to be opening up in the later years of the independence leader, have contracted considerably after power was passed on to the second generation. Unlike the 1pdoms, where 5 of the 6 comparable states (i.e., the ones not designated √) are still run by the original party, only 2 of these 6 (Singapore and Ivory Coast) are, and the renamed successor parties in Zimbabwe, Tanzania, Egypt, and Tunisia seem to be operating as the personal vehicle of the new leader (DeCalo, 1989).

Table 3e.i ranks these 6 states in order of the opposition parties' percentage of presidential vote and assembly seats, so that the most restrictive 1p-oth states appear last. In the 5 with presidential systems, three leaders (in Tunisia,

Table 3e
Power Sharing in Other One-Party Polities

i - Rankings of n=8 (of 12) 1p-others in most recent elections, 1990-1995

By dominant party % of Presidential vote		By dominant party % of Assembly seats		
√√Yugoslavia	54%, of Serb.Repub., '92 under wartime conditions	√√Yugoslavia '92 w/Serbia '93	73/138 123/250	52.8% 49.2% (w/37% vote)
√Iran	63%, but Pres. ≤ Ayatollah	√Iran	no parties	n.a.
Singapore	59%, but Pres. < PM	Ivory Coast	165/175	94.2%
Ivory Coast	84%	Singapore	77/81	95.1% (w/ 61% vote)
Zimbabwe	84%	Egypt	431/444	97.1% (boycotts;wartime)
Egypt	96%	Zimbabwe	118/120	98.3%
Tanzania	96%	Tanzania	244/244	100%
Tunisia	99%	Tunisia	163/163	100%

ii - 1p-others, party, recent electoral history; in order of openness

State	Party, Date Estab.	Last Election(Pres.,assy.), Dubious Tactics
√√Yugoslavia	SP, 1989	"Nationalist" successor to Communist Party; same leader. War elections.
√Iran	NO Parties	IRP dominated from 1979 to 1987. Now, indep. candidates < clergy.
Singapore	PAP, 1959	8/93P,8/91a, when opposition had 1 hour to file for quick-call election.
Ivory Coast	DP, 1960	12/90 - 1st contested election for Pres. in 30 yr. history.
Zimbabwe	ZANU-PF , 1987	3/95 - Govt. press control, subsidies for party work, etc.
Tanzania	CCM, 1977	Successor to independence-era TANU, same Chm. to 1990.
Egypt	NDP, 1978	Successor to Nasser's '62 party (to legit. '52 coup/rev.); war elections.
Tunisia	RCD, 1987	Successor party to independence era PSD; same exclusivist tactics.

Note: √ = special cases; other six are mass independence parties or their successors.

Tanzania, and Egypt) ran unopposed and got between 96 and 99 percent approval; the two with opponents (in Ivory Coast and Zimbabwe) each won with 84 percent of the vote. The percentages of seats in the representative assemblies for the dominant parties in all 6 states ranged from 94 percent (Ivory Coast) to 100 percent (Tanzania and Tunisia). Egypt is interesting among these states as an example of a military party system which evolved up from a modernizing coup-regime (mil^) during the years 1952 to 1977 to its present place among the civilian states on the CGSS; it has tightened up in recent years, however, holding its most recent elections during times of war (in 1990, during preparations for the war against Iraq; in 1992 and 1995, during the Islamic Fundamentalist insurgency), provoking boycotts from the main opposition in the first two instances (Barnett, 1992). **Table 3e.ii** identifies the parties and some of their electoral tactics.

The second category of 1p-oth polities includes the two special cases—designated √ on **Table 3e**—of Iran and Yugoslavia. Iran is somewhat of an anomaly in that it has *no* political parties. The prevailing Islamic Republican Party was deemed irrelevant and abolished at the request of its secretary general in 1987, but the dominant political power is still the revolutionary clergy who led this party and the 1979 revolution. In any event, the military is not the most significant actor, so Iran does not belong on the second page of the CGSS (Amjad, 1989). In Yugoslavia (whose placement characteristics actually overlap those of the next category), the ex-Communist Party seems to be running a one-party dominant system which tolerates other parties within the federation of Serbia and Montenegro. However, its involvement, since 1991, in the wars in Croatia and Bosnia stifles serious criticism, not to mention significant party organization, against the government. Ex-Communist President Milosevic's use of ethnic nationalism to perpetuate his party in office is reminiscent of the way South Africa's ANP used race and the apartheid ideology, and Iran's rulers use religion.

Finally, the third group of 1p-oth polities—*1p-other: ex-com* in the *Format* for 3ce—includes the 4 other former communist states whose systems are hard to describe at the current time. While China, Vietnam, North Korea, and Cuba have abandoned Marxism in the economic sphere, they still retain severe Leninist parties which brook no opposition parties (or even dissident factions within the vanguard party) in the political arena.

The *Excerpts* from the Data Bank for subsection 3e are for the special case of Iran, and for Zimbabwe as an example of the constricted opposition type of 1p-other system. (The *Excerpt* for 1p-oth: ex-com was presented in section 3c, with other communist states in transition.)

Format for 3de 1PP Data Banks

(to *vary* fm 1pdom to 1p-other:constricted & ex-com)
(ex-com, takes 3c format + format of prototype it most nearly approximates)
State - i. name and information on ruling party (date established, SG roles, etc.);
ii. result of more recent election: date, level (i.e., office: Pres, rep. assy, other); % vote and/or # seats; degree of choice.
iii. other information, including why polity choice is not higher (~mpr) or lower (mil*^°).

Format for 3d 1pdom Data Bank

State - i. name of party; historic information accounting for its dominance (date, circumstances of its founding, length of rule, etc.).
ii. date, level most recent election: Pres. &/or rep.assy.; % vote and/or # seats of 1pdom.
iii. # seats, information on *other parties; incl. tactics used to keep them from real power.*

Format for 3e 1p-other: Constricted Opposition Data Bank

State - i. name (etc., +) of party & Secretary-General (= Head of State often)
ii. date, level most recent election: Pres. &/or rep.assy.; (% vote,# seats)
iii. *restrictions on choice,* incl.: if candidates must be party members vs. party approved vs. independents; also, number of incumbents typically defeated; etc.
iv. reason for **1p-other** designation in dubious (i.e., 1pdom, mil^) cases.

Senegal - 1pdom

i. Socialist Party (PS); mass-based independence party of Leopold Senghor, founded in 1949 (fm. French Soc. P.). Its SG is his 1981 successor, Pres. Abdou Diouf; Exec.Cmtee. of 10, Politburo of 30.

ii. Presidential elections:

2/83 - incumbent Pres. Diouf 85%, Wade 14.8%, three others 0.2%

2/88 - incumbent Pres. Diouf 73%, Wade 26%, two others 1%.

2/93 - incumbent Pres. Diouf 58.4%, Wade 32.0% + claiming fraud.

Assembly elections:

2/83 assy.: PS 111 seats; SDP (Sen.Dem.P.) 8, Pop. Liberation P. 1. (TOT: 120).

2/88 assy.: PS103 seats; SDP 17 seats. (TOT.: 120)

5/93 Assy.: PS 84 seats; SDP 27 seats; others = 9 seats. (TOT.: 120)

iii. Fairly open vote, though rioting and unrest at election time resulted in state of emergency and (temporary) jailing of perennial opposition presidential candidate A.Wade and many of his SDP supporters in both 1988 and 1993. Combination of SMD & Prop.Rep. voting systems ensures some, but no where near 50%, of vote to opposition.

Situation more open than under Senghor (1960-81) when only the SP party was legal during 1963-74. But opposition "coalitions" declared illegal in 1985, and before 1988, no ID required to vote, no secret ballot, no opposition presence during vote count; these procedure are still scanty. Parties may not be based on "divisive" factors like language, religion, or ethnicity.

Malaysia - 1pdom

i. Malay.Natl.Front (Barisan Natl.). ~5% pop. mbrs.; secular, multi-racial (w/ quotas). Front composed of United Malay Natl.Org.(=UMNO), moderately Islamic Malays, plus ~14 (in 4/95 election) ethnically-based separate orgs. (to reflect: Chinese, Indians, + non-peninsula regional areas of Sabah, Sarawak).

ii. Leg. (>PM) Results, most recent elections:

	1982	1986	1990	1995
l: DAP=Democratic Action Party, ldr. Lim Kit Sang	16	24	20	9
(more blindly multiracial, so Chinese-dominated)				
c: MNF=Malay Natl. Front (of which UNMO)	(70)	(73)	(71)	(72)
total with all ethnic components added to UNMO	132	148	127	162
c: Semangat=Spirit of '46 (fd.'88 fm.UNMO)	n.a.	n.a.	8	?
r: PAS=Islamic Party (wins rural SMD seats w/ 40% vote)	5	1	7	?
regl: Bersatu (United) Sabah P.	0	0	14	?
independents, others parties in '95	8	4	4	21
	161	177	180	192

Votes of ethnic components of Malay Natl. Front in '82, '86, '90:

Malay Chinese Association 24,17,18;   Malay Indian Congress 4, 5, 6.

n=2 Sabah affiliates: Peop.U.(Beyaya =PBB)=10, 7, 10; United Sabah Natl. Org. = 0, 5 ,6;

n=4 Sarawak affiliates (n=~19-22 total seats):

Unit. Trad. Bumiputra P.(Sarawak Alliance)=8,10,10; Sarawak Natl. P. 6, 4, 3;

Sarawak United Peop. P.5, 4, 4; and Sarawak Dayak Party 0,4,4.

Other: Malay Peoples Movement (=Gera-Kan Rakyat Malay) 5, 5, 5 .

iii. PM in effect chosen by the 1500 delegates to the UNMO party conference every 4-6 years. UNMO maintains control through gerrymandering districts to favor Malays in countryside over Chinese in towns (1990: MNF got 70% seats with 53% votes; in 1995, 84% seats with 63% votes). Also, banning of outdoor rallies, keeping campaigns short (10 days, "so as not to inflame ethnic tensions") and, especially co-opting of regional (Sabah, Sarawak) and ethnic (Chinese, Indian) leaders and communities. This tactic is less successful with more religious Muslims (esp. in Kelantan), and with secular left, both of which are tolerated as long as they don't threaten UNMO control. Internal Security Act used twice in 30 years to remove opposition from state government control.

Semangat '46=Sprit of '46 - founded in 1988 by ex-PMs Tunku abdul Rahman and Hussein bin Om, as well as Razaleigh Hamzah, to challenge autocratic PM Mahathir - was first rival Malay-led organization with allies from opposition Islamic (F. Chior), Kelantan Christian (J. Pairin), and Indian groups. It has only been spottily successful.

Mexico - 1pdom

i. Institutional Revolutionary Party (PRI) - mass party (16 mill. mbrs.) dating from 1910s revolution; institutionalized in 1929, since which it has not lost a Pres. el., and only a few Sen. or Gov. elections (& only since 1989). World's longest continuing ruling party (since USSR collapse).

Got 90% all votes in all elections through 1960s; since then, declining (see Data Bank). Many tactics used to coopt other parties (see iii.), which if they win 1.5% vote get govt. subsidies. PRI wings: left: Carpizo, Camacho; right: Coloso, Zedillo, ex-Ag.Min. C. Hank G. and party pres. I. Pichardo P.

ii. elections, 8/94:	turnout: 77.7%	Pres.	$\geq$	(dir.+indir.)=LH + UH = Tot.
l:PRD=P. of Dem.Rev.(fd.'91=Cuathemoc Cardenas)		16.4%		5 + 66 = 71 + 9 = 80
c:PRI (fd.'29;Ernesto Zedillo P.de L.)		48.9%*		277 + 23 = 300 + 59 = 359
r:PAN=Natl.Action P. (fd.'39;Fernandez de C.)		26.1%		18 +101 = 119 + 24 = 143
n=~10 minor parties, esp. WP,PSP		8.6%		0 + 10 = 10 + 0 = 10
		100%		300 + 200 = 500 + 92 = 592

*48.9% lowest PRI pres. win ever; down from 50.7% fraudulent win in '88 (most observers say Cardenas won outright; even Mex.City Research Center says he lost by only 35-31%).

iii. Electoral "reform" tactics used to preempt other parties:

1986: #1 party stays in power even if < 51% vote. Other parties allocated 200/500 LH seats iaw 1pdom dictates; i.e. opp."minorities" get most of 200 remaining LH seats; i.e., 300 dir. el. SMD +200 PR seats for those not coming in 1st in ea. district, but having 1.5% of national vote.

1990: any party with ≥34% vote gets 50%+1 seats in assy.; coalitions (as '88 FDN) banned, for 9/91 el. No "joint cands.," no publiciz. of vote totals not same as Fedl.Election Council's; a crime to protest official count; no oppositon access to state TV; paid (tho unidentified) govt. "news" in private media. PRI majority on Fedl. Election Council (FEC) where Interior Minister = Chairman, as in Cuba.

1993: LH mininimum for opposition raised from 150 to 185 =30%, still <33% needed for constitutional amendment block; UH expanded fm. 64 to 128 (=31 states x4 ea., w/ 1 minority guaranteed; see Singapore) in 1994,'97. Extend to yr.2000 requiremt *parents* m/b born in Mex. keeps PAN's Fox out of '94 Pres. race.

1994 post-Chiapas: campaign financing limits (but so high PRI-dispensor of Gov.$ still favored); better (but not equal) opposition media access; end PRI-dom. FEC, create body of w/ non-partisan majority (but "Appeals Tribunal" still PRI-dominated, and Congress can overrule both); Spec.Prosecutor for election fraud. Nothing on voter rolls. See also 4c for ethnic reforms.

1/95 post-peso fall: cut govt.-PRI links, more campaign financing limits; elections for Mex.City Mayor; full independence of FEC under PRI critc F. Creel.

iii. Moves to allow opposition control at *local* levels: fm.1% in '85; to 5% of 2400 local govts. in '90; to 4000/19,000 el. pub. offs. in opposition hands, 11/92. '89 PAN Gov. of Baja Cal.Norte = 1st opp. "allowed" in 60 yrs. (but not apparent PRD Gov. wins earlier in Oaxaca and Guerrero in '89 or in '90 fm PDR in Mexico state). In '91, PAN win in Guanajuato. 2 fraudulent PRI wins (in Tabasco, 2/92; and in San Luis Patosi, 11/91) were overturned by Pres. In 7/92 state els., Govt. lets PAN win in Chihuahua (richer, northern state); but doesn't let PRD win in Michoacan (poorer, southern state), or in Sinaloa or Tamaulipas in 11/92 where PRI wins were dubious. 12/93 deal to allow PAN mayor of Merida for PRI Gov. of Yucatan. 2/95: PAN wins Jalisco Govt. outright. 5/95: Govt. allows PAN re-election in Guanajuato in return for PAN's not contesting fraudulent PRI win in Yucatan.

iii. Moves to co-opt on national level: appointment of "independent" (leave of absence) PAN member (Lozano) to Cabinet as Attorney General, 12/94; first time ever.

?*1pdom bec. 5b(prospective); + without Army acquiescence no pres. could govern; even though army has not held the office since '46, its power impt., as shown by textbook controversy on '68 student "massacre". Also, election campaigns often violent: ~250 FDN/PRD mbrs. killed since '88, many protesting state election fraud. Also, in '94: assassination of PRI pres. cand. Colosio (Mar.),and SG R. Massieu (Sept.).

Iran - 1p-other: special case

i. - <u>No parties</u> after 6/87, when main dom. party since 1979 rev. (Islamic Repub. P.=IRP) was abolished (along with all others) as "no longer necessary." But, "groups" rel. to various clerical factions (all claiming support of dominant revol. ideology) still run slates (see below). And, before that, many (~18) small parties tolerated under IRP sway. Today, all (not in exile) agree on basics of support for the 1979 rev. & its export, and domestic polit. repression of dissenters. Disagree only over degree of free market vs. more govt. support/protection of bazaari (see evolution of positions in ii & assurance of orthodoxy in iii below.

ii. <u>El.Results:</u> assy. n=270, 4 yr. term (1/3 vote to win district w/o run-off.); Pres. = 4 yr .term, 1 yr. after assy.
<u>4/88 assy</u> - 2000 screened, 1400-16000 cands; 188 got majority in Rd. 1; 5/88 run-off needed for 82 undecided seats. "Radical" clerics (i.e., for more state control over economy) seem to strengthen their (& PM Moussavi & Speaker Rafsanjani) position (~139/270) over private-enterprise mullahs. Rafsanjani moderates economic views after 5/88 Iraq war end & 5/89 death of Khomeini, and runs as pragmatist in..
<u>8/89 Pres.</u> - only 2 of 79 candidate applications approved by Coun. of Guardians; Assy.Spkr. Rafsanjani elected w/ 94.5% vote (15.7m./16.4m.voters) over assy. dpty. Abbas Shaibani (3.8%). Turnout: 69%.
<u>10/90 Assy of Experts</u> (n=83; els. Spiritual Ldr., interps. constitut.) - allies of Pres. Rafsanj. win nearly all seats; many opps. excluded fm running (by Counc. of Guards). Turnout: 1.8m/10m (successful boycott).
<u>4/92 assy</u> - 3240 applicants screened down to 2050 approved candidates by Couc. of Guardians (to get more economic reformers). Tho no parties, Fundamentalist pro-bazaari Society of Combative Clergymen win 29/30 Tehran seats. But pragm. spptrs. of Pres.Raf. (Assoc. of Militant Clergy) win ~200/270 overall.
<u>6/93 Pres.</u> - Low 57% turnout, 4 cands. chosen by Council of Guardians from 128 applicants. Winner: Pres. Rafsanjani with 63%v. over: Ahmd.Tavakoli 24%; Abd.Jasbi 9%; Raj.ali Taheri 2%. Lower turnout and winning margin indicates somewhat of repudiation of 4/92 assy. results and liberal economic program. His rivals for '97 are: Spkr. ali Akbar Nateq-Nouri (more pro-bazaari), and Rev. Gd. Chm. of NSC, ali M. Besharati.

iii. <u>Restrictions</u> on choice of both Pres. & assy. assured by vetting by Council of Guardians (2c.ii) of any candidates who dissent from basic Islamic revolution orthodoxy.

iv. **1p-other** bec. there are NO parties, and hence less organized participation than in the n=13 1pdom states. But many factions (allied with various religious leaders=mullahs) in ex-IRP, rep. assy., Council of Guardians, & Assy. of Experts. Not like Iraq or other mil^o polities because many civilian (esp. religious) polit. institutions, elections, and participation (voting age 15); low 5c, 5d scores; and paramilitary Rev. Guards have been merged in with regular army since end of Iraq war, death of Ayatollah Khomeini (1989).

Zimbabwe - 1p-other: constricted opposition

i. <u>ZANU-PF</u>=Zimbwe Afr. Natl. Union-Patriotic Front; '87 merger of: ZAPU-PF=old ZANU, and Nkomo's Zimbwe Afr. Peoples Union (ZAPU). Indep. leader Robert Mugabe is 1st Secy. & Pres., VP = Nkomo.
12/89: ZANU-PF 1st Party Congress; n=4800 dels. fm. local & prov. elections; C.Cmtee n=160; Politburo n=26 apptd. by SG Mugabe. 9/90- last major opp. party comes into ZANU-PF; C.Cmtee persuades Mugabe not to outlaw remaining small rival parties. But still press control, party operatives in govt., & new Cabinet Minister of Political Affairs with $15 mil. budget for ZANU-PF work.

ii. <u>4/90 election:</u>. 1st dir. pres. el. allowed by 1980 (UK-imposed) constitution - turnout 54%, (down from 95% in '85 Leg.>PM election). Results: <u>Pres.</u>(6-yr.term) - ZANU-PF's Mugabe 78%; Zimbwe.Unity Mvmt's Edgar Tekere 16%; others 6%. <u>Assy.</u> (5-yr.term) - ZANU-PF 117/120 seats, with 80% vote, ZUM 2s (16%v.); ZANU-Ndonga P (Sithole) 1s. + 30 apptd., all ZANU-PF giving it 147 of 150 total.
<u>4/95 assy. el.:</u> ZANU-PF 118 seats, in 57% turnout (only 65 of 120 contested); five major opposition parties boycott, claiming chaotic registration (100,000 turned away at polls), infiltration of their parties by state intelligence agents, no access to media, etc..

iii. <u>History of/restrictions on other parties:</u>
pre-'74: UANC (Muzorewa); ZAPU (Nkomo's *Ndebeles*); '87-ZANU-Ngdonga Party (Sithole); 12/89-ZAPUP (Ndelula); 12/89-ZPDP (Pasalk); '90-NDU. Most important now are:
5/89: ZUM=Zimb.Unity Mvmt. Fdr: Edgar Tekere (ex-SG ZANU); vs. Mugabe, 1-party-state, corruption, etc., but rallies banned, no mention in official press during campaigns. Strong near Mozambique border.
5/92: Forum f. Dem. Reform - calls for smaller Cab. of n=14 (vs. 32), re-estab. of UH, limited Pres. tenure. Leads to 3/93 "Forum Party"; wants devolution (esp. to Matabeleland & Bulawo); SG T. Dlodlo (Ndebele), Chm. E.Dumbutshena (Shona). State intelligence infiltrators provoke intra-party squabbling.
3/95: ZANU-PF primary elections defeated 30 incumbents, and several of Pres. Mugabe's candidates.
5/95: New Law allows $10 mil. in state election funds to parties which win 15 seats in assy. (only ZANU-PF).

iv.**1p-other** because opposition has only 2 of 120 seats in assy. which is weaker than Pres., not much in light of Mugabe's past 1party-only intentions, (and 30/30 ZANU-PF apptees. to assy.). Also: Govt. (i.e., party) controls media; its secret police harass political dissidents; and Govt. subsidy to ZANU-PF. 1995 primary results indicate some competition within ZANU-PF.

REFERENCES

Amjad, M. (1989) *Iran: From Royal Dictatorship to Theocracy.* Westport, CT: Greenwood Press.

Barnett, M. N. (1992) *Confronting the Costs of War: Military Power, State and Society in Egypt.* Princeton: Princeton University Press.

Berglund, S. and J. A. Dellenbrant (eds.) (1994) *The New Democracies in Eastern Europe: Party Systems and Political Cleavages.* Brookfield, VT: Edward Elgar.

Bremmer, I. and R. Taras (eds.) (1993) *Nations and Politics in the Soviet Successor States.* New York: Cambridge University Press.

Budge, I. and D. McKay (eds.) (1994) *Developing Democracy.* Thousand Oaks, CA: Sage.

Camp, R. A. (1993) *Politics in Mexico.* New York: Oxford University Press.

Clapham, C. (1993) "Democratisation in Africa: Obstacles and Prospects," *Third World Quarterly,* 14(3): 423–438.

Colburn, F. D. (1990) *Managing the Commanding Heights: Nicaragua's State Enterprises.* Berkeley: University of California Press.

Copper, J. F. (1994) *Taiwan's 1991 and 1992 Non-Supplemental Elections: Reaching a Higher State of Democracy.* Lanham, MD: University Press of America.

Damgaard, E. (1992) *Parliamentary Change in Nordic Countries.* Oslo: Scandinavian University Press.

Danopoulos, C. P. (ed.) (1992) *Civilian Rule in the Developing World: Democracy on the March?* Boulder, CO: Westview Press.

Dawisha, K. and B. Parrott (1994) *Russia and the New States of Eurasia: The Politics of Upheaval.* New York: Cambridge University Press.

Decalo, S. (1989) *Psychoses of Power: African Personal Dictatorships.* Boulder, CO: Westview Press.

Diamond, L. (ed.) (1994) *Political Culture and Democracy in Developing Countries.* Boulder, CO: Lynne Rienner.

Diamond, L. and M. F. Plattner (eds.) (1993) *The Global Resurgence of Democracy.* Baltimore: Johns Hopkins University Press.

Fortes, M. and E. E. Evans-Pritchard (eds.) (1987) *African Political Systems.* London: Routledge.

Friedman, E. (ed.) (1994) *The Politics of Democratization: Vicissitudes and Universals in the East Asian Experience.* Boulder, CO: Westview Press.

Hayao, K. (1993) *The Japanese Prime Minister and Public Policy.* Pittsburgh: University of Pittsburgh Press.

Higley, J. and R. Gunther (eds.) (1992) *Elites and Democratic Consolidation in Latin America and Southern Europe.* New York: Cambridge University Press.

Holmes, L. (1993) *The End of Communist Power: Campaigns and the Legitimation Crisis.* New York: Oxford University Press.

Horowitz, D. L. (1990) "Comparing Democratic Systems," *Journal of Democracy,* 1(4): 73–79.

Huntington, S. P. (1991) *The Third Wave: Democratization in the Late Twentieth Century.* Norman: University of Oklahoma Press.

Inkeles, A. (ed.) (1991) *On Measuring Democracy: Its Consequences and Concomitants.* New Brunswick, NJ: Transaction.

Jowitt, K. (1992) *New World Disorder: The Leninist Extinction.* Berkeley: University of California Press.

Kaminski, A. Z. (1992) *An Institutional Theory of Communist Regimes: Design, Function, and Breakdown.* San Francisco: Institute for Contemporary Studies.

Kurth, J. and J. Petras (1993) *Mediterranean Paradoxes: The Politics and Social Structure of Southern Europe.* Herdon, VA: Berg.

Legters, L. H., J. P. Burke, and A. Diquattro (eds.) (1994) *Critical Perspectives on Democracy.* Lanham, MD: University Press of America.

Lijphart, A. (1984) *Democracies: Patterns of Majoritarian and Consensus Government in Twenty-One Countries.* New Haven, CT: Yale University Press.

Liu, Y. (1993) *Patterns and Results of the Third Democratization Wave.* Lanham, MD: University Press of America.

Mainwaring, S., G. O'Donnell and J. S. Valenzuela (eds.) (1992) *Issues in Democratic Consolidation: The New South American Democracies in Comparative Perspective.* South Bend, IN: University of Notre Dame Press.

McFaul, M. (1994) *Understanding Russia's 1993 Parliamentary Elections.* Stanford, CA: Hoover Institution on War, Revolution and Peace.

Means, G. P. (1991) *Malaysian Politics: The Second Generation.* New York: Oxford University Press.

Motyl, A. (ed.) (1992) *The Post-Soviet Nations: Perspectives on the Demise of the USSR.* New York: Columbia University Press.

Nathan, A. J. (1990) *China's Crisis: Dilemmas of Reform and Prospects for Democracy.* New York: Columbia University Press.

Pei, M. (1994) *From Reform to Revolution: The Demise of Communism in China and the Soviet Union.* New York: Oxford University Press.

Pempel, T. J. (ed.) (1990) *Uncommon Democracies: The One-Party Dominant Regimes.* Ithaca, NY: Cornell University Press.

Pempel, T. J. (1992) "Japanese Democracy and Political Culture: A Comparative Perspective," *PS: Political Science & Politics* (March): 5–12.

Pinkney, R. (1994) *Democracy in the Third World.* Boulder, CO: Lynne Rienner.

Powell, G. B. (1982) *Contemporary Democracies: Participation, Stability, and Violence.* Cambridge: Harvard University Press.

Pridham, G. (ed.) (1994) *Transitions to Democracy.* Brookfield, VT.: Dartmouth.

Randall, V. (ed.) (1988) *Political Parties in the Third World.* Beverly Hills, CA: Sage.

Rothschild, J. (1993) *Return to Diversity: A Political History of East Central Europe since World War II.* New York: Oxford University Press.

Rozman, G. (ed.) (1992) *Dismantling Communism: Common Causes and Regional Variations.* Baltimore: Johns Hopkins University Press.

Sakwa, R. (1990) *Gorbachev and His Reforms 1985–1990.* New York: Prentice-Hall.

Scalapino, R. A. (1992) T*he Last Leninists: The Uncertain Future of Asia's Communist States.* Washington, DC: Center for Strategic and International Studies.

Sjolin, M. (1993) *Coalition Politics and Parliamentary Power.* Lund, The Netherlands: Lund University Press.

Somerville, L. (1986) *Angola.* London: Pinter.

Stokes, G. (1993) *The Walls Came Tumbling Down: The Collapse of Communism in Eastern Europe.* New York: Oxford University Press

Stromm, K. (1990) *Minority Government and Majority Rule.* New York: Cambridge University Press.

Sullivan, M. J., III (1991) *Measuring Global Values: The Ranking of 162 Countries.* Westport, CT: Greenwood Press.

Tiruneh, A. (1993) *Ethiopian Revolution 1974–87: A Transformation from an Aristocratic to a Totalitarian Autocracy.* New York: Cambridge University Press.

Urban, M. E. (1990) *More Power to the Soviets: The Democratic Revolution in the USSR.* Brookfield, VT: Edward Elgar.

Vanhanen, T. (1990) *The Process of Democratization: A Comparative Study of 147 States, 1980–88.* New York: Crane Russak.

Walker, R. (1993) *Six Years That Shook the World: Perestroika—The Impossible Project.* London: Manchester University Press.

Waller, M. (1994) *The End of the Communist Power Monopoly.* New York: St. Martin's Press.

White, S. (1990) *Gorbachev in Power.* New York: Cambridge University Press.

White, S., G. Gill, and D. Slider (1993) *The Politics of Transition: Shaping a Post-Soviet Future.* New York: Cambridge University Press.

Widner, J. A. (1992) *The Rise of a Party State in Kenya.* Berkeley: University of California Press.

Wightman, G. (ed.) (1994) *Party Formation in East-Central Europe: Post-Communist Politics in Czechoslovakia, Hungary, Poland, and Bulgaria.* Brookfield, VT: Edward Elgar.

Zloch-Christy, I. (1994) *Eastern Europe in a Time of Change: Economic and Political Dimensions.* Westport, CT: Praeger.

4

Culture and Political Systems:
Nations versus States

Culture will be used as the unifying rubric (Gellner, 1987; Rhoodie, 1993) to study those aspects of nationalism and ethnicity which are important, both as preconditions for the democratic institutions postulated as desirable in Chapters 2 and 3, and as the causes for violent conflict and resulting militarized governance to be studied in Chapters 5 and 6. *Cultural sub-nationalism* will be the term used to describe those expressions of group identity which present challenges to the political and territorial integrity of the state, a phenomenon increasingly prevalent in today's world (Stack, 1986; Young, 1993).

Culture and cultural sub-nationalism will be the first of two factors to be analyzed which will affect this study's characterization of political systems; the second, force and violence, will be covered in Chapter 5. As such, the next two chapters are transitional and supportive to the main theses of this work relating to political systems. Consequently, Chapters 4 and 5 are shorter than Chapters 3 and 6, and the *Excerpts* from the Data Banks pertaining to ethnicity and force and violence are also more limited.

Before analyzing the cultural concepts of nationalism and ethnicity at greater length, some terms delineating the full spectrum of possible manifestations of such behavior will be defined.

4a ETHNICITY, NATIONALISM, AND STATISM

Ethnicity will be defined here as that aspect of self-identity which gives a person membership in a politically significant group. The political significance of the group identity is important, because normal elements of group identification—race, language, religion, cultural traditions—will not be deemed relevant in this study unless they are employed by some political actors as a means of gaining power.

The smallest institution of group identity which might be so empowered is the family, in the sense of large, extended clans, which in many countries can still be politically significant. Tribe is another, comparable word used to describe people with similar traits, customs, and characteristics (Isaacs, 1975). What these concepts lack, however, is a sense of significant size and organization created for purposes of maintaining the group's distinctiveness as contrasted with other groups with a claim on their loyalty, and for purposes of wielding power in the wider public arena (Anderson, 1991; Eriksen, 1991).

A *nation* is generally larger than a tribe in size and, more importantly, has an explicit organizational apparatus dedicated to the purpose of maintaining the consciousness of the members of the group precisely as members of the group in the most public of settings. To this end, anthems, flags, clothes, and rituals—particularly at times of birth, adolescence, marriage, and death (and, in the United States, at the start of sporting events)—are often employed to reinforce the sense of the individual's identification with the group (Brass, 1985; Kristeva, 1993).

Finally, a *state* refers to political machinery created to organize and enforce (via the law) the public behavior of members of the group within a defined territory. One problem in today's world, mentioned in the Introduction and in Chapter 1, is that of the 187 sovereign states (i.e., those admitting to no higher legal authority) in the world today, many do not have a comfortable match between the institutional political machinery of the state, and large masses of national populations within its jurisdiction (Graubard, 1993; Smith, 1988).

Table 4a lists the level of ethnic homogeneity for the 100 states selected for further study in this book, defined as the percentage of the population of the largest ethnic group. Using terminology employed by Nielsson and Jones (1988) and Sullivan (1991: 249–252; 259–263), these states can be said to fall within four groups:

1. Extremely homogeneous *nation-states,* where 90 percent or more of the population belongs to the same ethnic group (n = 26 out of 100 states)
2. *State-nations,* relatively homogeneous countries with between 71 and 89 percent of the population belonging to the main ethnic group (n = 30 of 100)
3. States with relatively mixed ethnicity, where the largest group comprises between 51 and 70 percent of the population (n = 20 of 100)
4. Extremely heterogeneous states, where no ethnic group comprises more than 50 percent of the population (n = 24 of 100)

Several points need to be made with respect to **Table 4a**. First, in only a relatively few states is there much of a match between the main nationality group and the state (Minority Rights Group, 1990). The 26 percent in the top group, which includes only 10 states with 97 percent or more homogeneity,

Table 4a
Ethnic Homogeneity (percentage of most populous ethnic group)

Europe	Islamic Zone	Africa	Asia	West.Hemisph.

Extremely Homogeneous "Nation-States" (≥90% in largest group), n=26

Europe	Islamic Zone	Africa	Asia	West.Hemisph.
Italy,Portugal-99			S.Kor,N.Korea-100	
Germany-99			Japan-99	
Netherlands-99			Australia-96	Costa Rica-96
Poland-98	Libya-97			Haiti-95
Greece-97			Bangladesh-94	
Czech.Rep.-95	Tunisia-95			
Denmark-95				
Hungary-95			China-93	
Ireland-94	Egypt-90			El Salvador-91
France-94	Somalia-90		Philippines-92	Argentina-91

Relatively Homogenous "State-Nations" (71% to 89%, largest group), n=30

Europe	Islamic Zone	Africa	Asia	West.Hemisph.
Sweden-88	Syria-89	Rwanda-88	Cambodia-89	
Bulgaria-85	Yemen-86		Vietnam-88	
Russia-83	Israel-82(or 63)		Taiwan-87	
UK-82	Turkey-82		India-83 (or 72, 34,etc.)	USA-80
Romania-82	Azerbaijan-81		Thailand-78	Chile-80
		Zimbabwe-77	Singapore-75	
	Algeria-75		Sri Lanka-74	Jamaica-76
Ukraine-74	Iraq-75		Nepal-73	Dom.Rep.-73
Spain-71		S. Africa-75(or 20,14,8)	Myanmar-72	

Relatively Mixed Ethnicity (between 51 and 70% in largest group), n=20

Europe	Islamic Zone	Africa	Asia	West.Hemisph.
	Uzbekistan-70			Nicaragua-70
				Canada-70
4/92ff Yugo.-69	Georgia-69			Panama-69
	Saudi Arabia-67			Venezuela-67
	Jordan-62		Pakistan-65	
	Tajikistan-61			Colombia-63
	Iran-56			Mexico-58
Belgium-57	Morocco-53			Peru-53
	Sudan-52	Burkina F.-52		Cuba-51

Extremely Heterogeneous (≤50% in largest ethnic group), n=24

Europe	Islamic Zone	Africa	Asia	West.Hemisph.
			Malaysia-49	Guatemala-50?
		Zaire-43	Afghanistan-47	Brazil-50?
		Ethiopia-40	Indonesia-45	Ecuador-46
	Kazakhstan-40	Madagascar-38		
		Mozambique-36		
		Angola-35		
		Zamb.,Seneg.-35		
		Guinea-35		
		Nigeria-32		
		Cameroon-31		
		Ghana-29		Bolivia-30
		Ivory Coast-21		
		Kenya-21		
		Tanzania-19		
		Liberia-19		
		Uganda-17		
TOT: 20	20	20	20	20 (100)

Note: States underlined are minority rule states (n=16: 0+6+9+1+0, by zone); see Table 4b Categories 3 and 5.

roughly corresponds to the results of an earlier study (Connor, 1978: 382) which reported only 9 percent of states with a "perfect, near-100%" match of nation and state, plus 19 percent with an "almost perfect 90–99% match." The second group of 30 countries relies a bit more heavily upon the machinery of government to work at maintaining the national identity (Migdal, 1989), part of what is meant by the reverse neologism "state-nation." Finally, almost 50 percent of the world's important states (i.e., those 44 in the bottom two categories, with mixed or heterogeneous ethnicity) have a tenuous identification between the main national group and the state.

An explanation of these results raises a second point regarding **Table 4a**: The specific "core" ethnic group referred to by the percentage next to each state needs to be precisely identified in each case. In some instances, particularly in the top tier, this is obvious: Germans in Germany, Japanese in Japan, and so on. However, this is not so clear among the other states, and often a political judgement must be made concerning just which aspect of ethnicity— race, religion, language, some combination of the three, or some other identifying trait—is being emphasized in the identification of the core group (Fijalkowski, 1991).

In the case of the United States, for example, the 80 percent ethnic core group refers to that part of the population which is white and English speaking. At an earlier time, before all the European-American ethnic groups had "melted" into the mythological "pot" of white, English-speaking Americans, religion (Protestantism) or northern European Anglo-Saxon ethnicity might have been a more relevant core group. Today, it is race (especially for African Americans, also possibly Asian Amerians) and language (for first-generation Hispanics, among others) which represent the significant social and political divides.

Race and language are also significant in the Sudan, with the added divisive elements of religion and geography (the Arab, Islamic north vs. the black, often Christian or animist, south). It is only the language which separates the main societal groups in Canada (English and French) and Belgium (Dutch and French). In Sri Lanka, it is primarily religion which determines the ethnic division between the majority Sinhala (Buddhists) and the minority Tamils (Hindus). In the United Kingdom, the language issues have receded, yet the English have other ethnic traits which distinguish them from the Scots, Welsh, and (even the Protestant) Northern Irish. Within some Arab states with common Arabic language and Islamic religion (e.g., Syria, Iraq), the political "ethnic" dividing line relates to a difference within the religion between Sunnis and Shiites. And exacerbating all these ethnic differences in most of the countries mentioned is an economic differential which often goes back generations and serves to perpetuate the privileged position of the group with the greater historic power (Samaringhe and Reed, 1991; Connor, 1984; Ross, 1978).

A third point to complicate the issue of political analysis in ethnically divided states is deciding which of several increasingly embracing ethnic classifications is most significant. In India, there are several choices: the religious group of Hindus (83%); the large geographic group of Indo-Aryans (72%);

the "Hindi-speaking Hindus" (34%); or smaller ethnic–linguistic divisions like "Marathis" or "Bengalis" (8% each). **Table 4a** opts for the first, because of all the divisions, the Hindu–Muslim one is the most *politically* significant.

In South Africa, the most politically significant group (since the 1993 constitutional changes) is deemed to be black Africans (75%), not the Zulus (20%), the whites (14%) or the Afrikaans-speaking whites (8%). In Zaire, the 43 percent on **Table 4a** refers to the approximate total of the three largest Bantu-speaking tribes in the south and center, rather than any one of them. In south and central America, it is generally wiser to recognize the larger mestizo (Spanish mixed with American Indian) group than to emphasize either of its component parts.

Finally, 16 states on **Table 4a** are underlined to indicate minority rule; the group whose percentages appear on this table is *not* the group in control of the government. These countries, to be treated at greater length in section 4b, include Syria, Iraq, Jordan, Tajikistan, Sudan, and Kazakhstan in the Islamic zone; Rwanda, Zaire, Ethiopia, Madagasacar, Angola, Guinea, Kenya, Liberia, and Uganda in Africa; and Afghanistan in Asia. For these determinations, the group "in control" is the de facto most powerful group in the government (e.g., General Kagame in Rwanda, the Uzbek and Russian military in Tajikistan, etc.), regardless of any pro forma holders of presidential or prime ministership posts . For a greater explanation, see section 4b, especially Table 4b, Categories 3 and 5, and the second page of *Excerpts* at the end of the chapter.

4b ETHNIC CONFLICT WITHIN STATES

Table 4b presents a way of analyzing ethnicity in 50 of the 100 selected states by dividing them into five categories based upon increasing levels of problems related to ethnicity (Zimmerman and Jacobson, 1994). The number 50 is as arbitrary as the number 100 for the total number of states under scrutiny in this work, and is chosen to represent half the states under consideration. Since ethnicity is such a pervasive element in all countries except those few perfect nation-state matches referred to in the previous section, another 20 states which could arguably be included among the "top 50" with ethnic significance are included on Table 4b below the dotted line.

Category 1 identifies, as *ethnically interesting*, 13 states with an ethnic minority worthy of some political notice to the group or groups typically controlling the government. Category 2 displays 13 states with an ethnic minority, which creates significant policy problems for the government and defines these countries as *ethnically problematic.*

In ethnic *minority-rule* states, the government is controlled by members of a minority ethnic group; in 8 of these states, there is no armed or violent opposition to such rule (Category 3), but in 8 others (Category 5) the majority ethnic group has taken up arms against the minority government. There are actually 16 *ethnic-conflict* states (Gurr and Harff, 1994; Horowitz, 1985), where an ethnic group (either minority or majority) is involved in a civil war

Table 4b
Categories of Ethnic Analysis (n = 50: 13 + 13 + 8 + 8 + 8)

Europe	Islamic Zone	Africa	Asia	West.Hemisph.
	Category "1" - Ethnically Interesting States, n=13			
Belgium-57%			Malaysia-49%	Bolivia-30%
Ukraine-74	Iran-56%			
Romania-82	Saudi A. 67		Singapore-75	Canada-70
Bulgaria-85	Egypt-90		Taiwan-87	US-80
n=4	n=3		n=3	n=3 (13)
	Category "2" - Ethnically Problematic States, n=13			
		Nigeria-32%	Indonesia-45	Guatemala-50
Spain-71	Morocco-53		Pakistan-65	Peru-53
UK-82		S. Africa-75	Phil. I. 92	
Russia - 83	Israel-82(or 63)		China-93	
n=3	n=2	n=2	n=4	n=2 (13)

Europe	Islamic Zone	Africa	Asia	West.Hemisph.
	Category "3"- *Minority Rule* States , n=8 + 8 in Category"5"= *16*			
		Uganda-3		
	Syria-11.5	*Kenya-11*		
		Zaire-11		
	Jordan-37	*Guinea-15*		
	Kazakhstan-40	*Madagascar-32*		
	n=3	n=5		(8)
	Category "4" - States with Ethnic Conflict (5b), n=8			
ex-Yugo.-69	Georgia-69		Myanmar-72	
	Azerbaijan-81		Sri Lanka-74	
	Turkey-82		India-83	
	Somalia-90			
n=1	n=4		n=3	(8)
	Category "5" - *Minority Rule* States with Ethnic Conflict (5b), n=8			
		Liberia- ? ≤5		
	Iraq-20	*Ethiopia-10*		
	Tajikistan-32	*Rwanda/Bur.-12*	*Afghanistan 27.5*	
	Sudan-41	*Angola-26*		
	n=3	n=4	n=1	(8)
TOT: 8	15	11	11	5 (50)
of n= 20	20	20	20	20 (100)

Europe	Islamic Zone	Africa	Asia	West.Hemisph.
Other candidates for inclusion (n=20):				
France	Algeria	Zimbabwe	Vietnam	Ecuador
Czech.Rep.	Yemen	Senegal	Cambodia	Colombia
Greece		Cameroon	Bangladesh	Mexico
		Tanzania	Nepal	Panama
		Mozambique		Cuba
				Dom.Rep.
n=3	n=2	n=5	n=4	n=6 (20)

Notes: Numbers indicate percentage of largest ethnic group, or of ruling ethnic group(s) in minority rule
states.
Italics = minority rule states.

(CVW) or insurgency (NSG) against the government (see section 5b for explanation of the distinction between these two terms). Category 4 identifies 8 states where minorities are rebelling against majority rule. Category 5 covers rebellions in a different 8 states in which a majority population is protesting against the rule of a minority, presumably a more oppressive situation.

Four measures are used to put each of the 50 chosen states in one of the five identified categories. These include the following: (1) the size of the ethnic group(s) as a percentage of the total state population; (2) whether there has been any recent strife (involving deaths) specifically targeting ethnic groups in the state; (3) whether ethnicity is a relevant factor in any official policies of a positive or negative nature (e.g., affirmative action laws and human rights violations, respectively); and (4) whether there are any irredentist or separatist claims upon, or by, the state.

Analyses of these measures, some examples of which can be seen in the *Excerpts* at the end of this chapter, substantiate the results presented in **Table 4b**. Twenty-six of the 50 states fall in the first two categories, with a line drawn between the first 13 in the "ethnically interesting" Category 1, and the next 13 in the "ethnically problematic" Category 2. One of the major distinctions between these two categories is that all of the "problematic" states have had violent ethnic strife to the point of insurgency or civil war at some point during the past generation (e.g., Spain vs. Basques, Morocco vs. Saharui, Nigeria vs. Ibos, Indonesia vs. E. Timorese, Guatemala vs. Amerindians, etc.); whatever the ethnic problems of states in the preceding "interesting" category (e.g., Bulgaria's Turks, Iran's non-Persians, Malaysia's Chinese, Canada's Quebecquois, etc.), they seldom reach the level of violence of those in the second, "problematic" category.

Of greater political significance are the 24 states in the last three categories, with either minority rule or significant violent ethnic rebellion, or both. These include, in Category 3, 8 states with minority ethnic rule, but without major insurgency in recent years:

Syria's Alawite Shiites (11.5% population) over Sunnis (72%)

Jordan's Hashemites (37%) over Palestinians (62%)

Kazakhstan's Kazakhs (40%) over Europeans (50%, including 39% Russians, 6% Ukrainians, 5% Germans)

Uganda's Banyakole Bantus (3%) over southern Bantu Bagandans (17%) and various northern Nilotic tribes (55%)

Kenya's Kalinjins (11%) over Kikuyus (21%), Luos (18%), Luhyas (14%), and others (36%)

Zaire's Noro-Mangbetu-aZanda (11%) over Bantu-speaking tribes such as Mongo, Totela, BaLuba, and BaKongo (43%)

Guinea's Susus (15%) over Fulani (35%) and Malinke (25%)

Madagascar's Malayo-Indonesian highlanders (32%) over African coastal peoples (38%)

The percentages of population of the respective ruling minority groups can be found in **Table 4b** for these 8 states, as well as for the 8 states in Category 5; for all other countries the percentage given is of the largest, and governing, ethnic group. A summary of the name and population percentage of the main groups in Categories 3 and 5 is also provided on the second page of *Excerpts*.

Category 4 includes 8 states where minorities are in rebellion against regimes which are seen as drawn from and favoring the majority ethnic group. These insurgents include the following: Serbs, Croats, and Bosnian Moslems laying claim to areas where they are dominant in the former Yugoslavia; a similar situation involving the main clans of Somalia; Ossetians and Abkhazians versus Georgia; Armenians in Ngorno-Karabakh versus Azerbaijan; Kurds versus Turkey; Karen, Wa druglords, and other non-Burmese tribes versus Myanmar; Tamils versus Sri Lanka; and Kashmiri Moslems, Punjabi Sikhs, and various northeast tribal groups versus India.

Finally, Category 5 includes 8 states with minority rule in which the majority is in active rebellion:

Iraq's Sunni Arab government, drawn from 20 percent of the population, versus Sunni Kurds (20%) and Shiite Arabs (55%)

Tajikistan's government of dubious Tajik legitimacy, sustained by Uzbek (24%) and Russian (8%) military, versus most Tajiks (61%)

Sudan's Islamic, largely Arab, government, drawn from northern 34 to 48 percent of the population versus Christian and animist black southerners (52%)

Liberia's 1991 government, externally imposed by the Economic Organization of West African States, versus Bassa-Krahn followers of the 1980–1990 Samuel Doe government (16%), and Americo-Liberian supporters of 1848–1980 governments (4%); the leading Kpelle group (19%) is unorganized militarily

Ethiopia's Tigrean government (10%) over Oromos (40%), Amharans (29%) and others

Rwanda's Tutsis (12%, before 1994 genocide and return of exiles) over Hutus (88%), and a similar situation in Burundi

Angola's mulatto and Kimbundu MPLA government (26%) versus UNITA from Ovimbundu (35%), and others

Afghanistan's Tajik (27.5%) president (1992–1995) versus Pathans (47%) and Uzbek (7.5%) militia, historic holder of balance of power.

The categories of analysis summarized in **Table 4b** will serve as a guide to the *Excerpts* from the Data Bank associated with this study to be presented at the end of this chapter. Five states—Spain, Sudan, Kenya, Sri Lanka, and Bolivia (one from each category across the five zones)—will serve as examples of how ethnicity in political systems might be more thoroughly analyzed. Ethnicity in these countries will be displayed according to a *Format* which lists information for each state relating to the various parts of this chapter.

The *Format* includes, for those elements of analysis covered to this point: the size of the ethnic group(s) as a percentage of the total state population (a measurement that might be further broken down by religion or language, where appropriate); and whether there has been any serious recent conflict (defined as involving significant loss of life) specifically targeting ethnic groups in the state. This second factor might be further subdivided not only into ethnic struggles against the government (as in the 16 states in Categories 4 and 5), but also into ethnic strife among groups within the state and past wars in the state which had an ethnic dimension. These elements are all covered in the *Format* for *Excerpts* from the Data Bank, lines a and b, at the end of this chapter. But before analyzing this framework further, two other aspects of analysis of ethnicity—public policy and irredentism—will be discussed.

4c ETHNICITY AND PUBLIC POLICY

Chapter 2 identified ethnicity as a factor which is often built into states' institutional governing structures. Special seats in the representative assembly (2b) set aside for targeted minority groups, and concomitant voting rolls (2e) to ensure them, were noted in Jordan, Pakistan, and Singapore, for example. Ethnicity was also noted as the basis for many of the decentralized subunits (2c.iii) in about half (8 of 17) of the federal states and all 15 of the countries with autonomous zones (Snyder, 1982). **Table 4c** identifies some of the more notable of these ethnic sub-units and elaborates upon some of the decentralization policies in 8 of these 32 states.

Another power-sharing structure that might be mentioned here is the reserving of a special Cabinet-level Ministry (2c.ii) to address issues related to minority groups. Examples can be cited from Russia, for its Ministry of Nationalities for its 130 minorities (especially the 21 with autonomous republics), the Czech Republic (with respect to Gypsies), Romania (for Hungarians), and Brazil (for indigenous Amerindians). Many Islamic states have special Ministries of Religious Affairs to "promote" the activities and thereby co-opt the leaders of the majority religious population (Sullivan, 1991: 298). One-party former-communist states (like China and Vietnam) have special government organizations to register (and control) the religious activities of minority groups (Catholic, Buddhist, etc.) in their countries (Ramet, 1990).

This section will take this concept of ethnicity's impact in politics further into areas of official public policy and unofficial, but de facto, practice (Mikesell and Murphy, 1991; Montville, 1990). In the Data Bank associated with this project, these matters are covered in line 4c of the *Format*. Ethnic policies which serve to positively enhance the participation of minority groups in the governance structure are often elements which argue for the inclusion of such a state on the civilian page of the CGSS; policies which violate the human rights of such group members are often arguments for placing a state lower on the CGSS (Nevitte and Kennedy, 1986; McGarry and O'Leary, 1993).

The objective criteria of language and religion are at the heart of the most explicit policies related to ethnicity. The issue of whether the minority lan-

Table 4c
Ethnicities and Decentralized Government

States with Federated Subunits (n=8 of 17):

Russia n= 89 regions, including 67 geographic, and 21 ethnic republics with autonomy (see below).

Belgium = 3: French-speaking Walloons, Dutch-speaking Flemings, bilingual Brussels.

Yugoslavia = 2(+2a): Serbia (w/ 2 once-auton. provs. Kosovo Alb.Mosl., Vojvid.Hungs.) & Montenegro.

Nigeria = 1991 constitut. w/ 30 further subdivisions of the 1963 first 3: Hausa-Fulani (~15), Yoruba (~9), Ibo(~6). Earlier attempts at 12 (1970), 19 ('76), and 21 ('87) failed; see also Ethiopia, below.

Tanzania = 2: Mainland & more Moslem (ex-Arab-colonized) Zanzibar.

Pakistan = 4 provinces: Punjab, Sindh, Baluchistan, Northwest Frontier Khyber Agency.

India = 25 largely language-based states (incl. 6 Hindi-speaking of different ethnicity); 7 union territories.

Malaysia = 13: Peninsula; + 4 union (Sarawak, [Christian] Sabah, Melaka, Pahany); + 9 royal: Johar, Kedah, (Moslem) Kalantan, Negeri Sembilan, Perak, Perlis, Pulau Penang, Selangor, Terengganu.

NOT ETHNIC: Germany's 16; Australia's 6; + 7 in West.Hemisphere: US's 50; Mexico's 30; Brazil's 26; Colombia's 27; Argentina's 22; Venezuela's 20; and Canada's 10 (except for Quebec).

States with Important Autonomous Subunits (n=15 of 15):

Russia - 21: 16 former Soviet autonomous repubs. + 5 ex-oblasts; incl. esp. Tatarstan (oil), Bashkiria, N.Ossetia, Chechen (oil pipelines), Yakutia (gold, diamonds).

Italy - 20, incl.: German-speaking areas of Trentino-Alto Adige; most of others not ethnically derived, but as recently as 150 years ago, many of Italy's regions were distinct city-states (Naples, Venice, Lombardy, Sicily, Sardinia, etc.)

Spain - 17, incl. Basques (see below), Catalonia (Barcelona), Galicia, Andalusia; most of others not that ethnically different from Castillian core, but tradition of regionalism (Aragon, Valencia, La Mancha, etc.).

Portugal - Azores & Madeira (offshore Atlantic Ocean islands).

Ukraine - Crimea (Russians); (also many/majority? Russians in eastern Donbass region of Ukraine.)

Georgia - Abkhazia, S.Ossetia; also: Adjaria?.   Azerbaijan - Ngorno-Karabakh (Armenians).

Uzbekistan - 1 = Samarkhand & Bukhara (Tajiks).   Tajikistan (pre-war) - 1 = Gorno-Bardakshan (Pamirs).

Iraq - Kurdistan, legally 1970-75, de facto under external duress, 1991ff; also, Maadan (Shiite Marsh Arabs).

Ethiopia (1994) 7 + 2 = Amhara, Tigre, Sidamo, Shankella, Somali Hararge, Afar, Gurage + Addis Ababa (capital), and Oromia (recalcitrant region); 1991 division had 14 regions (see Nigeria, above).

China = 5: Sinkiang (Uigurs); Xizang (Tibetans); Guangxi Zhuang; Xingxia Hui; Inner Mongolia.

Bangladesh = 3: Chittagong Hills Chakma Buddhists; plus 2 others.

Sri Lanka = 2 (not 3): Main Sinhala & eastern mixed region; + ne Jaffna Tamil peninsula region.

Philippine I. = 1: Autonomous Region for Muslim Mindinao, in 4 of 13 provinces there (see 5b Excerpt).

Further Information on Ethnicity and Selected Decentralizations

Russia - *Tartarstan* delayed signing 3/92 Federal Treaty until 2/94, when it extracted full economic freedom, more control over resources, and taxes than other 20 regions, plus its own police, presidency, assembly, and constitution.

Spain - Euskadi *Basques* have more autonomy than Catalans; can collect own taxes and pass on share to central government proportionate only to central services rendered.

Tanzania - *Zanzibaris* (750,000, mostly Moslems) have disproportionate power: their own constitution and assembly; only foreign policy, defense, and Home Affairs are reserved for center. 8/93 Tanzania parliament accepted two "parallel" governments.

Pakistan - 4 provincial govts. in federation (see above) control their own electoral machinery. 60% of Pakistan population in Punjab province. N.W. Khyber Agency a very autonomous tribal territory *(Pathans):* no Pak. police permitted (9/93) there.

India - in Muslim-dominated *Kashmir*, non-Kashmiri Indians cannot own real estate, or inherit wealth. Marriage & all non-commercial laws under Sharia. Quotas for Muslims in government jobs.

Malaysia - opposition strong in Sabah (*Christian* PM Pairin until '94 ouster), and *Kelantan* (Parti Islam + Semangat '46). *Sarawak* produces 80% of Malaysia's timber exports (#2 export; #1 in world).

China - *Sinkiang* prov. = 16% land, 1.3% pop. (=16m., incl. 62% Hui Muslims vs. 38% Han Chinese). *Turkics* (fomerly east Turkestan, in China only since 1884) incl. 45% Uigur (+Kazaks & Uzbeks). Also, *Tibetan Buddhists* in Tibet; and more *Mongols* in China's Inner Mongolia than in Mongolia.

Canada - failed 1993 Constitution attempt to recognize *Quebec* as a distinct society w/ power over culture & immigration; promise never to have less than 25% seats in LH despite population shifts (25.4% now).

guage might be used in the schools is particularly sensitive in places such as Bulgaria (with respect to Turkish), Romania (Hungarian), Turkey (Kurdish), Algeria (Berber), and in several states of the former Soviet Union where Russian is now the new minority vernacular. France, which for centuries built one of Europe's oldest nation-states by insisting on Parisian French as the mode of instruction, has recently begun to allow local languages (like Breton, Occitan, Corsican, etc.) to be used in the classroom in the provinces. Singapore and Taiwan have at various times stipulated that Mandarin Chinese, and not local dialects, be used exclusively in schools. The question of whether minority-language groups can have their own newspapers (generally allowed), radio, and television stations (each progressively less likely) is also a public policy issue in many countries (Todorova, 1992).

Allowing religious laws to supersede state law for some family-related subjects such as marriage, divorce, and inheritance, is also an issue in places like India (which permits Muslim Sharia law to cover many of these matters, much to the consternation of fundamentalist Hindus), countries with significant Muslim minorities in Africa, and in Israel (where even greater deference is given to the Orthodox Rabbinate, to the point of allowing it to define citizenship and "who is a Jew" [Haynes, 1994; Janke, 1994]).

Affirmative action quotas for places in government jobs and universities are commonplace policies in India (with respect to castes), China (to the benefit of non-Han Chinese), Sri Lanka (to include Tamils), and Myanmar (to exclude Chinese and Indians). In Malaysia, the "New Economic Policy" specifically earmarks much government spending in the economy to be directed to firms owned by Malays, not Chinese. As these examples indicate, such quotas can be used either to enhance or retard the social and economic integration (and progress) of minority populations (Sowell, 1990; Banton, 1983; Wirsing, 1981).

Laws favoring settlers moving into contested lands can be cited in China (to subsidize Han Chinese moves into Tibet and Inner Mongolia), Malaysia (to favor Muslims moving into Christian Sabah), Indonesia (to facilitate Javanese going to other islands, especially Catholic East Timor), and Israel (to favor settlements in Gaza and the West Bank, especially during Likud Party administrations). More forcible evacuations, at the level of human rights violations, might be cited in the cases of Iraq (vis-à-vis Kurds, with 4000 villages destroyed and 1.5 million people resettled in the 1980s) and South Africa (3.5 million forced removals over a twenty-year period while attempting to implement its Bantustan policy of tribal homelands in the 1960s and 1970s).

Other human rights violations—such as torture, summary executions, suspicious "disappearances," and political prisoners—cited in the annual reports of Amnesty International, the U.S. State Department, and the various regional divisions of Human Rights Watch (see Chapter 7a) are invariably visited upon members of societies' ethnic minority groups in disproportionate numbers. During the existence of the Soviet Union, most political prisoners were Ukrainians, Jews, and other non-Russians; in the United States, capital punishment is chiefly reserved for blacks. Similar fates await Kosovo Muslims in Yugoslavia, Kurds in Turkey and Iraq, Bahais in Iran, and Amerindians in Latin America.

Since ethnicity can have such dire consequences, it might be noted that many states (e.g., Russia, Kenya, Tanzania, Malaysia) have laws against inflaming ethnic tension, or even making blatant ethnic appeals during election campaigns. Ethnicity is such a volatile issue that some states (e.g., Nigeria, Lebanon) have been unable to even conduct a census in which ethnic identity is asked of respondents. Similarly, citizenship, and the possibility of dual citizenship, is an extremely touchy issue, especially for Russians in the former Soviet states and places where foreign workers came years ago and now have children and grandchildren living in their adopted countries (e.g., Algerians in France, Turks in Germany, Palestinians in Kuwait, Mexicans in the United States, etc.).

Finally, there are examples of informal, but nonetheless real, control over certain aspects of society by particular minority ethnic groups in some countries. The military is a caste often populated by a particular ethnic (or geographic) group out of proportion to its percentage of the population (Pathans in Pakistan, Sikhs in India, Bedouins in Jordan, Turkics in Iran, Alawite Shiites in Syria, even blacks in the United States); oftentimes the officer class is of yet a different ethnicity (Russians in Kazakhstan, Punjabis in Pakistan, Southerners in the United States) (Ellwood and Enloe, 1980).

In many countries, there is a similar division of labor between a minority ethnic group which dominates in business and the economy (Chinese in Asia, South Asians and Arabs in Africa and the Caribbean, whites in American cities), and that which controls the government (generally from the majority population group). Examples of these policies or practices affecting minority groups can be found in line c of the *Excerpts* for the five selected states at the end of this chapter.

4d IRREDENTIST COMMUNITIES

Given the significance of ethnicity in the allocation of society's rewards and punishments, it is understandable why many people would prefer to live in a governmental jurisdiction where control is exercised by members of "their own kind." This desire raises the issue of *irredentism,* the attempt of an ethnic or nationality group to link up with its fellow-members in another state. Because of the transborder aspects of this activity, a study of this subject broadens the scope of inquiry from comparative to international politics (Moynihan, 1993; Midlarsky, 1993; Chazan, 1991) and involves such issues as separatist, refugee, expatriate, and migrant worker communities.

Tables 4d and **4d.i** identify and analyze the thirty-two main irredentist movements in the world today. Two factors are significant in making such a determination: demography and geography. The sheer number of people comprising a group is obviously important in determining whether this group is going to be politically signficant. While some small nations occasionally have

Table 4d

Main Irredentist Groups, by Size and Zone (n = 32: 8 + 8 + 5 + 11 + 0; estimated total size plus number outside "natural" home state)

Europe, n=8:

e-Russians - 146 million total including: 123m. in Russia (148m.) + 22-23m. outside: 11.6m. in Ukraine
 (52m.); 6.4m. in Kazak. (17m.); 1.7m. in Uzbek. (23m.); 1.3m. in Belarus (10m.); .9m. in Kyrgyz. (4.4m.);
 .9m. in Latvia (2.5m.), .9m. in Moldova (4.3m.), .6m. in Estonia (1.5m.), .5m. in Azerbaijan (7.3m.), etc.

Romanians - 22.0 mil. tot. including: 19.1m. in Romania (23m.) + 2.9m. in Moldova (4.3m.).

Hungarians - 12.5 mil. tot.; incl. : 9.8m. in Hungary (10.2m.) + ~ 3 m. outside in: 1.8m. in Romania (23m.),
 .6m. in Slovakia(5.4m.), .3m. in Vojvidina (Serbia (8.3m.)).

Serbs - ~10 mil., incl. 7.1m. (of 8.3m. pop.) in Serbia, .2m. in Kosovo (of Yugo.=10.8m.)) + 2.6 m.
 outside, incl.: .6m. in Krajina, Slavonia, etc., Croatia (4.5m.), and 1.4m. in Bosnia (3.5m.), .6m beyond.

e-Gypsies - 9 mil. total in world; 8 m. in Europe, incl.: 3m. in Romania(23m.); .85m. in Bulgaria (8.5m.); .85m.
 in Hungary (10.2m.); .65m. in Slovakia (5.4m.); .65m. in Spain (39m.); .5m. in France (58m.); .35m. in
 Portugal (10m) ; .2m. in Greece (10.5m.).

Catalans - 8 mil. total: 6m. in Spain (39m.) and 2m. in France (58m.).

Albanians - 6.0 m. tot. incl.: 3.5m. in Albania + 2.5m. outside Albania, incl.1.9 m. in Yugoslavia (10.8m.)
 Serbian province of Kosovo, .5m. in Macedonia (2.1m.), .2m. in Greece (10.5m.).

Irish - 5.2 mil. tot. incl.: 3.6m. in Ireland (3.6m.); + 1.6m. in N. Ireld.,UK(59m.), incl. .65m. RC & .95m. Prot.

Islamic Zone, n=8:

Azeris - 26 mil. total, including: 20m. in Iran (61m.) + 5.8m. in Azerbaijan(7.3m.), incl. .35m. in Nakhichevan
 enclave in Armenia (3.7m.).

Kurds - 22-26 mil. total, incl. 12-13m. in Turkey (61m.), 5.5m. in Iran (61m.), and 4m. in Iraq (20m.).

Uzbeks - 18 mil. total, including: 15m. in Uzbek.(23m.); + 1.3m. in Afghan.(18m.) 1.2m. in Tajikistan(5.8m.).

,e-Jews - ~13.4 mil. total incl.: 4.4m. in Israel (pop. 5.5m.); 9 mil. in diaspora, incl. 6 mil. in US.

Somalis - 12.6 mil. total, incl. ~8-9 m. in Somalia, 3.3 m. in Ethiopia(56 m.) .8 m. in Kenya(28 m.).

Tajiks - ~8.0 mil. total, incl. more (4.8m.) in Afghan. (18 m.) than in Tajikistan (3.2m. of 5.8m. pop.)

e-Armenians - 7.0 mil. total, including: 3.7m. in Armenia (3.7m.) + .4m. in Azerbaijan (7.3m; incl. .2m.in
 Ngorno-Karabakh); + 2.9m. in diaspora.

Palestinians - 5.7 mil. tot. incl.: 2.5m. in Jordan(4.1m.);1.9m. in Israeli Occupied Territories (1.1m. West Bank
 + 0.8m. Gaza Strip = future Palestine state); .75m. in Israel(5.5m.); .32m. in Lebanon (3.7m.); etc.

Africa, n=5:

Hausa-Fulani - 42.4 mil. tot., incl. 32.3m. in Nigeria (101m.), 6.1m. in Niger(9.2m.), 1.6m. in Mali (9.4m.), etc.

Hutus - 12.3 mil. total, incl. 6.8m. in Rwanda (7.8m.), and 5.5m. in Burundi (6.4m.), before 1994 refugees.

BaKongo - 8.0 mil. tot., incl.: 5.3m. in Zaire (44m.), 1.7m. in Angola (11.5m.), and 1m. in Congo (2.5m.)

Ewes - 3.3 mil. total, incl.: 2.2m. in e. Ghana (17.5m.) and 1.1m. in w. Togo (4.4m.), and ruling in neither.

Tutsis - ~2+ m. total, incl. 1.0-1.5m.(post-1994 take-over) in Rwanda (7.8m.), 1m. in Burundi (6.4m.).

Asia, n=11:

-Chinese - 1,171 mil. tot., incl.: 1,134m. in China (1,219m.); + claims on Taiwan (21m.), Hong Kong (6.0m.),
 Mongolia (2.4m.), Macao (.4m.); also upon: ex-SU Central Asian (Kaz.,Kyrg.,Taj.)(6.5m.), and India's
 Arunchal Pradesh (.9m.). See also "overseas (expatriate, non-irredentist) Chinese" (~40 mil.), esp. in:
 Thailand=7m., Malaysia 5m., Indonesia 5m.,Singapore 2m., Vietnam 1m.

Bengalis - 183 mil. total, including: 71 m. in India (931 m.) + 112 m. in Bangladesh (119 m.)

Punjabis - 120 mil . tot., including: 36 m. in India (931 m.) + 84 m. in Pakistan (130 m.)

Koreans - 68.4 mil. tot., incl.: 44.9m. in South + 23.5m. in North; + 1.8m. in China, .8m. in US, .7m. in Japan.

Tamils - 68.4 mil. tot., incl 65.2 m. in India (931 m.) + 3.2 m. in Sri Lanka (18 m.).

Nepalese - 30.4 mil. tot., incl: 16.6 m. in Nepal (23 m.) + 13.5 m. in India (931 m.) + .3 m. in Bhutan (.8m.).

Pathans - 21.2 mil. tot., incl. 13.3m. in Pak.(130m.) and 7.9m. in Afghanistan (18m.)

Kashmiris~13 m. incl. 4-6m. Musl. in Pak.(130m.) + 7.8m. in India(931m.), incl. 5.5m.Muslim, 2.3m. Hindu.

Baluchs - 6.3 mil. tot. incl.: 3.9m. in Pak.(130m.) + 2.2m. in Iran (61m.) + .25m. in Afghanistan (18m.).

Mongols - 6 m. tot. incl.: 4m. in Inner Mongolia Auton.Zone of China (1.2 b.) + 2m. in Mongolia (2.4m.pop.)

Papuans - 3.4 mil. tot. incl.: 2.2 m. in Papua New Guinea (4.1 m.) + 1.2 m. in Indonesia (198 m.).

Notes: e = nations with many expatriates in diaspora (Russians, Gypsies, Jews, Armenians, Chinese).
  Δ = special South Asian cases where religion dominates ethnicity (Bengalis, Punjabis, Kashmiris).
  * = more outside of home state than in it (Jews, Azeris, Tajiks, BaKongo, Pathans, Mongols).
  ( ) = 1995 population of state, rounded to nearest million for states with > 10 million population.

Table 4d.i

Analysis of Main Irredentist Groups (n = 29; without 3 South Asians divided by religion [Bengalis, Punjabis, and Kashimiris])

By Total Size	By # outside home state	By % outside home state
e-Chinese 1,171 million	Chinese 37.2m. + "overseas"	Kurds 100%
e-Russians 146m.	%-Kurds 24.0m.	Gypsies 100%
	Koreans 23.5m.	Baluchs 100%
Koreans 68.4m.	Russians 22.5m.	Palestinians 100%
Tamils 68.4m.	Azeris 20.0m.	Ewes 100%
		Hutus 100%
Hausa-Fulani 42.4m.	Nepalese 13.6m.	
Nepalese 30.4m.	?%-Pathans 13.3m.	*BaKongo 100% (v. 87.5% not in Congo)
Azeris 26.0m.	%-Hutus 12.3m.	*Pathans 100% (v. 62.5% not in Afghan.)
	Hausa-Fulani 10.1m	
Kurds 24m.	Jews 9.0m.	*Azeris 77%
Romanians 22.0m.	%-Gypsies 8.0m.	*Jews 67%
Pathans 21.2m.		*Mongols 67%
Uzbeks 18.m.	?%-BaKongo 7.0m.	*Tajiks 60%
	%-Baluchs 6.3m.	
e-Jews 13.4m.		Armenians 47%
Somalis 12.6m.		Nepalis 47%
Hungarians 12.5m.	%-Palestinians 5.7m.	
Hutus 12.3m.	Tajiks 4.8m.	
Serbs 10.0m.	Somalis 4.1m.	Albanians 42%
e-Gypsies 9.0m		Papuans 35.2%
Tajiks 8.0m.	Armenians 3.3m.	Koreans 34.3%
Catalans 8.0m.	%-Ewes 3.3m.	Somalis 32.5%
BaKongo 8.0m.	Tamils 3.2m.	Irish 31% (RC & Prot.)
	Uzbeks 3.0m.	
e-Armenians 7.0m.	Hungarians 3.0m.	Serbs 26%
Baluchs 6.3m.	Romanians 2.9m.	Catalans 25%
Mongols 6.0m.		Hungarians 24%
Albanians 6.0m.	Serbs 2.6m.	Hausa-Fulani 23.8%
	Albanians 2.5m.	
Palestinians 5.7m.		Uzbeks 16.7%
Irish 5.2m.	Mongols 2.0m.	Russias 16.3%
	Catalans 2.0m.	Romanians 13.2%
Papuans 3.4m.	Irish 1.6m.	Tamils 4.7%
Ewes 3.3m.	Papuans 1.2m.	Chinese 3.4%
Tutsis 2.0m.	Tutsis - none after 1994	Tutsis - none after 1994

Main (> 2m. population) *Separatist* Groups *within* a Single Country:
Punjabi Sikhs - 12 m.; vs. 8m. Punjabi Hindus in Punjab; vs. 35m. Punjabi Hindus in India (931 m.).
s.Sudan non-Moslem blacks - 8 m., from ~14m. blacks in Sudan (28m.) of which ~5m. animist, 3m. Christian.
Quebecquois - 6 m. French-speakers in Quebec (7m. total), or 8m. French-speakers in Canada (30m.).
Katangans - 5.7 m. BaLuba (=Kuba, Lunda) in Shaba province, protected by Zaire (44m.) vs. Kasai.
Tibetans - 4.6 m. total, including 2.0m. in Chinese Autonomous Zone + 2.6m. elsewhere in China (1.2b.).
In Myanmar (45 m.): Karens - 4.1m., Shan - 2.7m., Moslem Rohingyas - 1.3m., KaChin - .9m., etc.
Ovimbundu - 3.5 m. in Angola (11m.); plus a small number in Namibia.
Basques - 2.3 m. in Spain (39m.); plus a small number in France.

Notes: e = nations with many expatriates in diaspora (Chinese, Russians, Jews, Gypsies, Armenians).
    % = nations with no territorial state (Kurds, Hutus, Gypsies, Baluchs, Palestinians, Ewes).
    ?% = nations with no territorial state, arguable (Pathans, BaKongo).
    * = more outside of home state than in it (Jews, Azeris, Tajiks, BaKongo, Pathans, Mongols).

drawn the attention of the global community (Kuwaitis, East Timorese), there are no groups listed in Table 4d with less than 2 million people (see also Table 4d.i, column 1).

The second essential element in determining the significance of an irredentist nation is geographic contiguity: the fact of a nation being spread over two (or more) territorially connected political jurisdictions (i.e., states). At this point, it might be noted there are at least five groups, designated by e in **Table 4d** and in column 1 of **Table 4d.i**—Russians, Gypsies, Jews, Armenians, and Chinese—whose irredentist concerns for their ethnic kin go beyond those located merely across the national border. In fact, Jews, Gypsies, and Armenians are nations *most* of whose members live in an expatriate diaspora not territorially contiguous to their putative homelands. Russians and Chinese have many members of their nations just across the homeland borders, and many others farther afield (Snyder, 1984).

The zonal breakdown of the thirty-two groups identified in **Table 4d** reveals none in the Western Hemisphere and only five in Africa. In Latin America, 500 years of intermarriage between the Iberian colonists and the indigenous Amerindian tribes has created a distinct mestizo ethnic group and a general blurring of ethnic and racial lines in most of that continent. In Africa, the European concept of "nationalism," with its elements of size and organization, had not taken root before the large-scale arrival of the imperialists in the nineteenth century, so the major identifiable irredentist ethnic groups which exist (Hausa-Fulani, Hutu, BaKongo, etc.) are rather few in number and weak in political organization dedicated to the purpose of unification. The main ethnic problem on this continent is not drives for fusion among groups across state lines but rather the splintering of states from within.

The South Asian subcontinent presents an interesting situation, in which religion is a more signficant political determinant than ethnicity, especially for three significant linguistic groups (annotated Δ on **Table 4d**). The 183 million Bengalis are divided into about 112 million Bengali Muslims in Bangladesh and about 71 million Bengali Hindus in India's state of West Bengal. Of the 120 million Punjabis, 36 million, mainly Hindus, are in India and 84 million Muslims are in Pakistan. Though fewer in number, the 12 to 14 million Kashmiris are the most controversial politically: About 7.8 million reside in the two-thirds of the land of Kashmir controlled by India, and about 5.5 million of these are Muslim and 2.3 million Hindu; the rest (all Muslim) are in the one-third of Kashmir controlled by Pakistan (Mitra, 1994; Oommen, 1992).

A final South Asian group, the Tamils, is also divided between 2 states, although geography, not religion, is the reason (Little, 1993). There are 65 million Tamils in the southern Indian state of Tamil Nadu. On the offshore island of Sri Lanka are another 3.2 million Tamils; it is there that a movement exists which has been fighting for more than a decade for an "independent Tamil homeland." If it succeeds, it will achieve the status of 6 other nations listed on **Table 4d**: that of having a state with fewer of its nationals in it than outside it.

These groups—identified by * on **Table 4d** and in column 3 of **Table 4d.i**—include the following: Jews (4 million in Israel, 9 million in diaspora); Azeris (6 million in Azerbaijan, 20 million elsewhere, mainly in Iran); Tajiks (3 million in Tajikistan, 5 million in Afghanistan); BaKongo (1 million in Congo, 5.3 million in Zaire, 1.7 million in Angola); Pathans (8 million in Afghanistan, 13 million in Pakistan); and Mongols (2 million in Mongolia, 4 million in China). In these examples, it is not clear that the "obvious" state for the BaKongo is the Congo, or that for the Pathans is Afghanistan, but the difficulty in even making such an identification relates to the impact of colonialism in creating not only the artificial nation-states mentioned earlier in this chapter, but also these divided nations without their own states.

The French, Belgians, and Portuguese who divided the BaKongo nation in the nineteenth century were probably unaware of what they were doing; in those days, African "tribes" were simply carved up and ruled over without much concern for the wishes of the native inhabitants (Asiwaji, 1985; Miles, 1994). The case involving the Tajiks in the new Soviet Union was a more conscious policy of divide and conquer; in the 1920s, Stalin purposefully dismembered Turkestan and put the majority-Uzbek Khodzent area in Tajikistan, and took the majority-Tajik cities of Samarkand and Bukhara and placed them in Uzbekistan. The fact that most of the Tajiks (about 5 million of 8 million today) were in Afghanistan was beyond the Soviet Union's control; but the more numerous Pathans of Afghanistan (about 7.9 million of that country's 18 million population) are in turn fewer in number than the Pathans in Pakistan (about 13.3 million of a 130 million population), where they in turn are ruled by the majority Punjabis. The policy of Afghanistan as a buffer zone between the Russian and British Empires in South Asia goes back more than a century, but the aftereffects linger on to this day. In 1992 and 1993, the government of Afghanistan (with Tajik President Rabbani) was controlled by the minority Uzbeks and Tajiks; in 1994, the Uzbek militia shifted its support to the Pathan Prime Minister Hekmytyar; in 1995, yet another group of Pathans (the Taliban Student Militia) became ascendent. In Tajikistan, the Tajik government is effectively controlled by Uzbek and Russian military forces, while most Tajiks are in rebellion or in exile in Afghanistan.

At this point, it might be noted that the prime move for irredentism can come either from the main body in a political jurisdiction, or from the population separated from that polity. As with other matters related to ethnicity, such movement does not depend only upon the size of the group, but also on the degree of political effort expended on behalf of the movement (Breuilly, 1994). In an effort to determine just which groups might have the potential for a significant irredentist impact on the political systems of hosting states, **Table 4d.i** ranks twenty-nine groups (after eliminating the three large ethnic groups of South Asia, which are divided by religion) in order of (1) the size of the total group (home state plus external population); (2) the numbers of the group outside any obvious home state; and (3) the percentage of the group's population outside of the home state.

Some notable results of **Table 4d.i**'s display are as follows. The nations with the most people outside of their home borders (>22 million in column 2) are the Chinese (with 37.2 million in claimed areas of some 7 neighboring states, even before taking into account another 40 million farther away; the Kurds (24 million in 5 states—Turkey, Iran, Iraq, Syria, and Armenia); the Koreans (23.5 million who are probably only temporarily ideologically divided and whose populations are presented here as if the larger, richer south will eventually absorb the north in the manner of the two Germanys at the end of the Cold War in Europe); and the Russians (with 22.5 million, about half in the eastern Ukraine).

The Kurds are the largest of 5 nations not in sovereign control of any homeland of their own at this point in history (designated by % in column 2, and 100% in column 3). Gypsies (9 million), Baluchs (6.3 million), Palestinians (5.7 million), and Ewes (3.3 million) are the others. Two other groups (designated by ?% in column 2 of **Table 4d.i.**) also arguably have this status: Pathans and BaKongo. The Pathans (~21.2 million) do not clearly rule in Afghanistan, where 37.5 percent of the Pathans are found and where they are the largest group, with 43 percent of the population, nor in Pakistan where 62.5% of Pathans are found, but where they are less than 10 percent of the population. Allies of the BaKongo rule in the Congo, where they are the dominant tribe with 40 percent of the small 2.5 million population, but where only 12.5 percent of the total BaKongo group (8.0 million) are found. In addition to the Pathans and BaKongo, there are the four groups mentioned earlier (and designated by * in column 3) with more members outside of their home state than within it: Azeris, Jews, Mongols, and Tajiks.

A nation not in control of its own affairs has a choice of either seceding (i.e., separating out) from the main body of which it is a part, or of overthrowing it. In fact, a dispute over which of these goals is most appropriate led to a division within the rebel group of non-Muslim blacks in the Sudan in recent years (Deng, 1994). In neighboring Ethiopia, both goals were pursued simultaneously in 1991, when rebel groups led by minority Tigreans (approximately 10% population) and Eritreans (2%) successfully overthrew the ruling Amharan group (28%) by conspiring to allow the Eritreans to secede and the Tigreans to take over the central government; the true majority group in that country Oromos (40%) has never been represented in government (Jalata, 1993).

Before concluding this section, it should be noted that *separatist* movements by ethnic groups whose members are mainly within a single state have not been discussed here but will be mentioned in line 4d of the Data Bank *Excerpts* associated with this section, and discussed at greater length in section 5b if their efforts have resulted in armed struggle (Heraclides, 1991; Premdas, Samarasinghe, and Anderson, 1993). Among the largest (i.e., more than 2 million population, and listed at the bottom of **Table 4d.i**) such groups are the 12 million Punjabi Sikhs in India; the 8 million non-Muslim blacks in the southern Sudan; the 6 million French-speaking Quebecquois in Canada; the 5.7 million Katangans in Zaire; the 4.6 million Tibetans in China; the 4.1 million Karens and 2.7 million Shan (among others) in Myanmar; the 3.5

million Ovimbundu in Angola; and the 2.3 million Basques in Spain. None of these, however, have any significant number of sympathetic kinfolk providing support from across neighboring borders.

The case of the Sikhs (a south Asian religious group, neither Hindu nor Muslim) raises once again the question of which of the elements of ethnicity is most salient in defining a group's identification. In the Punjab, where most of the 12 million Sikhs are found, are also 8 million Punjabi Hindus. There are also 28 million Punjabis elsewhere in India (a large number in the state of Haryana, where they comprise most of the population of 16 million), not to mention the 84 million Punjabi Muslims in Pakistan. The problem, from the point of view of some Sikhs, is that they are not sufficiently in charge of their own affairs; the difficulty, from the perspective of India, is that even giving the Sikhs majority control of one of the twenty-six federal states of India (Punjab, after the creation of the new state of Haryana for Punjabi Hindus) was not sufficient to satisfy some Sikh leaders.

Similar situations in other countries, and their impact on their states' political structures, are best studied on a case-by-case basis and in the context of each state's particular modalities for power sharing. In an effort to incorporate these aspects of ethnicity into such analyses, this chapter's conclusion proposes a *Format* for presenting relevant data.

4e FORMAT AND DISPLAY OF DATA BANK EXCERPTS

The *Format* for 4abcd—Ethnic Group Data Bank, which precedes the *Excerpts* at the end of this section, follows the main divisions of this chapter, which have shown how (a) the size of the respective groups, (b) their record of intercommunal strife, (c) the government's public policies, and (d) the existence of irredentist communities provide the context for many of the violent conflicts to be covered in Chapter 5 and the militarized polities to be discussed in Chapter 6. But wars and military dictatorships cannot definitively solve the problems of interethnic relations. People continue to travel, do business, intermarry, and have children in other states, creating a kaleidoscope of constantly changing ethnic balances in countries around the world. Accordingly, the data base proposed here, and incorporated into relevant parts of Chapters 2, 3, and 6's analyses of civilian and military polities, must be regularly updated and maintained to keep pace with the changes in the real world.

By way of example, ethnic analyses of 5 states—1 from each zone, 1 from each ethnic category—selected from the Data Bank associated with this research, are displayed in accordance with the suggested *Format* in the *Excerpts* at the end of this chapter. In Category 1, Bolivia is the most extreme example of a Western Hemisphere state with a significantly sized, but politically quiescent, Amerindian population; the percentages of these indigenous peoples in each of the other Latin American countries is also given along with this *Excerpt*. Spain is a Category 2 country: It formerly faced a significant ethnic insurgency from a segment of its population; using the power-sharing political institution of autonomy (see 2c.iii), however, it has been able, in recent years, to quell and co-opt the Basque separatist movement.

Representing Category 3 is Kenya. In its second generation of leadership, control of Kenya's dominant party has been taken away from the majority Kikuyu of independence leader Kenyatta by President arap Moi's minority Kalenjin tribe; although the political system has become somewhat more militarized and repressive since the earlier era, it has not yet degenerated into civil war or insurgency. Category 4's Sri Lanka, on the other hand, has a significant minority group (the Tamils) which, until the most recent decades, was accommodated by a parliamentary system and some preferential policies; when the system changed to presidential and the preferences were removed, the Tamils, in order to achieve their political ambitions, took up arms to demand autonomy or their own state. Finally, in Category 5, Sudan is a country whose government, drawn from the 34 to 48 percent Arab (or mixed Arab) population which lives in the north, is using religion (imposition of Islam's Sharia law) to consolidate its control over fellow northerners who are not Muslims (e.g., the Nuba), as well as over blacks in the south, many of whom are Muslims but who do not wish to force the faith on their racial kinsmen.

Between Category 3 Kenya and Category 4 Sri Lanka is a list of all 16 minority-rule states, which identifies the name and percentage of population of the minority ruling group and of the other leading groups in each state. At the end of the *Excerpts* for the 5 prototype states is information on three particularly troublesome non-ruling irredentist ethnic groups without states of their own but of international political significance—Kurds, Palestinians, and Hutus. Data on them are drawn in shortened form (especially lines a and d) from the Data Banks of their relevant "oppressor" states: Iraq, Jordan, and Rwanda/Burundi, respectively.

Format for 4abcd Ethnic Group Data Bank

Top Line: **State - population + Ethnic Category (0,1,2,3,4,5;** incl. 5b conflict type**)**;
a. % ethnic group members, in order of largest to #3, #4,..... last important group; with
 names of troublesome groups, & **%, names of minority ruling groups.**
 .i = religion %s (including 2 types Moslems, 2 types Christians where relevant);
 .ii = language %s, (where available & relevant; i.e., aids in "a"; official > national langs.)
b.i = ethnic conflict between groups within the state
 .ii = ethnic struggle vs. state (see 5b);   .iii = past ethnic wars (see 5a=wars, historic)
c. impact/relevance of ethnicity; including (positive, negative):
 i. P=special policies (e.g., affirm. action in govt. jobs, univs.; use of local language in schools, media);
 ii. HRv=Human rights violations (see 7a);
 iii. note groups favored by colonials:
       Maronites, Copts, Fulani, Tutsi, Masai, Sikhs, Gurkhas, Tamils, VNmese (in Cambodia), etc.
d. irredentist & separatist claims (upon, or by, this state); see Table 4d.

Notes: **Bold Italics** = ruling minority group.
 Italics = insurgent or troublesome ethnic group.
 % underlined = most relevant ethnic percentage reflected in Table 4b.

Excerpts from Ethnic Group Data Bank

Bolivia - 7.4 million - Category 1
a. 30% mestiço; 60-65% *Amerindian* (incl. 30-37% Quechua, 20-25% Aymara; also:
 Guarani, Mojeno, Chimane); 5-10% European; 2% Amazonian; 3% other.
 .i) 95% Roman Catholic (nominal; only 15% practicing).
 .ii) three official languages: Spanish (spoken by less than 50%), Quechua, Aymara.
b. Amerindian 60-65% does not threaten 30% mestiço rule because of divisions within
 the larger racial group.
c. Amerindian leader Victor Hugo Cardenas (ex-leader, Tupac Katari Revolutionary
 Movement, 1985) elected VP (as c-r: MNR candidate) in '93; 1st time Amerindian on
 any national political ticket. Only since then has there been some relaxation of
 discrimination in law: e.g., govt. workers (esp. in education & medicine) permitted to
 wear traditional clothes; Indian organizations "not sanctioned by state" qualifying for
 loans; folk medicine legal; teaching in Indian languages; etc.

Note on Latin America: No countries are considered to have minority rule (Category
 3) because of the fluidity between races subsumed under the general heading of
 "mestiço" (= European + Amerindian). In some states the mestiço ruling class
 considers itself white, or the white rulers do not emphasize the differences. In other
 cases with a large Amerindian population, the mestiços and white have successfully
 kept the Amerindians divided among themselves into different "tribal groups."

Latin American *Amerindians* = 30 million total
By population size (in millions), by state: Mexico 9.5; Peru 8.6; Guatemala 4.6; Bolivia
 4.4; Ecuador 2.2; Brazil 1.5; Chile 1.2; Argentina 0.7; Colombia 0.3; Venezuela 0.2;
 Nicaragua 0.1.
In % of population, by state: Bolivia 60%; Guatemala 50%; Peru 40%; Ecuador 25%; El
 Salvador 20%; Mexico 10%; Chile 9%; Panama 8%; Honduras 7%; Nicaragua 4%;
 Argentina 3%; Brazil, Colombia, Venezuela,1% each.

Spain - 39.1 million - Category 2

a. ~71% Spanish (Latin-Mediterranean); 18% Catalan (7-8 mil., esp. around Barcelona); 8% Galician; 6% *Basque* (2.3m.). Also, .65 m. gypsies; and .5 million foreign workers, especially from north Africa.

b. ii) *Basques* in northeast particularly militant (5b:1968-1987) in pressing their demand for a separate state, starting in late 1960s under Franco, and persisting well into current era until finally appeased with high degree of autonomy.

   iii) regional separatism ended after Spanish Civil War (1936-39) won by Fascist Franco regime which consolidated power in center for a generation (1939-75).

c. i) autonomy (2c.iii) for 17 regions, including offshore Canary islands; two Moroccan enclave "possessions" (Ceuta and Mellila).

   ii) discrimination against gypsies (US Dept. of State Human Rights Report).

Kenya - 28.3 million - Category 3 (*Minority Rulers, %, in bold*)

a. 21% Kikuyu (especially in Nairobi & central province), 16-20% Luo (in west, Lake Victoria region), 14% Luhya (in west), **11% *Kalinjin,*** 11% Kamba, 9% other Bantu (than Kikuyu), 16% other (including 5% Kisii, 5% Meru, 3% Somali, 1% S.Asian, 1 % Turkana in n.w., Masai in s.w.). Total: ≥40 groups, 100 clans.

   i) 38% Protestant, 28% Roman Catholic, 26% indigenous, 6% Moslem.

b. n=~1200 dead since 10/91 in Kalinjin(+ Masai & Pokot)-inspired ethnic strife (in suspected Govt. effort to show "dangers of democracy"), esp. anti-Luo (& anti-Kikuyu) in Rift Valley (25% land). Estimates of casualties: Special Parl. Cmtee, 12/92: 800 dead; *NYTimes* 9/7/93: >1000 dead, 150,-200,000 displaced; *Economist* 11/20/93: 1500 dead; Economist 2/4/95: 10,000 Kikuyu displaced in 1/94.

c. Ethnicity dominates politics despite official discouragement of ethnic appeals via one-party state. Pres. Moi's Kalinjin (& smaller Rift Valley tribes: Masai, Pokot) favored in jobs; also, policy to "retake" Rift Valley land given by UK colonialists to favored Kikuyu. Kikuyu had 1st president (Kenyatta), & current leaders of opposition parties (Kibaki, Matiba); also dominate economy. Important Luo elites have been assassinated (Mboya '69, Ouko '90). Asians still do well in economy.

Minority Rule States (n=16: 8 from Category 3 + 8 from Category 5*)
by ruling group's name (% from Table 4b), in zones; (leading group's name and % from Table 4a)

Ruling Group	Leading Group
Syria - 11.5% Alawite Shiites	over 72% Sunnis
*Iraq - 20% Sunni Arab	over 55% Shiite Arab, 20% Sunni Kurd
*Tajikistan - 24% Uzbek + 8%Russian	over most of 61% Tajiks (-Govt. collaborators)
Jordan - 37% Hashemites	over 62% Palestinians
Kazakhstan - 40% Kazakhs	over 50% Europeans, incl. 39% Russians, 6% Ukrains.,5% German
*Sudan - 34-48% Arab	over 52% black
Uganda - 3% Banyakole	over 17% Baganda, 55% n. Nilotic/Sudanese
*Liberia - ≤5% ECOWAS-installed	over 19% Kpelle, 16% Bassa-Krahn, Gio-Manos, 4% Americos, et al.
*Ethiopia - 10% Tigre	over 40% Oromo, 29% Amharan, et al.
Kenya - 11% Kalinjin	over 21% Kikuyu, 18% Luo, 14% Luhya
Zaire - 11% Noro-Mangbetu-aZanda	over 43% Bantu-sp. tribes: Mongo+Totela,BaLuba,BaKongo,etc.
*Rwanda - 12% Tutsis	over 88% Hutus
Guinea - 15% Susus	over 35% Fulani, 25% Malinke, et al.
*Angola - 25% Kimbundu/2% mixed	over 35% Ovimbundu, 19% Bakongo, etc.
Madagscr. - 32% Malay-Indo.Hi-landrs.	over 38% coastals, others

*Afghan.- 35% Tajik(27.5) & Uzbek(7.5) over 47% Pathan

Sri Lanka - 18.2 million - Category 4 (CVW)

a. <u>74%</u> (~13 mil.) Sinhalese (Aryan), incl.: 43% lowland, 29% fm.Kandyan hills; 18% (~3.2m.) Tamil (Dravidian) incl.:*12% Jafffna Tamil* (~2.2m. incl. .6m. on peninsula), 6% Indian Tamil (~1.0m., fm.19th century plantations); 7% Moslem Moors (=Tamil-speaking Arabs).

   i. 72% Buddhist(official), 16% Hindu, 7% Christian,7% Moslem

   ii. Sinhala the official language; Tamil also "an" official language since '87; English a "link" language spoken in govt. & by elite 10%.

b. Civil war due to ethnic claims of the (esp. Jaffna) Tamils (see 5b CVW with 35,000+ dead). 27 pogroms vs. Tamils, 1956-83 (leading to 1977 vote to secede) w/ 40,000 dead (esp. 4000 d. in '83 riots). Tamils were favored by UK colonials; backlash by Sinhalese against them ever since.

c. Buddhism & Sinhalese favored since 1956 (2500th anniv. of Buddha) decrees of PM S. Bandaranaike; when he backed off enforcement, he was assassinated in '59. 95% of army & govt. bureaucracy is Sinhalese despite minority affirmative action policies for Tamils in '78 Constitution. UNP-installed presidential system of (1978-94) favored Sinhalese in first-past-post elections; SLFP promised parliamentary system (?with more PR elections) to give Tamils & Moslems greater chance, in 1995 (see 6a).

d. Irredentist interest of 65 million Tamils in southern Indian state of Tamil Nadu in their 3 million kinsmen in Sri Lanka.

Sudan - 28.1 million - Category 5 (CVW) (*Minority Rulers, %, in bold*)

a. 52% *black* (~14.6 m.) incl. 11% Dinka, and other Nilotics (Nuer, Mundari, Hausa, etc.) in south ; 14% non- or mixed- Arab, northern tribes including 4% Nubian (in center), 5% Beja (in east), 5% Darfur, etc. (west); **~34% Arab** (≤10 mil., probably less than 1/2 not mixed), incl. leading sects (parties) pre-military rule: Ansar (Umma P.) & Khatmia. Also: 2% foreign; 1% other. Total of 300 ethnic groups, 100 languages.

   i) 68% Sunni Moslem (~19 m., incl. some black) in north; v. 8 m.(=28%) w/ other beliefs; incl.: 19-25% indigenous (=~6 mil.); 7-18% Christian (~3.5m=12.4% many of whom have fled, & incl. RC=2m. [2/93 Pope visit], Anglican=1.2m.[12/93 Abp. visit]).

   ii) Arabic is only official language, despite some 44 other main langs. spoken in south.

b. i) In (w) Darfur prov., Furs v. Maharujas (+Libya, Sud.mil.), '87-90ff. Related to.....

   ii) Civil War (5b) & Human Rights violations (7a) due to race & ethnicity; esp. northern Arab Moslems vs. southern black Christians, animists. Religious persecution of Nuba (non-Arab northerners): 50,000 relocated Su.'92. 5b SPLA = Dinka,Nuer, Kakwa; & (sometimes) Toposas & DarFurs; i.e. black Africans. SPLA 7/92 split betw. #1 Dinkas on w. bank of Nile under Garang, and #2 Nuers on e. bank (Nasir)under Riek Mashar. 1993 Govt. attacks on Fur & Nuba in north were virtual genocide.

c. The 68% Moslem majority includes many blacks; the 52% black majority includes many Moslems. But dominant hegemonic group, **Arab Moslems** are not any majority (see Iraq). After 1969-72 Anya Nya war, southern third got autonomy, until 1983 partition of south into 3 smaller regions and introduction of Sharia Law. Its implementation on 32% non-Moslems (~21% animist, ~12% Christian) since 1983 provoked civil war in south, even though law enforced primarily in the north (i.e., not on southern Christians [~2.5 mil.]), esp. under Nimery til 1989 coup.

Iraq - 20.6 million - Category 5 (LAT) (*Minority Rulers, %, in bold*)
a. 74% Arab; 18-20% *Kurd* (~3.9 m.); Also: 2-3% Turkic/Turkman, 1-2% Persian, 1% Assyrian, .5% other.
   i) 58% Shi'ite Arab; 30-40% Sunni of wh. **20% Sunni Arab**, 16% Sunni Kurd (=~3.3 m.); also: 3% Shiite Kurd (555,000); 3-5% Christian, 2% other, including 10,000 Yazidi Kurd.
b. Periodic attempts to destroy Shiite and Kurdish cultures: (details removed from this EXCERPT)
c. Government drawn from minority Sunni Arabs since 1932 independence via UK and League mandate.
d. Separatist/Irredentist problems from Kurds. See also 4b-Turkey-Category 4, and below:
#Kurds - 22-26 mil. - Aryans, not Arabs; from Ottoman & Persian Empires; world's largest stateless
   national group (since independence of Ukraine in '91): 53% are in Turkey (=12.7 m.), 23% in Iran (5.5 mil.)
   18% in Iraq (4.0 mil.); + 6% (=1.4 m.) elsewhere, including: 4% in Syria (1 m), .1% in Armenia (.24m).
   Also: .5 million workers in Europe, 80% of them in Germany.

Jordan - 4.1 million - Category 3 (*Minority Rulers, %, in bold*)
a. 97% Arab, but ~62% Palestinian (2.4-2.8 mil.), only **~37% Hashemite** (incl. 12% Bedouin assimilated);
b. "Black" September 1970 rebellion of PLO:Fatah (Arafat) Palestinians crushed and driven into exile.
c. Politics grounded in ethnicity to ensure Hashemite Arab dynasty continues to rule over majority
   Palestinians, incl. 1.5 m. refugees absorbed in three main waves: 1948 and 1967, from Israel; and 1990-
   91, from Kuwait. Claim to .9 m. Palestinians of West Bank relinquished in 1988. Bedouins dominate
   army, (c.Asian) Circassians (<1% pop.) heavy in domestic security and intelligence.
d. Jordan caught up in problem of Palestinian irredenta. See below:
#Palestinians-5.4-6.0 mil. (in ≥75 states)
a. 14% of Israel(.75 mil.); 37-40% of Israel+Occupied Lands(1.9m.: 1.1m. W.Bank, 0.8m. Gaza); ~60% of
   Jordan(2.5m.); Kuwait pre-Gulf War 300,000 down to 20,000 in '92; 11% of Lebanon (.32m), 2% of
   Syria (.26m); + .25m in Saudi A. & 3 Peresian Gulf states, .15m in other Arab states, .15m in US
   (esp.Detroit), .175m other non-Arab states.
   i) Palestinians are 75% Sunni Moslem, 25% Christian.
c. Major forced emigrations: in '48 fm. Israel, in '67 fm. Jordan West Bank/Occupied Territories, in '70 fm.
   Jordan East Bank, in '82 from Lebanon, in '91/92 from Kuwait. ~2.6m. want to return to Israel.

Rwanda - 7.8 million - Category 5 (LAT) (*Minority Rulers, %, in bold*)
a. 88% Hutu; **12% (Wa)Tutsi** (~1 mil., before major changes of 1994: i.e. genocide of ~.5 m. Tutsis,
   exodus of ~2 m. Hutu refugees (esp. to Zaire=1.0m & Tanzania=0.5m.) after take-over by minority
   Tutsis, and influx of some 1 m. Tutsis returning from 1960s-exile in Uganda and Burundi). Thus, current
   (1995) statistics *could* be: 6.3 mil. pop. with 1.5 mil. Tutsis (23%) now ruling.
b. History of ethnic conflict linked with that of Burundi: 1959 rebellion of majority Hutu (RC-led) overthrew
   Belgian-favored (& Protestant) Tutsis in 1961, causing .1m. dead, ~.2 m. to flee. 1963 indep. incl. '61-
   66 war vs. UNAR Tutsi Inyanzim, ~17,500 dead. 9/90-4/94 war by RPF Tutsi exiles with 20,000 dead,
   before death of "moderate" Hutu president led to genocide vs. .5 m. Tutsi civilians by new Hutu govt. &
   militias before 7/94 overthrow and take-over by minority Tutsis. Total dead since 1959: ~1.5 million
c. Under Hutu-majority government (1963-94), strict quotas vs. Tutsis in education, govt.; I.D.'s, passcards
   to preserve Hutu dominance (esp. Akazu clan of Pres. Habyarimana,1973-94) over Tutsis who
   predominated in business, churches, & universities under Belgians.
d. Irredentist issues with neighboring minority-ruled Burundi. As of 1995, minority Tutsis rule in both states,
   majority Hutu in neither ; earlier Hutus had control in Rwanda, Tutsis in Burundi (see next):
Burundi - 6.4 mil. - Cat. 5 (LAT) (*Minority Rulers, %, in bold*)
a. 86% Hutu(Bantu; short, stocky farmers & laborers fm. south); **14%(Wa)Tutsi**(~1m.; Hamitic; tall, thin
   cattle-herders from Ethiopia in 16th century); 1% Twa(pygmy).
b. History of periodic massacres of majority Hutus esp. their elites, by ruling minority Tutsis: 1972, with 150-
   300,000 dead; 1988, with 25,000 dead; 10/93, with 100-200,000 dead, 1 mil. refugees (after 6/93 1st-
   ever Hutu Pres. ousted in coup + backlash). Total dead: 275-575,000.
   Total dead in both Rwanda & Burundi, 1959-94: ~1.8 - 2.1 million (of ~14 mil. population in 1995).
c. Ethnic favoritism retains Belgium-perpetuated minority rule & prevents "Rwanda 1959" (when 88% Hutu
   overthrew 12% Tutsi). All officers, most of 17,000 in army & civil service are Tutsis who also dominate in
   business, universities, courts; 13 of 15 governors. 6/93 Hutu president was only a figurehead, and he
   was assassinated by Tutsis in Army coup when he attempted repatriation of Hutus in exile.
d. Total Hutus in Rwanda-Burundi is ~12.3 mil. (87%), total Tutsi is ~2 m.(14%), of 14.2 official total
   population (1995).

REFERENCES

Anderson, B. R. (1991) *Imagined Communities: Reflections on the Origins and Spread of Nationalism*. London: Verso.

Asiwaji, A. I. (ed.) (1985) *Partitioned Africans: Ethnic Relations Across Africa's International Boundaries 1884–1984*. New York: St. Martin's Press.

Banton, M. (1983) *Racial and Ethnic Competition*. Cambridge: Cambridge University Press.

Brass, P. R. (ed.) (1985) *Ethnic Groups and the State*. New York: Barnes and Noble.

Breuilly, J. (1994) *Nationalism and the State*. Chicago: University of Chicago Press.

Chazan, N. (ed.) (1991) *Irredentism and International Politics*. Boulder, CO: Lynne Rienner.

Connor, W. (1978) "A Nation Is a Nation, Is a State, Is an Ethnic Group, Is a . . . ," *Ethnic and Racial Studies*, 1(4): 377–400.

—— (1984) "Eco- or Ethno- Nationalism?"*Ethnic and Racial Studies*, 7(3): 342–359.

Deng, F. M. (1994) *War of Visions: Conflict of Identities in the Sudan*. Washington, DC: Brookings Institution.

Ellwood, D. C. and C. H. Enloe (eds.) (1980) *Ethnicity and the Military in Asia*. New Brunswick, NJ: Transaction Books.

Eriksen, T. H. (1991) "Ethnicity versus Nationalism," *Journal of Peace Research*, 28: 263–278.

Fijalkowski, J. (1991) *Dominant National Cultures and Ethnic Identities*. Berlin: Free University of Berlin.

Gellner, E. (1987) *Culture, Identity, and Politics*. Cambridge: Cambridge University Press.

Graubard, S. R. (ed.) (1993) "Reconstructing Nations and States," *Daedelus: Journal of the Amerian Academy of Arts and Sciences*, 122(Summer): 1–272.

Gurr, T. R. and B. Harff (1994) *Ethnic Conflict and World Politics*. Boulder, CO: Westview Press.

Haynes, J. (1994) *Religion in Third World Politics*. Boulder, CO: Lynne Rienner.

Heraclides, A. (1991) *The Self-Determination of (Secessionist) Minorities in International Politics*. Portland, OR: Frank Cass.

Horowitz, D. L. (1985) *Ethnic Groups in Conflict*. Berkeley: University of California Press.

Isaacs, H. (1975) *Idols of the Tribe: Group Identity and Political Change*. New York: Harper and Row.

Jalata, A. (1993) *Oromia and Ethiopia: State Formation and Ethnonational Conflict, 1868–1992*. Boulder, CO: Lynne Rienner.

Janke, P. (1994) *Ethnic and Religious Conflicts: Europe and Asia*. Brookfield, VT: Dartmouth.

Kristeva, J. (1993) *Nations without Nationalism*. New York: Columbia University Press.

Little, D. (1993) *Sri Lanka: The Invention of Enmity*. Washington, DC: U.S Institute of Peace.

McGarry, J. and B. O'Leary (eds.) (1993) *The Politics of Ethnic Conflict Regulation*. New York: Routledge.

Midlarsky, M. I. (ed.) (1993) *The Internationalization of Communal Strife*. London: Routledge.

Migdal, J. S. (1989) *Strong Societies and Weak States: State–Society Relations and State Capabilities in the Third World*. Princeton: Princeton University Press.

Mikesell, M. W. and A. B. Murphy (1991) "A Framework for Comparative Study of Minority Group Aspirations," *Annals of the Association of American Geographers*, 81(December).

Miles, W. F. S. (1994) *Hausaland Divided: Colonialism and Independence in Nigeria and Niger.* Ithaca, NY: Cornell University Press.

Minority Rights Group (1990) *World Directory of Minorities.* London: St. James Press.

Mitra, S. K. (ed.) (1994) *Subnational Movements in South Asia.* Boulder, CO: Westview Press.

Montville, J. V. (1990) *Conflict and Peacemaking in Multiethnic Societies.* Lexington, MA: Lexington Books.

Moynihan, D. P. (1993) *Pandaemonium: Ethnicity in International Politics.* New York: Oxford University Press.

Nevitte, N. and C. H. Kennedy (eds.) (1986) *Ethnic Preference and Public Policy in Developing States.* Boulder, CO: Lynne Rienner.

Nielsson, C. P. and R. Jones (1988) "From Ethnic Category to Nation: Patterns of Political Modernization." Paper presented at International Studies Association Annual Convention, St. Louis.

Oommen, T. K. (1992) *The Shifting Salience of Religion on the Construction of Nationalism: India.* Working Paper 5.3, University of California Center for German and European Studies, Berkeley.

Premdas, R., S. W. R. Samarasinghe, and A. Anderson (eds.) (1993) *Secessionist Movements in Comparative Perspective.* London: Pinter.

Ramet, P. (ed.) (1990) *Catholicism and Politics in Communist Societies.* Durham, NC: Duke University Press.

Rhoodie, E. M. (1993) *Cultures in Conflict: A Global Survey of Ethnic, Racial, Linguistic, Religious and Nationalistic Factors.* Jefferson, NC: McFarland.

Ross, J. (1978) "A Test of Ethnicity and Economics as Explanations of Collective Political Behavior," *Plural Societies,* 9: 65–75.

Samaringhe, S. W. R. and C. Reed (1991) *Economic Dimensions of Ethnic Conflicts.* London: St. Martin's Press.

Smith, A. D. (1988) *The Ethnic Origins of Nations.* Cambridge, MA: Blackwell.

Snyder, L. L. (1982) *Global Mini-Nationalisms: Autonomy or Independence.* Westport, CT: Greenwood Press.

——— (1984) *Macro-Nationalism: a History of the Pan-Movements.* Westport, CT: Greenwood Press.

Sowell, T. (1990) *Preferential Policies: An International Perspective.* New York: William Morrow.

Stack, J. F.. Jr. (1986) *The Primordial Challenge: Ethnicity in the Contemporary World.* Westport, CT: Greenwood Press.

Sullivan, M. J., III (1991) *Measuring Global Values: The Ranking of 162 Countries.* Westport, CT: Greenwood Press.

Todorova, M. (1992) *Language in the Construction of Ethnicity and Nationalism: The Bulgarian Case.* Working Paper 5.5, University of California Center for German and European Studies, Berkeley.

Wirsing, R. G. (ed.) (1981) *Protection of Ethnic Minorities.* New York: Pergamon Press.

Young, C. (ed.) (1993) *The Rising Tide of Cultural Pluralism: The Nation-State at Bay?* Madison: University of Wisconsin Press.

Zimmerman, W. and H. K. Jacobson (eds.) (1994) *Behavior, Culture, and Conflict in World Politics.* Ann Arbor: University of Michigan Press.

5

Force and Violence in Politics

In addition to culture and ethnicity, a second factor affecting the classification of political systems relates to the use of force and violence in public policy. To measure the presence of this phenomenon in specific states, four issues will be addressed: (a) a country's recent history of warfare; (b) current violent conflict occurring in this state; (c) its record of coups d'état and other violent overthrows of the government; and (d) contemporary indicators of militarism (such as the size of the armed forces and military expenditures).

5a WAR: THE RECENT HISTORIC RECORD

The first issue relating to the presence of force and violence in a state's politics is its history of warfare. Since most of the 100 states selected for study in this work achieved their independence after 1945, the analysis of the historical record of war will focus on the most recent fifty-year era. **Table 5a** ranks states according to their experience in war since 1945, based upon a methodology developed in this author's earlier book (Sullivan, 1991: 32–33) which drew upon a data bank of some 140 wars based upon the work of the Stockholm International Peace Research Institute (1985ff), Sivard (1985ff), Laffin (1986ff), the Center for Defense Information (CDI) (1986), Brogan (1990), and Kende (1978).

This original research has been updated for this current study using media of record (*New York Times, The Economist*), Laffin and SIPRI through 1994, as well as CDI (1992), Clutterbuck (1993), Tillema (1991), Wickham-Crowley (1992) and Carter Center (1992). The results confirm the thesis that most wars in the contemporary era are civil wars (Enzensberger, 1994; Mueller, 1989), a point to be elaborated upon in section 5b.

Table 5a
States with Most Experience in War, 1945–1995 (scores indicate number of wars multiplied by number of total years at war)

Europe	Islamic Zone	Africa	Asia	West. Hemisph.
^° = 30/41(73%)--------------------------------------^° = 30/41(73%)				
			*India 375.25+	US 390
			Vietnam 322.5	
UK 258.75			China 320	
France 232	*Israel 224.00+			
	^Iraq 211.75+			
		S.Africa 156.5	*Philippine I. 162	
Portugal 148			*Indonesia 143+	
USSR/Russia 131.25+				
		^Ethiopia 112.25+		
		° Angola 99+		Cuba 96
	Iran 65	^Uganda 75	^Cambodia 76.5+	
	Yemen 62.5µ			
	Egypt 61.75+			*Guatemala 61.25+
	°Sudan 58+			
	^Syria 54			^Peru 54+
	°Somalia 52.5+	^Mozambique 52		*Colombia 52+
	°Algeria 52+		*Pakistan 49.5	
	^°Morocco 46+		°Myanmar 46.5+	*Argentina 40
	*Turkey 35+	°Rwanda/Bur.36+	*Sri Lanka 39+	
	^Libya 33.75		°Afghanistan 34+	
	°Georgia 27+	°Zaire 22.5		*El Salvador 26
*^°: 0/4	11/13	6/7	8/10	5/7

Europe	Islamic Zone	Africa	Asia	West. Hemisph.
^° = 13/31(42%)--------------------------------------^° = 13/31(42%)				
			Malaysia 18	*Nicaragua 18
Yugoslavia 15+		Zimbabwe 16	*Bangladesh 15	
Greece 10	^°Jordan 10	°Liberia 12+		
Spain 5.75	°Azerbaijan 7+	Tanzania 6	Taiwan 8	*Bolivia 4
		Cameroon 5	N.Korea 3	Ecuador 2
Nethrlds. 3	°Tajikistan 3+	°Nigeria 3	*S.Korea 3	Costa Rica 1
Hungary <1	Tunisia 2	*Madagascar 1		*Chile 1
Czechoslov. <1		Kenya 1		*Panama <1
Romania <1		^Burkina F. 1		Dom.Rep.<1
*^°: 0/7	3/4	4/8	2/5	4/6

No Wars

Europe	Islamic Zone	Africa	Asia	West. Hemisph.
^° = 7/28(25%)--------------------------------------^° = 7/28(25%)				
Swed.,Den.,Italy	Uzbekistan	Sen.,^Guinea	Austrl.,Jap.	Venez.,*Braz.
Ireld.,Belgium	Kazakhstan	IC,^Ghana	Singapore	Mexico,Jamaica
Germany,Poland	^° Saudi A.	Zambia	*Nepal	Canada, °Haiti
Ukraine,Bulgaria			*Thailand	
*^°: 0/9	1/3	2/5	2/5	2/7

Europe	Islamic Zone	Africa	Asia	West. Hemisph.
Total: 20	20	20	20	20 (100)

Notes: + = war continuing in 1995.
  *^° = designations of CGSS militarized polity states.
  μ = includes average of pre-1990 S. Yemen (19.5) and (N.) Yemen (103.5).

Names of the wars can generally be found in Sullivan (1991: 34–38), and for five selected states in the *Excerpts* at the end of this chapter. For each state, the calculations involve multiplying the number of its wars by the total number of years it has experienced war, with some half-weight discounting for periodic wars and insurgencies because it is judged that a state's commitment to such wars is less than that in a full-scale civil or international war. A + inserted after the total indicates that a war is still continuing at the time of this writing.

A periodic war is one which waxes and wanes over the years, with occasional periods of intense fighting alternating with periods of comparative quiet. An *insurgency* (to be discussed at greater length in section 5b) is a low-level civil war in which the non-governmental side does not hold significant territory for any length of time, and the deaths involved are less than 1,000 per year (Sivard, 1989: 22; Eckhardt and Azar, 1979).

With these definitions and methodology as background, some remarks can be made based on state scores and rankings on **Table 5a**. At the top of the table, with war-scores in excess of 100, are such historic imperial powers as the United States, the United Kingdom, France, Portugal, USSR/Russia, and China—most of which spent much of the last fifty years fighting to retain, or to succeed one another in, their respective empires. Also among the leaders by this measure are some aspiring regional powers—such as India, Indonesia, South Africa, Ethiopia, Iraq, and Israel—some of them former colonies which have had to fight to retain their new dominion over putative nations within them. Four non-states not displayed in Table 5a (Palestine, Kurdistan, Western Sahara, and Tibet) also have significant war-scores and help to account for the high ranks of the "oppressor states" against which they have struggled (respectively, Israel/Jordan, Turkey/Iraq/Iran, Morocco, and China).

Concerning the thesis of this book regarding forms of government, 30 of the 41 states (or 73%) with the highest scores in war experience have political systems on the second page of the CGSS. These are designated in **Table 5a** with either a * for militarized party states, a ^ for moderating military regimes, a ° for entrenched military regimes, or a ^° for monarchies, as these polity types were defined in Chapter 1. At the other extreme, only 7 of 28 (25%) of the states with no wars since 1945 have militarized political systems. An intermediary status exists with 13 of 31 (42%) of a middle group with minimal war experience over the last fifty years. Although no causality is inferred from these numbers, it is clear that states with significant experience in war are more likely to have militarized polities as this term is used in this work.

The methodology of annotating states in tables with *, ^, or ° will be used in this chapter on two other occasions (Tables 5c.iii and 5d) to show similar relationships between high degrees of militarism and low placement on the Comparative Government Spread Sheet.

5b CURRENT VIOLENT DOMESTIC CONFLICT

If past wars leave a legacy of militarized political systems, this result is even more evident for countries locked in the midst of present violent domestic conflict (i.e., civil war or insurgency). Most annual studies of war in the contemporary world (Laffin, SIPRI, Sivard) put the number of such conflicts at between thirty and forty at any particular time depending on how "civil war" is defined. **Table 5b** identifies 33 states as beset by the worst levels of violent domestic conflict at the time of publication (1995). As in Chapter 4, the number 33 is arbitrarily chosen, this time to represent one-third of the states in the Comparative Government Spread Sheet. Because the definition of "conflict" is somewhat broad, another 10 candidates for inclusion are listed at the bottom of the table. The 33 states selected for further discussion will be divided into four categories, in order to provide a more analytic framework for comparison.

The first, or mildest, category of conflict is that relating to latent (LAT) or periodic wars, which wax or wane over the years with occasional periods of intense fighting alternating with periods of comparative quiet but no affirmative moves toward resolution. Among the 6 states included in this category are Iraq, whose Kurds have been protected by the Gulf War allies (especially the United States) in an enclave in the northern third of the country since 1991; Somalia, where five years of clan warfare died down in 1994; Yemen, united since 1990 but where the most recent fighting between the leftist south and the conservative north was in May 1994; Rwanda, whose latest spasm of Hutu–Tutsi violence was in 1994; the archipelago of Indonesia, which is periodically beset by separatist efforts on at least three fronts, in East Timor, western Papua, and northern Aceh; and the Philippines, another island chain challenged by Muslims in the south and communists elsewhere (see the *Excerpts* at the end of this chapter).

The second category of internal violent politics is that relating to *waning* (WAN) conflict, defined here as one in which a "peace process" has been started, which generally includes a ceasefire in place, separation and regrouping of forces, some demobilization of troops (in preparation for the reintegration of the remainder into a new national army), and preparation for elections (including the setting of a date and the registration of voters)—all of the above under the aegis of some outside impartial international organization such as the United Nations or some regional alliance (Licklider, 1993). Among the 11 states in this situation in 1995 are the United Kingdom (whose northern Irish opponents declared a ceasefire in August 1994); Tajikistan (where a ceasefire and resulting presidential election in the fall of 1994 are being assured by the presence of Russian troops); Azerbaijan (where Russia mediated a ceasefire with the Armenians in Ngorno-Karabakh in June 1994); Morocco (versus Western Saharan POLISARIO movement since 1975, U.N.-sponsored peace process since September 1991); Israel (versus Palestinians since 1948

Table 5b
Major Current (Violent, Domestic) Conflict, as of December 1995 (n = 33: 6 + 11 + 6 + 10; by percentage of land/population controlled by non-government forces and/or date of last major outbreak)

Europe	Islamic Zone	Africa	Asia	West. Hemisph.
1. (LAT)*Latent or Periodic* conflicts to watch (1995ff), n=6				
	°Iraq(3/91)		°Indonesia('62,76,88)	
	Somalia (3/94)	Rwanda/Bur.(7/94)	°Philippine I. ('89,'92)	
	Yemen (5/94)			
	n=3	n=1	n=2	(6)
2. (WAN)*Waning* (talking toward ceasefire, moving twd. settlement, 1995ff), n=11				
	Tajikistan-50%(11/94)	Mozambique-50%(8/92)		
	Azerbaijan-20%(6/94)			
UK/	Morocco-16%(9/91)	Angola-25%(11/94)		El Salv.-20%(1/92)
N.Ire.-0%(8/94)	Israel-0%(9/93)	S. Africa-0%(8/90)	Cambodia-15%(10/91)	Nicaragua-5%(2/90)
n=1	n=4	n=3	n=1	n=2 (11)
- -				
3. (NSG)*Insurgencies* (=Little land held; and low intensity [<1,000 dead/yr.]), n=6				
	Egypt	°Ethiopia	°India	Guatemala
				°Colombia
				Peru
	n=1	n=1	n=1	n=3 (6)
4.(CVW)*Civil Wars* n=10				
°Russia-1%	Algeria-5%			
	Sudan-8%		Sri Lanka-15%	
ex-°Yugoslavia:	°Georgia-10%		°Myanmar-15%	
Croatia-30%	Turkey-30%			
Bosnia-70%		Liberia-95%	°Afghanistan-95%	
n=2	n=4	n=1	n=3	(10)
Tot.: 3	12	6	7	5 (33)
of n=20	20	20	20	20 (100)

- -

Europe	Islamic Zone	Africa	Asia	West. Hemisph.
Other (recent/prospective) candidates for inclusion (n=10):				
°Ukraine(Crimea,Donbass)	°Iran(Muj.,Kurds)	Uganda(northeast)	Bangladesh(Sh.Bahini)	Canada(Quebec)
Spain (Basques)	Jordan(Pals.)	Zaire (Shaba)	China (Tibet)	Mexico(Chiapas)
n=2	n=2	n=2	n=2	n=2 (10)

Note: ° = states in which there are more than one war against the government (n=12).

founding and especially versus PLO since its creation in 1965, peace process since historic "White House handshake" of September 1993); Mozambique (versus RENAMO guerillas since 1976, U.N.-sponsored peace process since August 1992); Angola (versus UNITA rebel movement since 1974 independence, ceasefire since November 1994); South Africa (five-year transition government following April 1994 first all-race elections); Cambodia (with Khmer Rouge still in control of 15% of territory despite peace process begun in 1991 and featuring a May 1993 election involving three other former combatant parties); El Salvador (whose March 1994 elections were intended to end fifteen years of armed struggle, and two years of a U.N.-sponsored transition to peace); and Nicaragua, in which two armed movements have been co-existing in an uneasy power-sharing relationship since 1990 (see the *Excerpts* at the end of this chapter).

The last two forms of current violent domestic conflict involve wars that are continuing, although at different levels of intensity. *Insurgencies* (NSG) are defined as wars in which the non-governmental side does not hold significant territory for any length of time and the deaths involved are less than 1,000 per year at the present time. As of 1995, these number 6: Egypt (whose Islamic Fundamentalist opposition have, since 1992, caused less than 1,000 deaths and hold no land); Ethiopia (where the Oromo majority, and some Amharans, are struggling against the post-1991 Tigre-dominated government); and India, whose various Kashmiri Muslim, Punjabi Sikh, and northeast (often animist and Christian) tribal rebels seldom evict the government from control of lands for any significant time despite horrific death tolls at times. Also, the generation-long civil wars in Peru, Colombia, and Guatemala have recently been downgraded to the level of insurgency in the research associated with this project; while the total number of deaths in each is significant (30,000 since 1980 in Peru, 20,000 since 1978 in Colombia, 135,000 since 1961 in Guatemala), the annual totals in recent years have not been at these rates.

Finally, the term *civil war* (CVW) will be used for that violent domestic political conflict in which the non-governmental side controls some identifiable percentage of territory or population and in which the deaths involved are more than 1,000 per year. This definition excludes states where rebels hold land but the government does not choose to contest such control (e.g., northern [Kurdish] Iraq, northern Somaliland, and western Cambodia, where the conflicts are considered latent or waning). With such restrictions, the number of active civil wars is thus about one-third of the total number, thirty to forty, often cited.

Ten such wars are noted in **Table 5b**: Russia (versus Chechnya in 1994–1995, and potentially against other restive ethnic republics, such as Tatarstan, Ingushetia, and North Ossetia in the future); ex-Yugoslavia (multisided, depending on definition of combatants—Croatian, Bosnian [and uncontested Slovenian and Macedonian] secessionists versus former Yugoslavia, Krajina and other Serb rebels versus Croatia, Serpska Republika versus Bosnia Federation of Croats and Muslims); Algeria (secular, modernizing military government versus Islamic fundamentalists); Sudan (Islamic, largely Arab, northern goverment versus southern [mainly Christian and animist] blacks); Georgia (versus Abkhazian and Ossetian secessionists, and sometimes between nationalist and more pro-Russian Georgians); Turkey (where another group of Kurds effectively controls 30% of the country); Liberia (where externally imposed ECOWAS [Economic Organization of West African States] government yielded power to a council of warlords in August 1995; Sri Lanka (decade-long struggle between majority Sinhalese Government and minority Tamils, especially in the northern Jaffna peninsula); Myanmar (generations-long war between Burmese central government and various tribal groups [Karen, Mon, etc.] since 1948 independence, and against other Burmans since 1988); and Afghanistan (multisided war between various Sunni Islamic mujaheddin, which ousted pro-Soviet regime in 1992, exacerbated by Pathan versus Tajik, Uzbek, and Hazara [pro-Persian, Shiite] differences).

It should be noted at this point that state placements in **Table 5b** are among the most fluid in any of the main categories of analysis in this work. Countries whose conflicts have been Latent for years may erupt into war without warning. This is also true for states which are in the Waning category, because a "peace process" has been started, and a limit of about five years (or one electoral cycle) is posited before moving an apparently quiescent state (like El Salvador or South Africa in 1995) out of this category.

In addition to the definitional differences among the 33 targeted major current conflicts, various other factors can be noted to delineate further distinctions among these states and to enhance understanding of the phenomenon of violent domestic political conflict. Four measures will be suggested here:

1. War deaths and casualty statistics are used by many (Small and Singer, 1982; Cioffi-Revilla, 1989) to measure the severity of war. In addition to the absolute numbers—which exceed more than 100,000 in the cases of Yugoslavia, Sudan, Somalia, Iraq's Kurds, Mozambique, Angola, Rwanda/Burundi, Liberia, Indonesia's East Timor, and Guatemala—relative measures relating to intensity (average number of deaths each year, or deaths as a percentage of population) could also be computed and states ranked accordingly.

2. The number of major militarized oppositional groups; among the 33 states under scrutiny, at least 12 (designated by ° in **Table 5b**) have more than one distinct (i.e., different ideological or ethnic) set of armed opponents.

3. The length of the conflict, based upon its starting date; the duration of these wars ranges from less than five years (in the case of states from the disintegrating USSR and Yugoslavia and the Islamic Fundmentalist uprisings in Egypt and Algeria, to more than thirty-five years (in Rwanda, Myanmar, India versus its northeast tribes, and Turkey and Iraq versus their respective Kurds).

4. Armed strength for each rebel group, a number which varies from about 1,000 in Guatemala, to more than 200,000 still fighting in Afghanistan years after the USSR and its puppet regime were driven out. A figure which is perhaps as significant as the number of combatants under arms is the percentage of the population which, though not in actual combat, offers political (and sometimes logistical) support to

these fighters. This statistic, however, is more difficult to estimate and is, indeed. the true "center of gravity" over which many insurgent wars are fought, according to theorists of this type of conflict (Odom, 1992; Thayer, 1990; Wolpin, 1981; Eckstein, 1965). The figure is estimated for some of the states in the *Excerpts* at the end of this chapter

Before concluding this section, it might be noted that 25 states appear on *both* Table 5b on current conflicts and Table 4b on ethnicity. This indicates that, today, most violent, domestic conflict (i.e., civil war) is ethnic based, as opposed to being ideological or otherwise political in nature (Sullivan, 1994; Gurr, 1993). In only 8 states with internal wars is ethnicity not a major determinant: Algeria, Egypt, Mozambique, Yemen, Cambodia, El Salvador, Nicaragua, and Colombia. In any case, the wars in 5 of these 8 countries are latent or waning, so the phenomenon of the non–ethnic-based ideological civil war might be less of a factor in international and comparative politics in the future.

Of more significance to this work is the connection between the states on **Table 5b** (especially those with active civil wars as defined above) and those in the most entrenched category of Chapter 6's militarized political systems. Of the 10 states in Category 4 of Table 5b, 6 are designated entrenched military (or mil°) regimes in Chapter 6d (not Russia, Yugoslavia, Turkey, or Sri Lanka). Among the 13 entrenched military regimes of the next chapter, only the coup regime of Nigeria is not accompanied by the violent domestic conflict covered in this chapter.

5c COUPS AND OTHER REGIMES OF VIOLENT ORIGIN

Civil wars sometimes result in the overthrow of a government and a change in regime. There are two other ways in which governments might be formed based upon violence—revolutions and military coups d'état. Because these three ways of employing force to create a government are often confused, it is important to define each phenomenon and to delineate the nuances which distinguish one from the other.

Civil wars, discussed in Chapter 5b, involve an armed struggle between two (or more) groups claiming to be the legitimate rulers of a state. If the established government loses such an encounter, it is common for some public policies to change (especially if a different ethnic group takes over), but apart from the allocation of government priorities, there is often not that much of a basic change in society (Andreski, 1992; Schutz and Slater, 1990).

A *revolution* is a different form of such struggle, in which the non-governmental side has as its goal not only the replacement of the government but a rapid and more complete transformation of society (Sederberg, 1994; Chaliand, 1991; Dunn, 1989). By this definition, there have been very few genuine revolutions in contemporary history. Perhaps only seven would qualify in this century: Mexico (1911–1919); Russia (1917); China (1927–1949); Cuba (1953–1959); Indochina (Vietnam, Laos, and Cambodia) (1946–1975); Iran (1978–1979); and Nicaragua (1977–1979). Even some of these "societal transformations" have been overturned or modified over time (Goldstone, 1994; Skocpol, 1994).

Two additional points should be made about revolutions. Except for Russia's, most of the examples cited took several years to occur, some as long as a generation. Successful revolutions generally are broadly based in popular sympathy; they gain this support by having the ideological dimension mentioned earlier, that is, the complete overturning of unpopular existing institutions and the establishment of a society based upon a totally new relationship between citizens and government (Midlarsky, 1986; Eisenstadt, 1978).

In contrast, a military *coup* is a rapid blow against the state which generally leaves most of society's basic structures untouched and changes only the top administrative strata of government. Most significant, it is perpetrated by the government's own soldiers from within the institutional military establishment, the very forces pledged to uphold the existing system (David, 1986; Farceau, 1994; Jackman, 1978).

Military coup regimes generally do not have a coherent economic or political belief system as part of their ideology. They often claim to intervene to maintain public safety or to preserve "law and order." Sometimes, self-styled "modernizing military regimes" eliminate corrupt institutions, like monarchies—as in Syria (1948), Egypt (1952), Iraq (1958), (North) Yemen (1962), Libya (1969), and Afghanistan (1973)—but do not follow through with rapid and thorough societal transformations. Hence, they are not considered revolutions and have generally been followed by subsequent coups. Because such administrations do not have any larger purpose, the result is often only self-aggrandizement of the junta leaders. It is this final factor, the longevity of the leadership, which most distinguishes the various types of regimes of violent origin to be discussed next.

Table 5c lists 26 examples of current (late 1995) regimes which came to power in violent removals of previous governments (i.e., coups, revolutions, civil wars) and are still headed by the leadership which perpetrated the original overthrow or some collaborative successor. The display identifies the dates when each came to power, and the major personalities involved (including the leader's rank at the time of the coup; most have since promoted themselves to general). Not included on this list are some states—like Angola, Mozambique, Zimbabwe, South Africa, and Cambodia—whose current leadership employed force *before* its accession to office was eventually negotiated (i.e., the actual transfer of power was not violent).

Scrutiny of some of the states listed on **Table 5c** will elaborate on some other aspects of this phenomenon. First of all, less than half (10 of 26) of the states listed on Table 5c are simple first-generation military coup regimes: Libya, Syria, Sudan, Algeria, Zaire, Ghana, Guinea, Burkina Faso, Nigeria, and Indonesia. The second most common source for a regime of violent origin (n = 5) would be states whose current government is the outcome of a civil war or revolution won by the opposition side: Romania, Azerbaijan, Ethiopia, Uganda, and Cuba. There are also 3 states on Table 5c where the

Table 5c
Regimes of Violent Origin, as of December 1995

State	Date of Coup	Leader	# yrs.
		Europe (n=1)	
Romania	Dec. '89	Army + CP/NSF's Ion Iliescu	6 yrs.
		Islamic Zone (n=9, incl. μYemen)	
Iraq	July '69/July'79	Gen.A.H.al-Bakr/Saddam Hussein	26 yrs.
Libya	Sept.'69	Col. Muammar Qaddafi	26 yrs.
Syria	Nov.'70	Lt.Gen. Hafez al Assad	25 yrs.
Yemen	May 1990	Gen. ali Abdallah Salih	5 (+12)yrs.
μN.Yemen	July '78-May 1990	Lt.Col. ali Abdallah Salih	12 yrs.
μS.Yemen	Jan.'86-May 1990	ali Salim (Saleh M.) al-Beedh	4 yrs.
Sudan	July '89	Brig. O.H.A.al Bashir < NIF SG H.Turabi	9 yrs.
Somalia	Jan. '91	Pres.Mahdi v.USC Gen.Aideed v.Egil in North	4 yrs.
Algeria	Jan. '92/Jan.'94	Gen. Khaled Nezzar/Pres.Gen.Liamine Zeroual	3 yrs.
Tajikistan	Dec. '92	Russia+pro-CP,Uzbek forces > Pres. Rakhmanov	3 yrs.
Azerbaijan	June '93	Col.S.Guseinov > Pres. H. Aliyev	2 yrs.
		Africa (n=9)	
Zaire	Nov.'65	Col. Joseph Mobutu	30 yrs.
Ghana	Dec. '81	Flt.Lt. Jerry Rawlings	14 yrs.
Guinea	Apr.'84	Col. Lansana Conte	11 yrs.
Uganda	Jan.'86	Maj. Yoseri Museveni	9 yrs.
Burkina Faso	Oct.'87	Capt. Blaise Campaore	8 yrs.
Liberia	Sept.'90/Mar.'94	ECOWAS+A. Sawyer/Collective Presidency	5 yrs.
Ethiopia	May '91	Col. Meles Zenawi	4 yrs.
Nigeria	Nov.'93	Gen. Shani Abacha	2 yrs.
Rwanda	July '94	Gen. Paul Kagame (>Hutu Pres.,PM)	1 yr.
		Asia (n=4)	
N.Korea	1947/1994	Marshall Kim Il Sung/son Kim Jong Il	48 yrs.
Indonesia	Mar.'66	Gen. Suharto	29 yrs.
Myanmar	Sept. '88/Apr.'92	Gen. Saw Maung/Gen.Than Shwe	7 yrs.
Afghanistan	May 1992	Pres.Rabbani v. Hekmytyar v. Dostam v. Taliban	3 yrs.
		Western Hemisphere (n=3)	
Cuba	Jan. '59	Commandante Fidel Castro	36 yrs.
Peru	Apr. '92	Pres. Alberto Fujimori + Army	3 yrs.
Haiti	Sept. '94	US Army + Rev. Jean-Bertrand Aristide	< 1 yr.

Violent-Origin Regimes include: traditional coups (n=10); opposition winners of civil wars or revolutions (Romania, Azerbaijan, Ethiopia, Uganda, Cuba); foreign-installed (Tajikistan, Liberia, Haiti); plus still-contesting armies (Somalia, Afghanistan); "peaceful" pass-alongs within junta (Iraq, Algeria, Myanmar, N.Korea, Yemen) with bequeathed power designation /; and "constitutional coups" (Peru).

Definitions:
coup - establishment forces; usually quick, bloodless (< 1,000 dead); change in top admininistration only.
civil war - opposition forces; generally long and > 1,000 dead; change of government policies.
revolution - opposition forces; generally long and > 1,000 dead; goal of total change of society.

Notes: *^° = CGSS designations for militarized polities.
μ = Two Yemeni states before 1990 unification.
< and > indicate whether military person named is less (<) or more (>) powerful than other figure noted.

military most influential in the seizure of power was that of a foreign country or countries: Tajikistan (1992), Liberia (1990), and Haiti (1994). There are yet 2 other countries where the struggle between contending armies is still under way (Somalia, Afghanistan) and there is no generally recognized government (see Chapter 6d's collapsed states).

There are also cases where power has been passed on peacefully to other members of the original junta (Iraq, Algeria, and Myanmar, with dual dates and leaders' names separated by a / in **Table 5c**, and North Korea, where the son succeeded the father, who was installed by the Soviet Army during World War II). These should be contrasted with truly revolutionary regimes which set up civilian party structures which provided for relatively peaceful transition to a new generation of leaders—for example, USSR, China, Vietnam, and Iran.

Finally, there are the cases of Yemen and Peru. Yemen is a variation of the peaceful passing of power; two earlier coup regimes in the north and south united in 1990, keeping as president the leader of one of the original coups, who has yet to be legitimated in any popular referendum. Peru is an example of a "constitutional" coup, or one in which the elected president collaborated with the military to suspend civilian political institutions and rule by decree, giving him an unfair advantage in the rewriting of the constitution and subsequent reelection. An earlier example of such a coup plus prolonged rule was the Philippines (1972–1986).

Regardless of which means of force produced the regime, **Table 5c.i** and **Table 5c.ii** provide a way to analyze and measure the impact on political systems of such violent-origin regimes. On Table 5c.i, the "frequency ratio" divides the number of violent takeovers by the number of years a state has been independent, as far back as 1945. The other column on Table 5c.i gives the "percentage of violent-origin regime years" a state has experienced over this same period of time. Finally, Table 5c.ii averages these two numbers (times 1,000) into a "composite violent origins" measure. (As with the wars in sections 5a and 5b, name identification of the regimes and their years in office can be found in the Data Bank associated with this project, examples of which are in the *Excerpts* at the end of this chapter.)

With this explanation of methodology, some concluding remarks about regimes of violent origin can now be made. Some 204 forceful overthrows of government have been identified in **Table 5c.i** (see zonal summaries at end of Table), most of which (i.e., 77, or 38%) have occurred in the Western Hemisphere (specifically, Latin America), where 16 of 20 CGSS states have been affected. Europe is the region least susceptible to such violent changes of regime—only 11 of 204 cases, affecting only 7 states. The Islamic zone, Africa, and Asia have each had between 38 and 40 such transfers of power; they are, however, the sites of most *recent* regimes of violent origins: Of the 26 such governments currently ruling and listed in **Table 5c**, 22 are in these three zones.

According to the left side of **Table 5c.i**, Thailand leads the world in number of coups (10.5; a half weight is assigned when power is passed peacefully

Table 5c.i
Violent-Origin Regime Measures (n = 59/100, through 1995)

Frequency Ratio (# since 1945, or independence year)				% Regime Years (+ = continuing at present time)		
State	ratio	Data	Indep./Base Yr.	State	% Yrs.	Data

Europe (n=7 states*, 11 violent overthrows)

State	ratio	Data	Indep./Base Yr.	State	% Yrs.	Data
Portugal	.050	2.5/50	1945	Spain	.600	30/50
Greece	.050	2.5/50	1945	Portugal	.580	29/50
Czech.	.040	2/50	1945	Greece	.140	7/50
Hungary	.020	1/50	1945	Czech.	.140	7/50
Poland	.020	1/50	1945	Romania	.102	6+50
Romania	.020	1/50	1945	Hungary	.100	5/50
Spain	.020	1/50	1945	Poland	.080	4/50

*None in 7/7 in northern Europe region; Italy,Bulgaria,Yugo.; Germany,Ukraine,Russia (n=13 states).

Islamic Zone (n=13 states*, 39.5 violent overthrows)

State	ratio	Data	Indep./Base Yr.	State	% Yrs.	Data
Tajikistan	.750	3/4	1991	Syria	.939	46+/49
Georgia	.250	1/4	1991	Algeria	.909	30+/33
Azerbaijan	.250	1/4	1991	Sudan	.769	30+/39
Syria	.160	8/50	1946	Tajikistan	.750	3+/4
Sudan	.128	5/39	1956	Somalia	.742	26+/35
µYemen	.115	4.5/39	1945/67	Iraq	.740	37+/50
Algeria	.091	3/33	1962	Iran	.700	35/50
Iraq	.090	4.5/50	1945	µYemen	.667	26+/39
Turkey	.060	3/50	1945	Libya	.590	26+/44
Somalia	.057	2/35	1960	Azerbaijan	.500	2+/4
Iran	.040	2/50	1945	Egypt	.360	18/50
Egypt	.030	1.5/450	1945	Georgia	.250	1/4
Libya	.023	1/44	1951	Turkey	.220	11/50

*None in: Uzbek.,Kazak.; Israel,Saudi A.,Jordan; Morocco,Tunisia (n=7 states).
µ=Average figures for N.Yem.,1945-90, & S.Yem., 1967-90 in 5c.i;
   2 Yemens' 5c.ii's avg. of 21 yrs. extended after 1990 since leader is same person.

Africa (n=10 states*, 38.5 violent overthrows)

State	ratio	Data	Indep./Base Yr.	State	% Yrs.	Data
Nigeria	.200	7/35	1960	Zaire	.857	30+/35
Burkina F.	.171	6/35	1960	Burkina F.	.829	29+/35
Uganda	.152	5/33	1962	Rwanda	.788	26+/33
Ghana	.132	5/38	1957	Uganda	.727	24+/33
Rwanda	.121	4/33	1962	Nigeria	.714	25+/35
Madagascar	.100	3.5/35	1960	Ghana	.632	24+/38
Ethiopia	.080	4/50	1945	Madagascar	.600	21/35
Liberia	.040	2/50	1945	Ethiopia	.420	21+/50
Zaire	.029	1/35	1960	Liberia	.300	15+/50
Guinea	.027	1/37	1958	Guinea	.297	11+/37

*None in: IC,Sen.; Cam.,Kenya,Tanz.; Zambia,Zimbwe.,S.Af.,Ang.,Moz. (n=10 states).

Table 5c.i *(continued)*

Frequency Ratio				% Regime Years		
State	ratio	Data	Indep./Base Yr.	State	% Yrs.	Data

		Asia (n=13 states*, 38.0 violent overthrows)				
Thailand	.210	10.5/50	1945	N.Korea	1.000	48+/48
Bangladesh	.167	4/24	1971	Taiwan	.826	38/46
Afghanistan	.110	5.5/50	1945	Thailand	.780	39/50
Myanmar	.096	4.5/47	1948	Bangladesh	.750	18/24
Cambodia	.073	3/41	1954	Myanmar	.723	34+/47
Pakistan	.063	3/48	1947	Indonesia	.617	29+/47
S.Korea	.043	2/47	1948	S.Korea	.553	26/47
Taiwan	.033	1.5/46	1949	Pakistan	.521	25/48
N.Korea	.031	1.5/48	1947	China	.520	26/50
Vietnam	.024	1/41	1954	Cambodia	.512	21/41
Indonesia	.021	1/47	1948	Afghanistan	.440	22+/50
Philippines	.020	1/47	1946	Vietnam	.390	16/41
China	.020	1/50	1945	Philippines	.286	14/49

*None in: India,Nepal,SriLanka;   Japan,Malaysia,Singapore,Australia. (n=7 states).

		Western Hemisphere (n=16 states*, 77 violent overthrows)				
Guatemala	.200	10/50	1945	Cuba	1.000	50+/50
Haiti	.190	9.5/50	1945	Haiti	1.000	50+/50
El Salvador	.180	9/50	1945	Nicaragua	.900	45/50
Bolivia	.160	8/50	1945	El Salvador	.780	39/50
Argentina	.150	7.5/50	1945	Panama	.640	32/50
Ecuador	.140	7/50	1945	Guatemala	.640	32/50
Peru	.120	6/50	1945	Argentina	.540	27/50
Brazil	.100	5/50	1945	Bolivia	.500	25/50
Panama	.100	5/50	1945	Peru	.500	25+/50
Dom. Rep.	.080	4/50	1945	Brazil	.460	23/50
Venezuela	.070	3.5/50	1945	Dom.Rep.	.380	19/50
Nicaragua	.060	3/50	1945	Chile	.320	16/50
Colombia	.040	2/50	1945	Ecuador	.300	15/50
Cuba	.050	2.5/50	1945	Venezuela	.220	11/50
Chile	.020	1/50	1945	Colombia	.080	4/50
Costa Rica	.020	1/50	1945	Costa Rica	.020	1/50

*None in: Mexico;   Jamaica, Canada, US. (n=4 states).

Zonal Summary

Europe	7/20 states	11.0/204 violent overthrows (5.4%)
Islamic Zone	13/20 states	39.5/204 violent overthrows (19.4%)
Africa	10/20 states	38.5/204 violent overthrows (18.9%)
Asia	13/20 states	38.0/204 violent overthrows (18.6%)
Western Hemisphere	16/20 states	77.0/204 violent overthrows (37.7%)

Notes: For regimes starting before 1945 and extending after that year, overthrow is counted in left column, but only the years since 1945 are counted in right column.

Half weight is assigned when power is passed peacefully from one group in a junta to another. Regardless of how many months in a year a regime rules, right column counts a full year.

For Latin American states whose independence goes back to nineteenth century and military rule is a tradition, regimes are listed beginning with those succeeding the first period of civilian rule after 1945.

Table 5c.ii
Composite Violent-Origins Measure

Europe	Islamic Zone	Africa	Asia	West.Hemisph.
	^° = 35/42(83%)------------------------^° = 35/42 (83%)			
	°Tajikistan 750.0			°Haiti 595.0
	^Syria 549.5		N.Korea 515.5	Cuba 525.0
	°Algeria 500.0	^Burkina F. 500.0	*Thailand 495.0	*El Salvador 480.0
		°Nigeria 457.0	*Bangladesh 458.5	*Nicaragua 480.0
	°Sudan 448.5	°Rwanda 454.5		
		°Zaire 443.0		
		^Uganda 439.5	Taiwan 429.5	*Guatemala 420.0
	^Iraq 415.0		°Myanmar 409.5	
	°Somalia 399.5			
	°Yemen 391.0			
	°Azerbaijan 375.0	^Ghana 382.0		*Panama 370.0
	Iran 370.0	*Madagascar 350.0		*Argentina 345.0
			*Indonesia 329.5	*Bolivia 330.0
Portugal 315.0				
Spain 310.0	^Libya 306.5		*S.Korea 298.0	^Peru 310.0
			^Cambodia 292.5	
			*Pakistan 292.0	
			°Afghanistan 275.0	*Brazil 280.0
	°Georgia 250.0	^Ethiopia 250.0	China 270.0	
*^°: 0/2	10/11	8/8	8/11	9/10
	^° = 6/17 (35%)----------------------------^° = 6/17 (35%)			
				Dom.Rep.230.0
				Ecuador 220.0
	Egypt 195.0		Vietnam 207.0	
		°Liberia 170.0		
		^Guinea 162.0	*Phil. I. 153.0	*Chile 170.0
Greece 95.0	*Turkey 140.0			Venezuela 145.0
Czech. 90.0				
Romania 61.0				*Colombia 60.0
Hungary 60.0				
Poland 50.0				Costa Rica 20.0
*^°: n=0/5	1/2	2/2	1/2	2/6
	^° = 9/41 (22%)------NO violent origins------^° 9/41 = (22%)			
Ireld.,UK,France	Uzbek.,Kazak.	Ivory Coast	*India,*Nepal	Mexico
Belgium,Nethrlds.	^°Saudi Arabia	Senegal,Cameroon	*Sri Lanka	
Sweden,Denmark	*Israel	Kenya,Tanzania	Japan	Jamaica
Italy,Bulgaria	^°Jordan	Zambia,Zimbwe.	Malaysia	
Germany,Yugo.	Tunisia	°Angola,^Mozambq.	Singapore	USA
Ukraine,Russia	^°Morocco	South Africa	Australia	Canada
n=13	n=7	n=10	n=7	n=4 (41
TOTS: 20	20	20	20	20 (100

Note: *^° = designations of CGSS militarized polity states.

from one member of a junta to another), followed by Guatemala (10), Haiti (9.5), and El Salvador (9). Three countries—North Korea, Cuba, and Haiti—have been under regimes of violent origin for all of the time since the start of this study (1945), and Nicaragua, Syria, and Algeria for more than 90 percent of that time (see the right side of **Table 5c.i**). Tajikistan has the highest composite score (750.0 on **Table 5c.ii**), a number which is somewhat skewed owing to its base number of years since independence being only four. The other high scorers in both frequency and duration of such regimes are Haiti, Syria, North Korea, Algeria, Burkina Faso, and Thailand.

With respect to the main theme of this book, **Table 5c.ii** shows that 35 of 42 (or 83%) of the states in its top tier are also found on the second page of the Comparative Government Spread Sheet (employing the *^° annotating methodology introduced at the beginning of this chapter.) In the 41 states with no record of violent overthrows of government, there are only 9 states (or 22%) from CGSS, page 2—Israel, Saudi Arabia, Jordan, Morocco, Angola, Mozambique, India, Nepal, and Sri Lanka.

5d CONTEMPORARY MILITARISM

It would seem that current statistical indicators pertaining to the military would be a final factor relating to force and violence in a country's politics, and the annual publications of Sivard, SIPRI, the International Institute for Strategic Studies (IISS) in London, and the U.S. Arms Control and Disarmament Agency (ACDA) provide a wealth of data relating to countries' armed forces and military expenditures. State standings according to these measures do not change much from year to year.

However, absolute numbers relating to this information generally reflect either the size of the country's population (in the case of armed personnel) or its wealth (in the case of defense spending). Research whose tabular results are not reproduced in this study shows this situation also obtains in the case of four relative measures: armed forces per 1,000 people, military expenditures as a percentage of gross national product, military spending per soldier, and military spending per capita (U.S. Arms Control and Disarmament Agency, 1995: 33–35). In all these cases, large countries have large armies, and wealthy countries have high military spending (and the large armies that this buys), regardless of political system. The United States (civilian mpr) is notable in this regard, having higher military spending than the next 8 countries combined.

However, there is one relative measure which does correlate with polity types: military spending as a percentage of Central Government Expenditures (CGE). Employing the *^° annotation methodology used earlier in this chapter), **Table 5d** shows that 66 percent, or 33, of the 50 states with highest military expenditures/CGE ratios, are militarized polities. More than half of the states with the highest ratios (greater than 10%) are in the Islamic zone (n = 16) and in Asia (n = 15), where the percentages of countries on the milita-

Table 5d
Military Expenditures/Central Government Expenditures, 1993

Europe	Islamic Zone	Africa	Asia	West.Hemisph.
	^° = 33/50(66%)------------------------------^° = 33/50(66%)			
	°Sudan 46.0e%		°Afghanistan 43.0e%	
	^°Saudi A. 41.0			
Yugoslavia 30.0e%		^Mozambiq. 32.0e%	Taiwan 28.0	^Haiti 30% ('94)Δ
	^Syria 26.2		N.Korea 26.7e	
			*Pakistan 26.3	
Russia 24.3e	^°Jordan 23.5	°Rwanda 24.1	Singapore 26.0	*Argentina 24.8%
	^Iraq 20.7e		°Cambodia 24.6e	
	*Israel 20.1		°Myanmar 22.2e	
	^°Morocco 19.5	°Angola 19.9e		USA 20.1
	*Turkey 19.5	°Liberia 18.5e	Vietnam 19.7e	
			*India 18.8	
	^Yemen 17.7e	^Burkina Faso 17.1	*S.Korea 18.1	
			*Sri Lanka 16.8e	
			China 16.2	*Colombia 16.5e
	°Azerbaijan 15.5e	Zimbabwe 15.0	*Thailand 15.9	
Greece 13.6e	^Li bya 14.7e		Malaysia 15.5	^Peru 13.3
	°Tajikistan 12.7e	Tanzania 12.5		
	Iran 12.4	Senegal 12.1e	*Phil. I. 12.6	
Romania 11.4	°Georgia 10.9e	^Ethiopia 10.9		
	Egypt 10.5e			
	Tunisia 10.3			*El Salvador 10.1
*^°: 0/4	13/16	6/9	9/15	5/6
	^° = 17/50(34%)------------------------------^° = 17/50(34%)			
UK 9.4	°Algeria 9.1	Cameroon 9.3	Australia 9.9	*Guatemala 9.4
Bulgaria 8.2e		^Uganda 8.8	*Bangladesh 9.2	*Chile 9.2
		Kenya 8.7		
France 7.3e		Zambia 8.7e		Canada 8.1
Poland 7.1		°Zaire 8.6		
Czech.Rep. 6.8				Venezuela 7.8
Portugal 6.0e				Ecuador 7.8
Sweden 5.9e				*Nicaragua 7.7
Spain 5.8				*Bolivia 7.6
Hungary 5.7		S.Africa 8.2		Dom.Rep. 6.9
		*Madagascar 7.0e	^Indonesia 6.7	
		^Guinea 6.5e	Japan 6.1e	
Germany 5.4e		^Ghana 5.0	*Nepal 5.5	Cuba 5.1e
Denmark 4.8				
Netherlands 4.3e				Jamaica 3.4
Italy 4.2e		Ivory Coast 4.0		Mexico 3.0
Belgium 3.6e		°Nigeria 2.7		*Brazil 2.7e
Ireland 3.0e	°Somalia 2.5e			Costa Rica 1.4
Ukraine 2.5e	Kazakhstan 1.9e			*Panama 0.0
	Uzbekistan 1.8e			
*^°: 0/16	2/4	6/11	3/5	6/14
n=20	n=20	n=20	n=20	n=20 (100)

Sources: US Arms Control and Disarmament Agency (ACDA), *World Military Expenditures and Arms Transfer* (WMEAT) 1995 for 1993 data, page 34; Δ=NY Times (9/94) for Haiti, before return of Aristide.
Notes: *^° = designations of CGSS militarized polity states.   e = extrapolated from ACDA, WME

rized page of the CGSS are 81 percent (13 of 16) and 60 percent (9 of 15), respectively.

Thus, it seems, as might be expected, that the role of the armed forces in militarized political systems not only influences the shape of these states' politics, but also redounds to the particular benefit of the military as an institution in these societies, a matter which can be a self-perpetuating phenomenon. As a consequence, some of these states seem destined to remain on page 2 of the Comparative Government Spread Sheet for a long time.

5e FORMAT AND DISPLAY OF DATA BANK EXCERPTS

The *Format* for 5abcd—Force and Violence Data Bank, presented with the *Excerpts* at the end of this section, follows the main divisions of this chapter which have shown how (a) the historical experience of war, (b) the presence of current violent domestic conflict, (c) the legacy of coups d'état and other regimes of violent origin, and (d) contemporary militarism, help to provide the justification for the placement of half of the 100 countries in the Comparative Government Spread Sheet on its second page of militarized polities.

By way of example of how some of these data might be used in Chapter 6 (Militarized Political Systems), analyses of force and violence in 5 states— representing each of the four zones with states on page 2 of the CGSS and drawn from countries experiencing progressively more extreme examples of current conflict (i.e., the rising categories of Table 5b)—are in the *Excerpts* from the Data Bank associated with this research and displayed in accordance with the *Format*. The states selected for presentation include the Philippine Islands (LAT), Nicaragua (WAN), Egypt (NSG), Turkey (CVW), and Liberia (CVW).

Before discussing these country choices, it should be mentioned once again that the placements in Table 5b are among the most fluid in any of the main categories of analysis in this work, a factor that will be clear if reference is made to some of the *Excerpts*. For example, turmoil in the Philippines has been on the downswing since the authoritarian President Marcos was succeeded in 1986 by the more accommodating Aquino and Ramos regimes; but the various Communist and Muslim rebels still occasionally engage in forays of violence against the government. The U.S.-inspired war in Nicaragua (November 1981 through February 1988) has been officially over since the 1990 election there, but remnants of the Contra and Sandinista forces retain military muscle in their respective geographic and political sanctuaries. The Islamic Fundamentalists in Egypt are often compared to those in Algeria, but in Egypt they control no territory and the deaths are less than 800 in three years, so their activity is designated an insurgency. The civil wars cited are in 2 countries with particular ties to the United States: Turkey, which uses NATO military aid and bases to prosecute the war against its Kurds; and Liberia, which has been in turmoil since the 1980 overthrow of its elite class of descendants of American slaves, who founded the country in 1848.

Format for 5abcd Force and Violence Data Bank

a. war: historical experience (from Table 5a and substantiating Data Bank)

b. conflict, current (violent, domestic). Vary Format to include:
  for LAT: links to 5a periodic* war dates; 5b rebel groups now becoming polit. parties.
  for WAN: schedule from ceasefire to final accord dates; 5b groups becoming parties.
  for NSG and CVW: for *each* group (1, 2, 3...) list as much of a,b,c as is available.

  LAT,WAN,NSG,or CVW (**%** = amount of rebel control [indicate locale using
  geographic abbreviations: n.e., s.w., cent., etc.; ~0% for NSG]), size of govt. forces (&
  military expenditure effort, if known), w/ relevant dates, total deaths, etc. (if not in 5a);
  vs. for *each* group (1, 2, 3...) list:

  a) name of group & its leader(s); founding date (&/or date starting war); information on
  origins, including: if faction of earlier group, its ideology (includes *ethnicity*);
  b) estimated armed strength & support, both local (using geog. abbrevs.; % land
  and/or % population there; ties to legal parties), and foreign (see ideology, line a).
  c) deaths and other war progress information (e.g., refugees, details of major battles,
  etc.) related to *this* group.

c. coup d'etat (or other violent-origin regime) measures (from Table 5c).

d. contemporary militarism (from Table 5d); + any other measures from ACDA, SIPRI,
  etc., especially as compared with other states in same zone; other relevant political
  history.

Excerpts from Force and Violence Data Bank

Philippine Islands - LAT ('89,'92)

a. 6 wars (incl. 3 mainly periodic), 36 years; 162.0 war experience

Phil. 1st indep. (pro-US) Govt. v. "communist" Huks, 1945-54*, esp.	1950-52	9,000 dead
Philippines vs. Moros (Muslims), 1972-89*, especially	1972-76	45-60,000 d.
Philippines vs. communist Natl. Peoples Army, 1969-92*, especially	1969-86	30-40,000 d.

b. **LAT** ('88,'92) - ~100,000-man army vs. communist NPA since 1969, vs. Moro (Muslims) since 1972.
  Both movements dwindling after amnesties, co-options (and captures) since 2/86ff democratic era of
  presidents Aquino and Ramos; **vs.**

1.a) New Peoples Army, of (Maoist) Communist Party, founded 1969; among leaders: A. Zumel; S.
  Occampo; R.Salas, captured '86; R. Baylosis, captured '86, escaped s '88; J. M. Sison, released by
  Aquino in '86, in exile in '94.
  b) estimated armed strength approximately 10,000 (4/94, *Economist*), down from high of 25,000,
  +10,000 in home militias and in control of 7000/42,000 villages (16%), before 1986 government change.
  c) Xmas '93 "truce" declared by seldom-active NPA; 3/94 amnesty offer lures in leader L. Mabilangan.

2.a) *Muslims* on southern islands (~13 provinces, esp. on Mindinao, Sulu and Palawan) in various groups,
  1972ff, including: MNLF=Moro National Liberation Front & Bangsa Moro Army (n=15,000 at height, aid
  from Libya); Ldr. Nur Misuari (in exile in Libya); active from 1972 to '76 ceasefire, autonomy promise; 1989
  constitution estabs. Auton.Region for Muslim Mindinao, accepted by 4 (of 13) provinces. Occasional
  eruptions since (during 1989 constitut.referendum, 1993 elections); 1/94 latest ceasefire agreement.
    Other groups: Moro Islamic Liberation Front (leader H. Salama); armies of Sultan M. ali Damaporo
  (1990), Abu Sayyaf terrorists (1994).
  c. Regimes of violent origin: n=1, 14 years (Marcos, 1972-86; constitutional coup).
  d. Army of107,000, military expenditures of $1.2 billion, 11.6% of CGE are all in bottom half of Asian zone
  (12th, 13th, and 14th of 20 states, resp'y; ACDA, WMEAT 1995 for 1993 data) since wars became latent.

Nicaragua - WAN (5%; 2/90)

a. 2 wars, 9 years; 18.0 war experience.

Sandinista Natl.Lib.Front Revolution vs. Somoza dictatorship	1977-79	35,000 dead
Sandinista Govt. vs. US CIA + counterrevolutionary "contras"	11/81-2/88	30,000 dead

b. 2/88 ceasefire (after US Congress cut-off of contra aid) led to **2/90** elections which resulted in 4/90 cf + demobilization accord; **WAN** because still 30,000 arms unaccounted for (1994) and essentially "power-sharing" between two armed groups:

1. contras - major force in Unified Nic. Opposition which won (temporarily) a majority in assy. in 2/90, and backed winning independent Pres. candidate Violeta Chamorro. Once had 16,000 armed, paid by US CIA/Oliver North; after demobe, given 770 sq.mi. in s.e. **(5%)**. "Re-contras", n=~1000 under Cmdr. Indomable (J.A.Moran Flores), until his exile; renewed fighting (n=800 dead), 1991-93; esp. in Sumer1993, when Northern Command 3-80, n=350, in n.w. El Zungano prov. under El Chacal (J.A.Talevera) kidnapped 37 SNLFs, incl. 2 MPs.

2. Sandinista Natl.Lib.Front - 1979-90 govt. allowed to retain control (for a while) of police under R. Vivas (til 8/92), Army Intelligence under Col. Lenin Cerna (til 9/93), and Defense Ministry under Gen. Humberto Ortega, brother of SNLF leader Daniel (til 2/95), with Army's size cut from ~65,000 to ~15,000. Encouraged by unrepentant SNLF founder T. Borge & director V.Tinoco, some dismissed Sandinista soldiers re-start: under Pedrito the Honduran; & in National Dignity Command which kidnapped VP Godoy & Assy.Speaker (ex-contra) A.Cesar, 8/93, thwarting re-contra demand for removal of Def.Min. Humberto Ortega, but not of Intelligence head Cerna who is ousted at this time.

c. Regimes of violent origin: n=3, 45 years (1945-1990). During Somoza family dynasty (1935-79), all three Somozas--the main political powers despite occasional elections of front-men--were assassinated.

d. Army of15,000, military expenditures of $36 million, 7.7% of CGE are all in bottom half of Western Hemisphere zone (15th, 16th, and 11th of 20 states, resp'y; ACDA, WMEAT 1995 for 1993 data) since end of contra war. Army one-fourth, expenditures one-half their 1980's sizes.

Egypt - NSG (0%)

a. 6 wars +1 NSG, 9.5 years; 61.75 war experience.

Egypt (+Jord.,Syr.,Leb.,Iraq) v. Israel Independence	1948	9,000 dead
Egypt v. Israel, UK, France for Suez Canal	1956	3,000 dead
Egypt (+Jord., Syr.) v. Israel (Six Day War)	1967	70,000 dead
Egypt v. Israel "War of Attrition"	1967-70	5,000 dead
Egypt (+Syria) v. Israel ("Yom Kippur/Ramadan War")	1973	16,000 dead
Egypt v. Libya (border)	1977	minimal death
Egypt v. Islamic Fundamentalist Insurgency	2/92ff	700+ dead

b. **NSG** (0 %, esp. in south and in Imbaba suburb of Cairo; with dead: 2/92ff: ≥700 (7/95), esp. Govt. officials, *Coptic Christians,* secular notbles, & tourists w/ 1000+ wounded; damage to $4 bil./yr. tourist industry); 10's of 1000's (of ~425,000) Govt. troops in southern Dairut & Asyut where rebels strong (& 20% of pop. is *Copt*). Losing popularity after 1,000's arrested, ~50 executed in 1993-95; **vs.** Islamic Fundamentalists (n=~40 cells, w/ n=~35 linked to #2), & n=3+ main groups, incl:

1. Muslim Brotherhood - oldest group from 1920s indep. struggle; founded1928, outlawed 1954-87.

2.a) Islamic Group - 1977 break-off fm. too moderate #1, its youth wing. Unclear leader; spiritual guide Sheikh Omar Abdelrahman in self-exile in US, w/ Sudan passport (perhaps obtained with CIA help in return for anti-Soviet Afghan work.) Linked to assass. of Rabbi Kahane in Brooklyn in '91, & bombing of World Trade Center, NYC, 2/93. Chief lawyer: Montasser al-Zayat, Mil.Cmdr. T.Y.Hamman, killed 4/94.

b) n=10,000 full time, incl. 800 Afghan war vets returned in '92 and ~2500 trained in Sudan by Iranian Revolutionary Guards. Broader support than #1 or #3 (with schols, clinics, social work, etc.), esp. after #3 assassinated Pres. Sadat, 9/81, when it in sympathy launched uprising in Asyut (soon crushed with 44 Govt. dead). 6/92: starts campaign to intimdate secular cultural leaders; 10/92ff: targets tourists in Luxor.

3. Islamic Jihad (Holy War Org.) - founded, '81, assassins of Sadat; then penetrated and dismembered by Govt.; re-emerged in '93, (as Vanguards of the New Holy War Conquest). Leader Ayman al-Zawarhi, MD, trained in Afghanistan by Iran; more violent, secretive than #2 (paramilitaries, infiltrators of army). Also follow Sheikh Omer Abdelrahman, tried for "encouraging" Sadat assassination, but acquitted. Suspected in assassination attempt on Mubarak in Ethiopia in 7/95.

c. Regimes of violent origin: n=1.5, 18 years. 7/52-9/70 - Gen. Naguib & ('54ff.) Col. Nasser - 18 years

d. Army of 424,000 is 3rd largest in Islamic zone, a function of large population; $1.670 billion military expenditures (7th in zone), equal to ~10.5% Central Govt. Expenditures (13th), are somewhat less due to country's relative poverty.

Turkey - CVW (30%)

a. 2 wars +1 NSG; 14 years; 35.0 war experience

Turkey + N.Cyprus (secession/partition) v. Cyprus	1974	5000 dead
Turkey left v. right "terrorism"(NSG) before mil. coup	1976-80	6000 d.
Turkey v. Kurds, periodic since 1920s, but esp.	1984ff	17,000+ dead

b. **CVW (30%**, esp. in south east provinces: 1 in '84, 14 in '92, 24 in '94); 220,-300,000 Govt. troops & local militias under St.ofEmerg. Governor Unal Erken, in 1994 offensives; $8 bill. effort since 8/84 **vs.**

  1.a) PKK=Kurdish Workers (Labor) Party-Leader, since 1978: Abdullah (Apo) Ocalan in Syria (Damascus HQ + Bakaa Valley). Marxist; founded in 1974 by Nemesi Kilu. Movement of 6 mil. Kurds in south east claims support of most of 12.7 mil. Kurds in Turkey (pop.61 mil.) of wh. 3m. in Instanbul slums, incl. many of 2m. refugees from war in southeast..

  Fm. 4a: 22-26 mil.Kurds in 5 states fm. old Persian & Ottoman empires where they had autonomy: Turkey=53%, ~13 mil.; Iran=23%, ~5 mil.; Iraq=18%, 4 mil.; Syria=4%, 1 mil.; & Armenia .2m. About 6 major insurgs. in 76 yrs. since 1919 League promise of homeland broken after 1920's discovery of oil in Kirkut (UK Iraq). Only Turkey's want a separate state; Iraq's two (Ldrs: Talabani of PUK, Barzani of KDP) would settle for "real autonomy"; Iran's (Ldr. Qassemlou, assass. by Govt.,7/89) for "social justice".

  b) n=15,000 (NYT,Econ.'94) + 1500 in Iraq, 1500 in Iran, 1000 in Syrian HQ; support/sanctuary of Syria (refugees), Iran (since '92), & Iraq (Saddam, but not rightist Iraqi Kurds, n=6000; see Iraq 5b). (+ See legal (Kurdish) Peoples Labor Party , often running on Soc.Dem.Peop.P. slate, in 6a Data Bank.)

  c)Toll: 16,-18,000 dead, 8/84 to 7/95, incl. 3000 in '94. 1500 villages demolished, incl. 800 since 1990. Point: getting more intense, especially since military given freer hand in 1993.

  2. Other groups: Armenians (ASALA); leftists (TWPLA,Rev.Left,etc.); Islamic Fundumentalists (Hezbollah, Islamic Action,etc.) - all latent for several years as of 1995.

c. Regimes of violent origin: n =3, 11 years; 5/60-3/66 - Gen. Cemal Gursel - 6 yrs.; 3/71-2/73 - Gen. Nihat Erim junta - 2 yrs.; 9/80-11/83 - Gen. Kenan Evren - 3 yrs.

d. Armed Forces of 814,000 are largest in Islamic zone, military expenditures of $7.075 billion are 2nd highest. Mil.Exp./CGE of 19.5% is 8th (of 20) in highly-militarized zone.

Liberia - CVW (95%)

a. 2 wars; 6 years; 12.0 war experience

Liberia CVW - I: Sam.Doe v. Chas.Taylor v. Prince Y.Johnson	12/89-11/90	40,000 dead
Liberia CVW - II: ECOWAS v. Taylor NPM, ULIMO, LPC, etc.	4/92ff	110,000+ dead

b. **CVW (95%**, nominal govt. barely controls capital) 4/92ff, with 110,000+ dead; 1-1.25 mil. refugees + .5 - .75 mil. displaced of 2.5 mil. pop.; hence, 60-80% pop. affected; in multisided war, including:

  1. ECOMOG(W.African Econ.Org.'s Military Observer Group), n=10,000 troops, under Gen. A.Mukhtar, fm. ~7 of 16 W.Af. states, esp. Nigeria=40% (v. Iv.Coast, other French-speakers); 11/90 intervntn. (& 1st ceasefire) to stop ex-Govt. S. Doe vs. rebels Prince Yormic Johnson (killer of Doe, 9/90; fdr.of brief IFOL faction of NPF) vs. Chas. Taylor. 11/90-3/94 ECOMOG + Govt.of Amos Sawyer controlled capital; after 1993 with a restructured Armed Forces of Liberia which soon broke away as...

  1a. AFL, ldrs. Gens. H.Bowen & M.Wright,w/ own agenda; ex-Doe Bassa-Krahns, trained in S.Leone.

  2. NPF=Chas. Taylor's Natl. Patriotic Front, fd. 12/89, w/ few 100. Ex-Doe Cab. Min. overthrew Doe in 1st war. De facto Govt., 11/90-4/92. But by 3/93, n=10,000, its once 95% land control down to 70% & HQ moved fm. Gbarnga (n.c., near Guinea) to Zwedru (n.e. near Iv.Coast whence supplies (which also come from Burkina Faso & Libya). *Americo-Liberian* leader of *Gio* and *Mano* tribesmen.

  2a. IFOL=Indep.Frt.o'Lib. faction of NPF, n=500, 7/90-10/92 under Pr. Johnson before exile to Nigeria.

  3. ULM=Ulimo=United Liberia Movement - fd.'92; SG Jos. Taybior, Gen.Alhaji Kromah; ex-Doe *Krahns*(animists) + minority *Mandigos* (Muslims), in n.w. Lofa Cty. near S.Leone, fighting Taylor's NPF. Libyan support; training in Guinea. HQ:Tubmanburg, n. of capital. 5/94 Muslims exile to S.Leone.

  3a. ULIMO-II, 1994 faction under mil.Cmdr. Roosevelt Johnson (*Krahn* vs. ULM ties to Islamic Fundmtlsts.).

  4. Liber.Peace Council - Fall'93 group fighting NPF in e.coast Gr.Bassa & Sinoe Counties, cutting NPF link to Iv. Coast; ldrs.G.Boley fm. US, ex-Doe Cab.Min, *Krahn*, and T. Woewiyu. Won't sign 9/94 ceasefire.

8/19/95: agreement to share power in Natl.State Council (of warlords) under Chm. Wilton Sankawulo and including Vice Chm. Taylor of NPF, Kromah (ULM), and Boley (LPC), among others. 12th such ceasefire in war, so delay now to 5b(WAN) until more movement toward scheduled 8/96 election.

c. Regimes of Violent Origin: n=2, 14+ years
  4/80-9/90 - M/Sgt. Samuel K. Doe - 10 yrs.; 9/90ff - ECOWAS + Amos Sawyer, et al. - 4+ yrs.

d. Military statistics from ACDA, SIPRI, etc. not meaningful, because country has devolved into anarchy since collapse of ECOMOG/Sawyer govt. in 1994 and time of data collection.

REFERENCES

Andreski, S. (1992) *Wars, Revolutions, and Dictatorships: Studies of Historical and Contemporary Problems from a Comparative Viewpoint.* Portland, OR: Frank Cass.

Brogan, P. (1990) *The Fighting Never Stopped: A Comprehensive Guide to World Conflict since 1945.* New York: Vintage Books.

Carter Center (1992) *State of World Conflict Report 1991/1992.* Atlanta: The Carter Center of Emory University, International Negotiation Network.

Center for Defense Information (1986, 1992). *A World at War.* Washington, DC: Center for Defense Information.

Chaliand, G. (1991) *Revolution in the Third World: Currents and Conflicts in Asia, Africa, and Latin America.* New York: Penguin.

Cioffi-Revilla, C. (1989) *The Scientific Measurement of International Conflict: Handbook of Data Sets on Crises and Wars, 1495–1988 A.D.* Boulder, CO: Lynne Rienner.

Clutterbuck, R. (1993) *International Crisis and Conflict.* New York: St. Martin's Press.

David, S. R. (1986) *Third World Coups d'État and International Security.* Baltimore: Johns Hopkins University Press.

Dunn, J. (1989) *Modern Revolutions: An Introduction to the Analysis of a Political Phenomenon.* Cambridge: Cambridge University Press.

Eckhardt, W. and E. Azar (1979) "Major World Conflicts and Interventions, 1945–1975," *International Interactions* 5(1): 75–110.

Eckstein, H. F. (1965). "On the Etiology of Internal Wars," *History and Theory,* 4: 133–163.

Eisenstadt, S. N. (1978) *Revolution and the Transformation of Societies: A Comparative Study of Civilizations.* New York: Free Press.

Enzensberger, H. M. (1994) *Civil Wars: From L. A. To Bosnia.* New York: The New Press.

Farceau, B. W. (1994) *The Coup: Tactics in the Seizure of Power.* Westport, CT: Greenwood Press.

Goldstone, J. A. (1994) *Revolutions: Theoretical, Comparative, and Historical Studies.* Fort Worth, TX: Harcourt Brace.

Gurr, T. R. (1993) *Minorities at Risk: A Global View of Ethnopolitical Conflicts.* Washington, DC: U.S. Institute of Peace Press.

International Institute of Strategic Studies (IISS) (annual) *Military Balance.* London: International Institute of Strategic Studies.

Jackman, R. W. (1978) "The Predictability of Coups: A Model with African Data," *American Political Science Review,* 72(4): 1262–1275.

Kende, I. (1978) "Local Wars 1945–1976," *Journal of Peace Research,* 15(3): 250–268.

Laffin, J. (annual) *The World in Conflict War Annual.* London: Brassey's Books.

Licklider, R. (ed.) (1993) *Stopping the Killing: How Civil Wars End.* New York: New York University Press.

Midlarsky, M. I. (1986) *The Disintegration of Political Systems: War and Revolution in Comparative Perspective.* Columbia: University of South Carolina Press.

Mueller, J. (1989) *Retreat from Doomsday: The Obsolecence of Major War.* New York: Basic Books.

Odom, W. E. (1992) *On Internal War: American and Soviet Approaches to Third World Clients and Insurgents.* Durham, NC: Duke University Press.

Schutz, B. M. and R. O. Slater (1990) *Revolution and Political Change in the Third World.* Boulder, CO: Lynne Rienner.

Sederberg, P. C. (1994) *Fires Within: Political Violence and Revolutionary Change.* New York: HarperCollins.

Sivard, R. D. (annual) *World Military and Social Expenditures.* Leesburg, VA: World Priorities.

Skocpol, T. (1994) *Social Revolutions in the Modern World.* New York: Cambridge University Press.

Small, M. and J. D. Singer (1982) *Resort to Arms: International and Civil Wars, 1816–1980.* Beverly Hills, CA: Sage.

Stockholm International Peace Research Institute (SIPRI) (annual) *SIPRI Yearbook: World Armaments & Disarmament.* Stockholm: SIPRI.

Sullivan, M. J., III (1991) *Measuring Global Values: The Ranking of 162 Countries.* Westport, CT: Greenwood Press.

——— (1994) "Ethnicity and War in the Post–Cold War Era," Paper presented at the annual convention of the International Studies Association, Washington, DC.

Thayer, C. (1990) *War by Other Means: National Liberation and Revolution.* New York: Unwin Hyman.

Tillema, H. K. (1991) *International Armed Conflict since 1945: A Bibliographic Handbook of Wars and Military Interventions.* Boulder, CO: Westview Press.

U.S. Arms Control and Disarmament Agency (ACDA) (1995) *World Military Expenditures and Arms Transfers, 1993–1994.* Washington, DC: U.S. Government Printing Office.

Wickham-Crowley, T. P. (1992) *Guerrillas and Revolution in Latin America: A Comparative Study of Insurgents and Regimes since 1956.* Princeton, NJ: Princeton University Press.

Wolpin, M. D. (1981) *Militarism and Social Revolution in the Third World.* Totowa, NJ: Allanheld, Osmun.

6

Militarized Political Systems

Having completed the analysis of culture, ethnicity, force, and violence, it is now time to return to polity types and to focus on the remaining 50 countries in the world from the second page of the Comparative Government Spread Sheet. All these states have a signficant militarized component, in comparison to the 50 civilian political systems studied in Chapter 3. Geographically, the focus of analysis moves from Europe to the developing world, especially the Islamic zone, 15 of whose 20 states are represented (Deegan, 1994), and Africa, Asia, and Latin America, where more than half of all states are covered (Diamond, Linz, and Lipset, 1987; Welch, 1987).

Militarized polities are characterized by a high degree of military influence over the political system, to the point where civilian political institutions are of lesser importance than they were in the CGSS, page 1 (Caspar, 1995; Clapham and Philip, 1984; Thomas, 1985; Perlmutter, 1981; Wendt and Barnett, 1993). This situation exists in countries where there has been a history of warfare, particularly civil war (see Chapters 5a and 5b), and in states where there is a tradition of military coup rule (see 5c). Even if such phenomena are not present today, the lingering manifestations of this legacy are often still found in such measures of contemporary militarism (see 5d) as high levels of "defense" spending and large numbers of significant political actors from the military establishment.

Because the key leaders in such countries are often military (or retired military) officers, there are generally links between the military and the police, and states of emergency or martial law are frequently invoked by the government when it is challenged by political opponents. In such an environment, it is not unusual for such opposition similarly to take a militant form, providing a plausible justification for the government's resort to force.

Governments which are characterized by such activity generally rewrite the rules for political participation (i.e., their countries' constitutions) in ways which legitimate (retroactively) their policies (Binnendijk, 1987; Goldman, 1990; Maniruzzaman, 1987). This process usually follows a predictable pattern involving several elements which are summarized in **Table 6abcd**.

First, some evidence of public electoral approval is sought, even if this is only a plebiscite on a constitution which justifies the coup regime itself (including a referendum on its leader as "head of state or government"). Under conditions of martial law, it is fairly easy to compel a significant percentage of the population to turn out for such an exercise and give such consent. It is not even necessary to have a political party as a vehicle to execute this initial legitimation, for no organized opposition political forces are allowed to take part. Even regimes in the midst of civil wars or the recent products of a military coup (polity types 6d) can take these minimal steps of institution-building.

The longer such a regime stays in office, however, the more it becomes necessary for it to start acting politically and building a base of support. This usually takes the form of giving "the people" (more precisely, those centers of societal power and interest groups favored by the regime) representation in an elected popular assembly. Oftentimes, only "independent" candidacies are permitted, because these are more susceptible to intimidation than political parties. If the regime is serious about prolonging its rule, however, it is at this point that a party composed of its supporters must be built. With such machinery, the regime can then seek additional mandates for its presence and its policies. A form of referendum on a single list of candidates is the easiest type of electoral exercise to control. A government engaged in such activities could thus be in CGSS political system 6d or 6c.

When the regime has a bit more confidence in its support and in its party structure, it can tolerate opposition candidates (though not any significant party organization mobilized behind them), or a choice of candidates, all of whom are members of (or approved by) the ruling party (still polity type 6c). It usually takes some time before the regime's civilian political institutions have matured to the point where other parties organized in support of opposition candidates are permitted—and this only at the representative-assembly

Table 6abcd
Institution-Building in Militarized Regimes

	Polity Type
0 - None of the following.	
1 - plebescite on constitution including referendum on existing Head of State/Govt.	6d=mil°
2 - election for a representative assembly; could be with:	
a. no parties (i.e., "independent" candidates only); b. one party (the govt.'s) & its single list	6cd
c. one party with choice of party-member candidates or party-approved candidates	6c=mil^
d. more than one party allowed, but win no seats	6bc
3 - other parties allowed and actually win some seats in assembly,	
but system still structured so they have little chance to rule.	6b=*1pd
4 - other parties allowed to run cands. for executive office, sometimes even win;	
but legacy of military rule is such that govt. yields armed forces significant autonomy.	6a=*mpr

level and seldom to contest the executive leadership itself—similar to Chapter 3's one-party dominant systems, but with a heavy military overlay (CGSS categories 6c or 6b, depending on the level of military influence).

Finally, the military might recede from overt political participation. Other parties are allowed to run candidates for executive offices and even win some of them. But the legacy of military rule is pervasive to the point that the elected government (type 6a) still must yield to the military considerable autonomy over its own institutions (e.g., control over its own budget and the selection of the heads of the armed services and sometimes even of the Defense Minister).

These steps can be varied in their particulars (Danopoulas, 1987; Pion-Berlin, 1990; O'Donnell, Schmitter, and Whitehead, 1986), as the discussion and Data Bank *Excerpts* of examples of military regimes in sections a, b, c, and d of this chapter will show. In general, however, the process can be summarized according to the four steps presented in **Table 6abcd**. Further details concerning the characteristics of the respective political systems can be found in the *Format* for 6abcd—Militarized Polity Data Banks for each of the four polity types, especially as they might vary (see phrases in italics) from the *General Format* for all four militarized polities. As one moves down the list of *Formats*, the salience of civilian political institutions (elections, parties, representative assemblies, etc.) becomes less, and the presence of elements of militarism (wars, coups, etc.) becomes greater. (As in Chapter 3, states will be chosen from zones and polities as surrogates for others in these categories, and the *Format* subheadings are explicitly denoted in the *Excerpts* for the more restrictive polity types.)

Reversing the order of coverage so that the military regimes with the greatest political sophistication (which are furthest along in the process of institution-building) are analyzed first would yield the order for the sections of this chapter for the first four of the militarized polity types: *mpr, *1pd, mil^, and mil°.

6ab MILITARIZED PARTY SYSTEMS (MILP*)

The *militarized party* category represents a transitional classification between the civilian and military parts of the Comparative Government Spread Sheet. In theory, the MILP* could be divided into two types—*mpr and *1pdom, corresponding to the two prototypes of Chapter 3—depending on the number of significant political parties active in the system. At the present time, however, there are no *1pdoms and 20 *mprs. These are reproduced from the CGSS at the top of **Table 6ab**.

6a Militarized Multiparty Republics (*mpr)

In *militarized multiparty republics*, there is multiparty civilian political activity, but it is deemed not as significant in determining governmental power sharing as in the 50 civilian-party states. Here, either the shadow of civil war looms over the political system, or for some other reason the military, instead

Format for 6abcd Militarized Polity Data Banks

General Format (to vary from *mpr to *1pd to mil^ to mil°)
State - polity type
i. data on any elections to executive branch   and/or   ii. to representative assembly
iii. information on political institution building, especially party structure
iv. why state placed here and not higher or lower in CGSS, using Chapter 5abcd
   militarism data, and Political Histories.

Format for 6a - *mpr Data Bank
State-*mpr + note if PRES., PARL., or MIXED; and electoral type
i. most recent election data on party distributions (seats in assy., % vote for presidential candidates, etc.).
   See 3a format (noting *'s for governing parties not needed in many weak assys. [v. strong. pres.]) plus...
ii. why ***mpr** and not mpr, using 5abcd militarism data (v. *mprs* in this region/zone), and Political Histories;
   especially lingering effects of past wars (5a) ,or coups (5c), or latent paramilitary party groups (5b).

Format for 6b - *1pdom Data Bank
State-*1pd - i. recent election data, esp. on assy. seats held by, & restrictions upon, *non-dominant* parties
iii. name of, and other information on, *dominant* party (date estab., name SecGen, ideology, etc.)
iii. why ***1pd** and not 1pdom (higher) or mil^ (lower), using 5abcd militarism data (v. *1pps* in this region/zone)
   and Political Histories, especially past wars, coups, or latent paramilitary groups.

Format for 6c - mil^ Data Bank
State-mil^ - i. information on executive branch referendum/legitimation, if any.
ii. information on representative assembly, including date and degree of choice in elections.
iii. info. on party strength, including time between *coup* & party(s) legalization.   Note any *transition schedules* to civilian rule, (mp)elections, etc.
iv. why **mil^** and not 1p civilian or *1pd (higher) or mil° (lower), using 5abcd data (v. comparable states in this
   region/zone), and Political Histories, esp. any paramilitary party groups, deaths in political violence, etc.

Format for 6d - mil° Data Bank
State- mil° - i. executive branch referendum/legitimation, if any.
ii. information on representative, or constituent, assembly (if any), especially election restrictions
iii. "lack of" party information; starting date of most recent on-going *coup or civil war*
iv. other military history information from 5abcd data banks, esp. 5b current conflict data, including: govt. &
   opposition armed strength, % of land held, deaths in political violence, etc.

---

of being the ultimate guarantor of national institutions, is a proximate arbiter of who rules. More to the point for this study's focus on the significance of political parties in defining political systems, the parties which exist in most *mpr states are generally less vibrant than those found in the mpr polities. They are also more numerous and younger, two factors which account for their weakness.

The 20 *mprs can be analyzed with respect to the political institutions mentioned in Chapters 2 and 3 (viz., the way in which their chief executive is chosen, the strength of their representative assemblies, and the number of parties sharing power in government coalitions). According to **Table 6ab**, thirteen chief executives are directly elected in strong presidential systems,

Table 6ab
Militarized Party Systems (MILP*)

Islamic Zone	Africa	Asia	West.Hemisph.

6ab. MILP*= Militarized Party Systems = *s: (n=2 0: 20+0)

Islamic Zone	Africa	Asia	West.Hemisph.
Turkey		India,Pakistan	Argentina,Brazil
		Bangladesh	Chile,Bolivia
	Madagascar	Nepal,Sri Lanka	Colombia
Israel		Thailand	Guatemala
		S.Korea	Nicaragua
		Philippine I.	Panama,El.Sal.
Sbtot. 2	1	8	9 (20)

Political Institutions in 20 *mprs, 12/95

Parties in Government

parl. multiparty coalition govts., n=6

Israel 6/92	India 6/91,Pakistan 10/93
Turkey 6/93	Thailand 7/95,Nepal 11/94

parl. simple majority rule, n=1
Bangladesh 3/91

presidential system, n=13

Madagascar 2/93	S.Korea 2/93	Arg.5/95,Braz.12/94, Chile 12/93
	Phil. Is. 5/92	Colombia 6/94, ΔBolivia 8/93
	Sri Lanka 5/93	Guatemala 6/93, El Salv.3/94
		Panama 5/94, Nicaragua 4/90

Parties in Representative Assemblies

Number (& Abbrev.Names) of *Main* Political Parties	% of Assy. Seats Held by Main Parties	Total # of Parties w/ Seats in Assy.
Brazil -8+ (DSP,PFL,PMD,NR,SDP,DLP,LP,WP)	Madagascar - ?137/137=100%	India 23
Thailand - 6+ (JUP, NP,DP,SAP,MF,AP)	Nicaragua 90/92=97.8%	Argentina 22
Philippines - 4+ (NPC,LP,LDP,NUCD)	El Salvador 82/84=97.6%	Brazil 19
Chile - 4+ (IDU, NRP,CDP,PFD)	Thailand 338/360=93.8%	Bangladesh 19
India - 4+ (CP,BJP,JD,LF)	S.Korea 279/299=93.3%	Nicaragua 17
Colombia - 4+ (LP,SCP,NSM,M-19)	Panama 61/67=91.0%	Israel 15
Guatemala - 4+ (UCN,MAS,PDC,PAN)	Turkey 402/450=89.3%	Thailand 10+
El Salvador - 4+ (ARENA,PDC,PCN,CD)	Sri Lanka 199/225=88.4%	Chile 10+
Turkey - 4+ (TPP,MP,SDP,IWP)	Nepal 179/205=87.3%	Pakistan 10+
Panama - 4+ (PRD,MOLINERA,CDP,PA)	Brazil 438/498=86.9%	Guatemala 8+
Bolivia - 3+ (ADN,MNR,MIR)	Guatemala 99/116=85.3%	Panama 8+
S. Korea - 3 (DLP,DP,UNP)	India 453/542=83.6%	Nepal 8
Bangladesh - 2+ (BNP,Awami Lg.)	Chile 100/120=83.3%	Bolivia 7+
Israel - 2+ (Labor, Likud)	Argentine 208/257=80.9%	Colombia 7+
Pakistan - 2+ (PPP,ML)	Philippines 196/201=79.6%	El Salvador 6+
Nepal 2+ (Con.P.,Un.Comm.P.)	Colombia 128/161=79.5%	Sri Lanka 6+
Sri Lanka - 2+ (UNP,SLFP)	Bolivia 122/157=77.0%	Philipines 5+
Argentina - 2+ (JP,RCU)	Pakistan 157/207=75.8%	Turkey 5+
Nicaragua - 2+ (SNLF,UNO)	Bangladesh 227/300=75.6%	S. Korea 3
Madagascar - ≤2 (AF,AREMA)	Israel 76/120=63.3%	Madagascar 2+
Average: 3.4+ main parties, with 86.35% seats		Avg: 10.5+ parties

Notes: Δ = Bolivia presidential only if winner gets >50 percent of votes; otherwise assembly decides.
+ = many parties are coalitions of several parties which may not last beyond one election.

and four of the remaining seven, where the head of government is selected by the assembly, have strong heads of state (the presidents in Turkey and Pakistan, the kings in Thailand and Nepal), making them more akin to mixed than to parliamentary systems. Only Israel, India, and Bangladesh are in the traditional parliamentary mode, but Israel is changing to a directly elected Prime Minister in 1996, and Bangladesh's ruling party campaigned calling for a presidential system. In short, the *mprs have more power tilted toward the executive branch, as compared to their civilian counterparts, where 9 of 13 mprs were clearly parliamentary.

With respect to parties in representative assemblies, **Table 6ab** indicates there is an average of more than ten parties holding seats in each of the *mpr assemblies, with 6 of the 20 states having more than fourteen parties represented. In fact, many of the assembly party numbers are often approximations; when a + is annotated after the number, the party count often includes coalitions of parties which have formed only for a single election. Even the main parties, numbering between four and eight in more than half the states, hold, on average, only 86 percent of the seats in the assemblies. Comparable numbers for the 13 (civilian) mprs in Chapter 3 would show the main parties holding 96.5 percent of seats, and a total of only six parties represented in the assembly on average.

Although their institutional forms are those of the multiparty republic, many of these *mprs resemble the military regimes to follow in the relative weakness of their parties and assemblies. In some *mpr states like Brazil (with eight main parties), and Thailand (with six), parties are often vehicles for the aspirations of individual military officers or other strong personalities, and often do not survive the passing of such personages from the political scene. Despite the recent record of efforts at building (or restoring) civilian political institutions, the legacy of military rule (or war) predominates. The historical record of wars (see 5a) and coups (see 5c) is more important in placing these states here than the evidence of elections, parties, and representative assemblies which, taken alone, might argue for some as having evolved into civilian party states. As compared with Chapter 3's 25 mprs and ~mprs, the 20 *mprs all have either a recent or a long history of military coup rule, war, or both.

Table 6ab.i ranks these 20 states according to their war experience score and their coup regime data from Chapter 5. This record shows that 12 of the 20 states have historically been beset by war (i.e., for fifteen years or more since 1945) and only 3 have never experienced war at all (Brazil, Thailand, and Nepal). Nine of the states appear on Table 5b among the countries considered to be still plagued by current, violent domestic conflict. The present generation of leaders (i.e., those coming of age since 1970) has experienced some form of war in an additional 5 states. The record of military rule (see 5c) is similar. Sixteen of the 20 countries (all except Israel, India, Sri Lanka, and Nepal) have been governed by coup regimes, with more than half of these states having had at least three coups, and more than half of their years since 1945 under juntas. For 16 of these states it is has been less than a gen-

Table 6ab.i
Legacy of Militarism in Militarized Multiparty Republics (*mpr)

5a - war experience score		5c.i-# of coups/freq.ratio		5c.ii-coup regime yrs.	
India	375.25+	Thailand	10.5/.210	Nicaragua	.900
Israel	224+	Guatemala	10/.200	El Salvador	.780
		El Salvador	9/.180	Thailand	.780
Philippines	162	Bolivia	8/.160	Bangladesh	.750
Guatemala	61.25+	Argentina	7.5/.150	Guatemala	.640
Colombia	52+	Brazil	5/.100	Panama	.640
Pakistan	49.5	Panama	5/.100	Madagascar	.600
Argentina	40	Bangladesh	4/.167	S.Korea	.553
Sri Lanka	39+	Madagascar	3.5/.100	Argentina	.540
Turkey	35+	Pakistan	3/.063	Pakistan	.521
El Salvador	26	Turkey	3/.060	Bolivia	.500
Nicaragua	18	Nicaragua	3/.060	Brazil	.460
Bangladesh	15	S.Korea	2/.043	Chile	.320
Bolivia	4	Colombia	2/.040	Philippines	.286
S.Korea	3	Philippines	1/.020	Turkey	.220
Panama	1	Chile	1/.020	Colombia	.080
Madagascar	1				
Chile	1	Israel	0	Israel	0
Brazil	0	India	0	India	0
Thailand	0	Sri Lanka	0	Sri Lanka	0
Nepal	0	Nepal	0	Nepal	0
Avg. (w/o Ind.,Isr.): 28.2		Avg: 3.87		Avg. .429	

Date of Last War (5ab)
Still (see Table 5b), n=9
Sri Lanka - CVW
India-NSG
Guatemala - NSG
Turkey-CVW
Israel-WAN(9/93)
Colombia-NSG
El Salvador-WAN(1/92)
Nicaragua-WAN(2/90)
Philippines-LAT('89/92)
Other, n=8
Panama - 1989
Bangladesh - 1989
Argentina - 1982
Pakistan - 1977
Chile - 1974
S.Korea - 1953
Bolivia - 1952
Madagascar - 1948
Never/Not Applicable, n=3
Nepal
Thailand
Brazil

Date of Last "Coup" Regime (5c)
Panama - 1994 (end of US installed regime)
Guatemala - 1993
Madagascar - 1993
Thailand - 1992
S.Korea - 1992/87
Nepal - 1991 (end of absolute monarchy)
Nicaragua - 1990
Bangladesh - 1990
Chile - 1989
Pakistan - 1988
Philippines - 1986
Brazil - 1985
El Salvador - 1984
Argentina - 1983
Turkey - 1983
Bolivia - 1982

Colombia-1957

Never/Not Applicable, n=3
Sri Lanka
Israel
India

Source: 5abc Data Banks with one-half value for half-war numbers as well as years for Table 5a.

eration since the last period of coup rule. For all this legacy, however, the average number of years at war (28.2) or under military rule (42.9% of the time) is less than that of the countries placing lower on the military page of the CGSS (see section 6cd).

Finally, there is an interesting geographic clustering of *mpr polities. Seventeen of the 20 *mprs are found in Latin America and Asia. Of the 9 Latin American states (Rouquie, 1987; Zagorsky, 1992), 5 are from South America and 4 of them are notable for their history of coup-regime rule (Argentina, Brazil, Chile, and Bolivia); 4 are from Central America, 3 of which have a recent history of violent civil war (Guatemala, El Salvador, and Nicaragua). Of the 8 Asian countries (Baxter, 1985; Bedeski, 1994; Choudhury, 1988; Bungbongkarn, 1988), 5 are from South Asia; 2 of these have considerable experience with domestic insurgencies (India and Sri Lanka), and 2 with military rule (Pakistan and Bangladesh).

The tradition of coup rule also characterizes South Korea, Madagascar, and Panama; whereas domestic insurgency is more the reason for the inclusion of Colombia and Israel in this category. The combination of both civil war and coup rule is present in the history of Turkey and the Philippines (Hale, 1994; Kessler, 1989).

The placement of Israel and India on the militarized page of the CGSS might be controversial: India is often portrayed as the "world's greatest" (i.e., largest in population) democracy, and Israel as the "only democracy in the Middle East." However, since their respective independence dates, they have both been beset by war with significant parts of their populations (Israel with Palestinians, India with Kashmiri Muslims and various northeast tribes (Austin, 1994; Sprinzak and Diamond, 1993).

Thailand and Nepal are interesting as examples of former monarchies which have moved up in CGSS (page 2) placement over time. Thailand's absolute monarchy was abolished in 1932, and the king has had to share power with the military (more than with civilian parties) in the years since—at least 10 coup regimes totalling some thirty-nine years since 1945. Nepal's monarch has been forced to share power with civilian parties only since 1991; the experience with multiparty politics is too short, and the strength of its king as arbiter between the parties is still too strong, to warrant placement of Nepal on the first page of the CGSS.

Data Bank *Excerpts* at the end of subsection 6b include Israel, Pakistan, and South Korea (as examples for India and 7 other Asian states [including west Asia]), and Brazil and El Salvador (from the Latin American zone).

6b Militarized One-Party Dominant Polities (*1pd)

Before leaving the militarized party category, a few words should be said about the possibility of *militarized one-party dominant polities.*

In the ten years during which the CGSS has been maintained in conjunction with this research, at least a half-dozen states have periodically fallen into this category. In the political participation section of *Measuring Global Values* (Sullivan, 1991: 370), Bangladesh, Madagascar, Taiwan, and Indonesia were listed as *1pd. South Africa and Sri Lanka were other possible inclusions. Of the 6 suggested states, 2 (South Africa and Taiwan) appear on CGSS, page 1 as 1pdom in this work; Bangladesh, Sri Lanka, and Madagascar are designated *mpr; and Indonesia as mil^.

South Africa's pre-1991 militarism was designed to maintain its unique apartheid system, which excluded the 85 percent non-white population from the political arena. As far as whites were concerned, the political system was in civilian hands, tightly controlled between 1948 and 1991 under the (one-party) dominance of the Afrikaner National Party. Since 1991, a similar dominant but greatly expanded coalition embracing the two main parties (ANP and ANC) has guided the transition which will continue until 1999. In like manner, the one-party Kuomintang regime in Taiwan was under martial law and allowed no dissent for thirty-eight years after its retreat from control of mainland China in 1949. Since 1988, however, the military has been less in evidence, and civilian opposition has been tolerated within 1pdom limits. Its placement seems more appropriate on the same page (and higher up on that page) of the CGSS as China. (For further explanations of these two states, see Chapter 3d.)

Today, Madagascar, Bangladesh, and Sri Lanka are more robustly multiparty (hence, *mpr) than they have been in the recent past. Madagascar is a classic case of a coup regime which attempted to guide a one-party dominant system between 1975 and 1992. However, when it finally permitted a free electoral choice in 1993 following an all-party national conference, the opposition Active Forces coalition so dominated the results that there is some question as to whether one *1pdom polity has been replaced by another. Today, Madagascar is the weakest of the *mprs in terms of having two fully viable parties. Similarly, in Bangladesh, when the eight-year coup regime of General Ershad ended in 1990 and held its first elections, his one-party vehicle lost to the parties (both also formed around earlier leaders who had come to power through violence) which had existed prior to his rule. In Sri Lanka, the civilian mpr tradition was somewhat strong, but the United National Party ensconced itself in office for seventeen years (1977–1994) by changing the system from parliamentary to presidential, tampering with the electoral cycle, and becoming more militarized as the Tamil insurgency spread. Eventually, however, the other main political party was able to reorganize and regain control of the government.

Finally, Indonesia, despite having a multiplicity of parties, is still under the government of its original coup leader (General Suharto, since 1966) and, in that respect, is more akin to Syria, Iraq, and other moderating military regimes, where the military's dominant party allows other weak parties representation in an assembly (or in the ruling front), but no significant influence over the executive branch of government. It is to such states that this study next turns.

Excerpts from Militarized Multiparty Republics Data Bank

Israel - *mpr: parl.

	Coalition:	GRAND	8p(r)	3p(lc)
n=25+, ~15+ w/ seats;	120/2=61 to *	6/84	11/88	6/92
fl:Hadash=Dem.Frt.f.Peace & Equality (Communists; mainly Arab)		4	4	3^
l: Other Arabs - theoretically could win12 seats, but despite tots. of.....(7)			(6)	(5)
are divided: 40% vote Jewish parties; 25% Fundmtlsts boycott				
Mada=Arab Democratic P. - leader, A.W.Darawsheh		1	1	2^
Progressive (United Arab) List for Peace - ldr., M. Miari		2	1	0
left of Labor partners (='92 Peace Bloc: pro-Palestin. self-determ.)		(12*)	(10)	n.a.
merged in '92 to become Meretz (Democratic Israel). ldr., Sh.Aloni		n.a.	n.a.	12*
l:Ratz (Citizens Rights Mvmt.; ldr.Shulamith Aloni ex-Educ.Min.)		5*	5	n.a.
l:Shinui (=Change; ex-Dem.Ctr.f.Peace; free market; rich; ldr.,Rubinstein)		3*	2	n.a.
l:Mapam (=United Workers; post-Marxist, pro-planning; ldr., Tsaban)		4*	3	n.a.
cl:LABOR Alignment - 150,000 registered mbrs. includes:		38*	39	44*
Yahad (=Labor; Rabin, Peres); Telem (=State Renewal); Dem.Mvmt f.Change				
religious parties - hold balance in assembly with total seats of..............(12*)			(18*)	(17)
Shas(=Sephrdc Torah Guardians,fd.'84; for I.D. cards; ldr., Deri)		4*	6*	6*^in & out
NRP=Natl. Relig. Party (prefers grand coalitions, dir.el.PM)		5*	5*	6
1992 United Torah Judaim (=next 2 +other parties; Ravitz,Verdiger)		n.a.	n.a.	4
Agudat Israel (Brooklyn Hasidics; Rabbi Schneerson; no pork)		2*	5*	n.a.
Degel HaTorah (=Torah Flag; non-Hasidic)		0	2*	n.a.
1984 only: Kach (Kahane; outlawed after '85 law vs. for racial appeals)		1	0	0
Ometz=Courage(1*) Morasha (1), Tami =Mvmt f.Isr.Tradition(1)		3	0	0
cr:LIKUD, incl.:Herut(=FreeCntr.,Shamir),Gahal,Modai Libls,State List		41*	41*	32
ldr., Netanyahu, ex-PM Shamir; dovish Levy defects, 6/95; hawk ldr., Sharon				
rgt-of Likud, non-religious,but for annexation of Occupied Territories: (5*)			(5-7*)	(10)
Tehiya (=Revival/Renaiss.Mvmt; Y.Neeman, ex-Stern mbr.G. Cohen)		4*	3*	0
Tzomet(=Crossroads; pro-el.change; anti-relig.pref.;exArmyChf R.Eitan)		1*	2*in&out	8:3(2*)+5
fr: Moledet (=Homeland; fd.'88, for expulsion of Arabs; Gen Ze'evi)		0	2*	3 :1+2
	TOTAL:	120	120	120
	Governing Coalitions:	108*	64-66*	56*^-62*

1% Prop.Rep. threshold meant sometimes took 10 months to form govt., always coalitions (usually w/ relig. parties). Up to 1.5% in '92 (~40,000/3.4 mil. votes for seat). Direct election of PM in '96 (2 votes: 1 for party list, 1 for PM (needs 50% or else runoff). El.changes passed in '91: 55-32 (no party discipline, free, vote).

Labor ('48-77 ruling party) has both hawks (ex-PM Rabin, Hillel, Bar-Lev) & doves (PM Peres, Pres.Weizman). 1992 (first) open primary leadership results (70% turnout): Rabin 40.6%, Peres 34.5%, Kessar of Histradut Labor Union 19%, MP Namir 6%.

Likud 2/92 ldrship results among C.Cmtee n=2800: Shamir 46.5%, dove Levy 31.2%, hawk Sharon 22.3%.

Religious parties hold the balance; all are firm on religious laws; 3 are flexible on land (most Zionist NRP is not). NRP controlled Chief Rabbinate, from1948 until 1993(loss). Non-Zionist Shas (fd.'84, for Orthodox fm. n. Af. under relig. ldr. Rabbi O. Yosef) has been partner of both Likud & Labor.

^Shas - Interior Minister A. Deri (hard on internal security, dove on peace), indicted for corruption 9/93, had to leave Cab. When party left COalition, 2/95, Labor's 62-58 majority govt. dropped to 61^-59 with 5* Arabs holding the balance for peace accord (hurts legitimacy among Jews, makes progress on 9/93 agreemt. w/ Pal. Authy. more difficult). CO picked up more Jewish support when 2 split from Tzomet, 12/94.

*mpr because of state of war with 19 (of 21) Arab states since '48; (peace with Egypt i 1979; with Jordan in 1994). Six major wars & 7th highest war experience score in world (see 5a Data Bank). Occupied Territory since '67; last local elected-governments there in '76 dismissed in '82. 5b(NSG) Intifada (Uprising) 12/87 to 9/93 peace accord (see 5b[WAN]; ~300 dead since then, through 7/95.)

~17,000 soldiers dead in six wars since '48. Country formed in violence (Haganah, Irgun, Palmach, & Lehi "5b groups") vs. UK in 1946-48. Many ex-military in politics: ex-PM Rabin, Pres. Weizman, ex-Pres Herzog all ex-Generals; as are heads of Tzomet & Molodet, & 10 MPs (out of 95, if Arabs, women, & Orthodox exemptees are removed); also candidates for mayor in 12 cities, 5/93. Most males must perform annual reserve duty into middle age. Point: despite vibrant democracy (especially among 82% Jewish majority population in 1947-67 borders), politics is heavily militarized in near-garrison state. Assassination of PM Rabin shows move to peace with Palestinians may increase militarism and concerns for security.

Excerpts from Militarized Multiparty Republics Data Bank *(continued)*

Pakistan - *mpr: parl.

		Coalition:	2p	2p; Δmin	1pmin.
n=2+ parties	207/2=104 to*		11/88;	10/90; 4/92Δ	10/93
I:Peoples Democ. Alliance (founded, 9/90), incl:			n.a.	50	85*
c-l: PPP=Pakistan Peoples P. (Bhutto)			93*(38%v)		
eth: *Mohajir* Qaumi Mvmt. Urdu-sp.,rich, in Sindh; Idrs: Tariq,Hussain.			14*	14* (-14)Δ	boycott
r-c: IJI=Islamic Dem.Alliance (fd.'88; Idr.,ex-PM Sharif, n =6 incl.:			56	105*(-8Δ)	n.a.
c-r: Pak.Muslim League (Jinnah'47; Zia/Junejo'86ff, Sharif)			in IDA	in IDA	72
r:Jamaat-i-Islami(*Sunni* Funds.; Maulana Dakhwashti), w/ IDA '88-93;			8	(6*) (-6Δ)	9
only party to support Zia in '79; Ldr. Qazi Hussain Ahmed					
Others, n=~40 incl. ethnic parties of *Pathans, Baluchs, Sindhis...*			19	17	41 (36^)
and Jamiat-i-Ulemai-Islami (Idr. Maulana Fazlur Rahman; w/ PPP,'93ff)					
Independents			27	21	0
TOTAL: (w/o 10 non-Muslim appointees)			207	207	207
			*=107	*=125; 97Δ	121*^

ΔMQM pullout of COalition over Sindh trouble, 7/92; 6+8 IDAs pullout in 4/92 for not fast enough Islamic.
Election turnouts dropping:1970 (1st free, leading to creation of Bangladesh)=67%; '77=55%; '85
(independents only)=52%; '88=43%; '90=48%; '93=40%.
Parties: two main strands - secular left under Bhuttos from Sindh; pro-military right from Punjab. Also,
n=dozens of smaller ones fluid in make-up. Gen.Zia's Movement for Return to Democracy ((1985-88) with
his PM Junejo & Chm. Jatoi eventually coopted into IDA and then Muslim League. Both platforms by '90
called for: Islamic society, no corruption, free enterprise.
UH (n=87),less impt., indir. el., 2/90:PPP 5; IDA 23; IDA allies 14; Others (local notables predominant) 45.
Prov. assy. els, 10/93: PPP won in Punjab & Sindh; and its Pres. cand. Farooq Leghari won in LH+UH, 274-
168, after assys. approved constit. amndmt. to limit Pres. powers (vs. excesses of Gen. Zia years ('77-88)).
*mpr bec.: 5c= 3 coups, 25 yrs.total.; avg. mil. govt.=8 yrs., avg. civ. govt. = 2 yrs. PM cannot call State of
Emergency w/o approval of NSC=Pres.,PM,CMs of 4 provs., + service chiefs. Five wars; war-experience
score of 49.5 is 7th in Asian zone. Kashmir territory dispute with India is permanently militarized. Also,
prime sponsor/base for US+Islamic Fundamentalist war vs. SU in Afghan.,1981-89. Since return to
democracy in '88, 3 elections, 5 govts. Violent politics: >1,000 dead in incidents involving parties in 1994.

S. Korea - *mpr: PRES (> assy)

Presidential Elections: (No Run-Offs)	12/87(87%t.o.)	12/92
l-c: PPD/DP=Kim Dae Jung	26.4%	34%
c: NPRD/DLP = Kim Young Sam	27.2%	42%*
c-r:UNP/ UPP(Unit.Peop.P./Unif.Natl.P.)=Chung Ju Young	n.a.	16%
r: DJP=Roh Tae Woo	36.2%*	see DLP
f-r: NDRP (Kim Jon Pil)	8.0%	see DLP
Others	2.2%	8%

Assy. els.: 299/2 = 150 to control Assy.	4/88 Assy (89% t.o.)	4/88 1/90	3/92 Assy(73% t.o.)
l-c: PPD/NDP=P.f.Peace & Dem./NewDem.P.; K.Dae Jung	70 (55el. + 16apptd, 19%v)		99 (74el+25appt)
c: UNP=Unificat. Natl. P. (1/92, Hyundai's C.J. Young)	n.a.		31 (23+8)
c-r: NPRD= New P.o'Reunif.&Dem.; in s.w.: civilian; K.Y.Sam	59 (46 + 13, 24%)	^ *	see DLP
r-c: DLP:Dem.Lib. Party (Roh,Sam,Pil,1/90 merger)	n.a.		149*(110+39)
r:DJP=Dem. Justice P.; military: Pres.Chun, Roh Tae Woo	125 (86+39,34%)	* *	see DLP
f-r:New Dem-Repb.P.; old military: Pres.Park,Kim Jong Pil	35 (27 + 8, 15%)	^ *	see DLP
Others, independents	10 (w/ 8% vote)		20el. (of which 2*)
TOTALS:	299 (224 el.+75 apptd.)		299 (227 el.+ 72 app)

1987 constit. resulted in most democratic,highest turnout, pres.election ever. Assy's new SMD system
favors rural areas; bonus seats ("apptd.", above) give even close party winners a sizable edge in seats.
1/90 merger of DJP, NPRD, & NDRP into one large Dem.Lib.P. giving system look of 1pd (219/299s = 73%
>67% needed to am.constitution). In reply, opp. PPD merged with another (n=5 seats) to form NDP.
3/91-new DLP wins 1st local els. in 30 yrs; 8/91 regionals-DLP wins 564/866 (65%s, 40%v) council seats.
*mpr bec. of history of mil. rule (26/26 yrs. after Syngman Rhee indep. leader installed by US Army, 1948-
60); '87-92 Pres. Roh was member of last (1981-87) junta; '92ff Pres.Kim Young Sam's first PM was ex-
mil. General. Parties tend to form around strong (often military) personalities, not ideas (see Thailand).
K.Y.Sam is first civilian Pres. since Rhee; even he harassing losing candidates. 1980 Kwang Ju massacre
of democracy-demonstrators (n=200 dead) delayed return to civilian rule by 7 years.

Brazil - *mpr, PRES (> assy)

Pres. els., 5 yr. term (runoff if not 50%v.); t.o.: 88%, 82%	11/89 Rd.1,Rd.2,		10/94	
Other left (Communists, Greens, etc.)	10.0%		n.a.	
l: PT=Worker's P.- Lula da Silva	16.8%	47%	27.0%	
l-c: PTD=Dem.Labor P- Brisola	16.2%		3.2%	
c-l:PSDB=Soc. Dem. P.- Covas, Pres.Cardoso	11.4%		54.3%*	
c-r: PRN=Natl.Reconst.P.- Pres.Collor de Mello, Gomes	28.5%	53%*	0.6%	
r-c:PMDB=Dem.Movement P.-Guimares,Quercia	4.0%		4.4%	
Other right (PFL, PDS, PDC, PPR, PRONA, etc.)	13.1%		10.5%	
	100.0%	100%	100.0%	

Assy. els., 4 yr. term, n=503-13/2=252-7 to control assy.	10/90 LH,	UH	10/95 LH,	UH
f-l:PCdB=Communist P. (Friere)	5	0	10	0
l: PT=Workers P. (Lula; fd. '78; unions, RC left)	35	1	49	5
l: PTB=Labor P. (Vargas,Gonzaga; fd. '45)	38	8	31	5
l:PSB=Socialist Party	11	1	15	1
l-c:PDT=Dem.Labor P. (Brisola; fd. '79; older Goulart socs.)	47	5	34	5
c-l:PSDB=Soc.Dem.P.('88 PMDB's for 4-yr Pres.; Pres.Cardoso)	37	10	62	11
c:PP='90 PTR + '90 PST + '94 PRN defectors	4	0	36	6
c:PL=Liberal Party	16	0	13	1
c-r:PRN=Natl.Reconstruction P. ('89 Pres.Collor vehicle)	40	3	1	0
r-c:PMDB=Dem.Mvmt.P. ('80, mil. majors; Neves, Pres.Sarney)	108	22	107	21
r:PFL=Liberal Front P. ('84 ex-mil.spptrs; VP Sarney,Chaves)	82	15	89	19
fr:PPR=PDS+PDC=Dem.Socs.(43 in '90)+Xtn.Dems.(22 in '90)	65	7	52	6
Others (n=~6):	15	4	14	1
	503	76	513	81

*mpr bec. mil rule from 1964-85, and NO sentiment to try military for HR violations, as in Arg.,Chile, etc. In '88 constitut., mil. has right to intervene in natl. affairs (fm. its Natl.Def. Coun.,2c.ii position), controls (a parallel) nuclear policy, space, intelligence, Amazon dvlpmt. (incl. road building), strike breaking, homeless street children-clearing. Military heads of state corps. (shipping, telephone,steel,etc.) Anti-democracy mil. academy curriculum. 25,000 mbr. Military Club=pressure group for pay parity (w/ civilian politicians). Military esp. strong vs. weak parties where loyalty is very fluid (law guarantees incumbents place on party ballots; 1/2 MPs in late '80s had switched parties). Kubitschek, '56-60, only dem.el.civilian to finish term in last 65 years. In 100 yrs. of republican rule, military for 40. Since 1822 independence: 1 king (til 1889), 2 dictators (incl. Vargas,1930-45), 5 deposed presidents, 7 constitutions. Coup attempt as recently as 2/94.

El Salvador - *mpr, PRES (> assy)

Pres. els., 5 yr. term (runoff if not 50%v.)	3/84Rd.1,Rd.2		3/89	3/94 Rd. 1, Rd.2	
l: CD=Ruben Zamora	illegal		illegal	25%	32%
c-r: PDC=Duarte, Chavez Mena	40%	55%*	36.6%	see Others	
r: PCN=Garcia, Moran Castanada	19%		4.2%	see Others	
r: Other right, incl. 2 Protestant Fundmtlsts. in '94	11%		5.4%	26%	
f-r: ARENA= d'Aubuisson,Christiani, Calderon Sol	30%	45%	53.8%*	49%	68%*
TOTALS:	100%	100%	100%	100%	100%

Assy. els., 3 yr. term, n=84/2=43 to control assy.	3/85	3/88	3/91	3/94
l: CD=Democratic Convergence (n=3 Soc.Dem.parties; ex-5b)	illegal	illegal	8 (12.1%v.)	22 (-7^)
c-r: PDC=Christian Dem. Party ('84 Pres. Duarte)	33	23	26(28.0%)	18
r: PCN=Party of Natl. Conciliation (old right)	12	7	9 (9.0%)	4
f-r: ARENA=Natl. Republican Alliance (ex-death squads)	13	30	39 (44.3%)	39
Others	2	0	2	1
TOTALS:	60	84	84	84

^Since '94, 7 moderate CD's under Villalobos have defected.

*mpr due to history of military rule and civil war. 5c composite coup frequency/duration ratio is 2nd highest in Hemisphere (9 coups, totalling 39 years since 1945). Most recent civil war (1979-91, with 75,000 deaths, 90% due to military) polarized politics leading to rise of ARENA party (former sponsor of death squads) from far-right of political spectrum before the war to assembly plurality in 1988, presidency in 1989, and control of 200/262 town councils in '94. Duarte (1984-89) was first civilian president (thanks to US pressure) since 1931. Left parties were excluded from political process until after civil war ended in 1991.

6cd MILITARY REGIMES (MIL°)

In the next two categories of military regimes, the influence of force and violence in politics overwhelms that of political parties or other institutions of government even more blatantly than in the militarized party states. They will be discussed together in an integrated manner, and the *Excerpts* will be deferred to the end of the double section, as in Chapters 3de and 6ab.

In the 14 *moderating military* states (mil^) of subsection 6c, the military is the predominant political actor. Although the ruling junta may have begun to build a political party and allow a direct national election to a representative assembly, the political history of these states, as well as their indicators from categories 5a (war) and 5c (coups), are more persuasive than any party activity in placing these countries here and not higher in the Comparative Government Spread Sheet. In short, the mil^ states' efforts at regime legitimation and power sharing are deemed less convincing than those of the countries covered before this point.

Nevertheless, these polities have proceeded further in institution-building than the 13 *entrenched military* states (mil°) of subsection 6d, where the political process is so broken down that the state is engulfed in civil war, or a military dictatorship is so repressive that it has not yet allowed parties or a representative assembly.

Table 6cd shows that among these 27 mil^ and mil° military regimes, the African and Islamic zones are most in evidence, with 11 and 10 states, respectively, comprising 79 percent of the total (Ayittey, 1992; Mansour, 1992). Coup regimes are more represented in the moderating military category, whereas states beset by civil war are more common among the entrenched military states. However, there is some overlapping of these two factors among the two military regime systems; indeed, a common reason for a coup is that a government is not prosecuting a civil war well (Pinkney, 1990; Kennedy, 1974).

Table 6cd summarizes the data from Chapter 5 relating to the legacy of militarism (i.e., war and military coup experience) for both the mil^ and the mil° polities. Table 6c and Table 6d present evidence of civilian political institutions in these states. The order of subject matter in these tables—first the military legacy, then the political institutions—is the reverse of that in section 6ab, where the political institutions were more significant than the military legacy. When compared with the similar measures in Tables 6ab and 6ab.i, the progressively rising military-legacy indicators and declining civilian-institution measures of the upcoming tables can be clearly seen.

For example, except for India and Israel (whose fifty-year records of regular elections ensure their high CGSS placement), the average number of years of war for the *mpr states was 28.2 (Table 6ab.i), as compared with 58.7 for the mil^, and 47.0 for the mil°. (Data for the 3 ex-Soviet states, independent for only four years, are not comparable and so are not included in the mil°

Table 6cd
Military Regimes (MIL°)

	Islamic Zone	Africa	Asia	West.Hemisph.
		6c. mil^= moderating military (n=14)		
	Iraq	Ghana,Guinea		
	Syria	B.Faso,Zaire		Peru
	Yemen	Ethiopia,Uganda		
	Libya	Mozambique	Indonesia	Haiti
Sbtot.	4	7	1	2 (14)

		6d. mil° = entrenched military (n=13)		
	Georgia,Tajik.Δ	Liberia		Δ=ex-USSR
	AzerbaijanΔ	Nigeria	Cambodia	
	Sudan		Afghanistan	
	Algeria	Rwanda	Myanmar	
	Somalia	Angola		
Sbtot.	6	4	3	(13)

Legacy of Militarism in MIL° regimes

moderating military regimes (mil^), n=14

5a - war score/current 5b status			5c.i-# of coups/freq.ratio		5c.ii-coup years	
Iraq	211.75+	LAT(3/91)	Haiti	9.5/.190	Haiti	1.000
Indonesia	143+	LAT('88)	Syria	8/.160	Syria	.939
Ethiopia	112.25+	NSG	Burkina Faso	6/.171	Zaire	.857
			Peru	6/.120	Burkina Faso	.829
Uganda	75	0 since '85	Uganda	5/.152	Iraq	.740
Yemen	62.5	0 since '94	Ghana	5/.132	Uganda	.727
Peru	54+	NSG	Yemen	4.5/.115	Yemen	.667
Syria	54	0 since '82	Iraq	4.5/.090	Ghana	.632
Mozambique	52+	WAN(8/92)	Ethiopia	4/.080	Indonesia	.617
Libya	33.75	n.a.	Libya	.590		
Zaire	22.5	0 since '78	Zaire	1/.029	Peru	.500
Burkina Faso	1	n.a.	Guinea	1/.027	Ethiopia	.420
Ghana	0	n.a.	Libya	1/.023		
Guinea	0	n.a.	Indonesia	1/.021	Guinea	.297
Haiti	0	n.a.	Mozambique	0	Mozambique	0
Average: 58.7			Average: 4.03		Average: .630	

entrenched military (mil°), n=13

5a -war score/current 5b status			5c.i-# of coups/freq.ratio		5c.ii-coup years	
Angola	99+	WAN(11/94)	Nigeria	7/.200	Algeria	.909
Cambodia	76.5+	WAN(10/91)	Afghanistan	5.5/.110	Rwanda	.788
Sudan	58+	CVW	Sudan	5/.128	Sudan	.769
Somalia	52.5+	LAT(3/94)	Myanmar	4.5/.096	ΔTajikistan	.750
Algeria	52+	CVW	Rwanda	4/.121	Somalia	.742
Myanmar	46.5+	CVW	ΔTajikistan	3/.750	Myanmar	.723
Rwanda	36+	LAT(7/94)	Algeria	3/.091	Nigeria	.714
Afghanistan	34+	CVW	Cambodia	3/.073		
ΔGeorgia	27+	CVW			Cambodia	.512
			Somalia	2/.057	ΔΔAzerbaijan	.500
Liberia	12+	CVW	Liberia	2/.040	Afghanistan	.440
ΔΔAzerbaijan	7+	WAN(6/94)	ΔGeorgia	1/.250	Liberia	.300
ΔTajikistan	3+	WAN(11/94)	ΔΔAzerbaijan	1/.250	ΔGeorgia	.250
Nigeria	3	n.a.	Angola	0	Angola	0
Average w/o Δ: 47.0			Average w/o Δ: 3.15		Avg/ w/oΔ: .590	

Source: 5abc Data Banks, with one-half value for half-war numbers, as well as years for Table 5a.
Note: Δ = ex-Soviet republics.

averages). Regarding coups d'état (see 5c), the duration measure is more significant than the frequency ratio, because while the *mprs have had, on average, as many coups as—or more coups than—the military regimes (3.87 as compared with 4.03 for the mil^ and 3.15 for the mil°), they have generally returned the political process back to civilians more quickly. The *mpr average for duration of coup regime years was 0.429, compared with 0.630 for the mil^ and 0.590 for the mil°.

It might seem surprising that the above data indicate that the moderating mil^ military regimes have higher 5a (war) and 5c (coup) scores than the entrenched mil°s. However, for the latter states the *current* conflict measure (5b) is more significant. Of the 13 mil° states, 6 are in the midst of civil wars, designated CVW under "current 5b status" in **Table 6cd**. Six others have recently completed such hostilities and are indicated by WAN or LAT. On the other hand, of the 14 mil^ polities, only 5 appear among the current 5b measures at all, and 3 of these conflicts are latent or waning, and 2 are at the lower NSG level. Five have had no measurable violent domestic conflict (as this term was defined in Chapter 5) at all, and 3 of the remaining 4 have had no such activity for more than a decade (i.e., since before 1986). Before discussing Tables 6c and 6d, the next two polity types will be analyzed separately.

6c Moderating Military Regimes (mil^)

Table 6c displays the 14 mil^s in order of greatest sophistication of political institutions (i.e., those listed first being closest to inclusion in category 6ab, MILP*). It shows that, despite the presence of some leaders who have monopolized power for a considerable period of time, there are generally elections, representative assemblies, and political parties, with the varying degrees of constriction typically imposed in dominant-party polities.

With respect to parties, recent multiparty electoral experiences have occurred in Peru (1995, 1990, 1985, 1980), Yemen (1993, the first time ever) and Haiti (1991, also the first time without fraud, and 1995). One-party dominant systems prevail in Indonesia, Syria, and Iraq (each of some long standing), and in Burkina Faso, Ghana, Guinea, and Mozambique (of more recent vintage).

Attempts at negotiated power sharing between parties characterize two of the moderating military regimes. The one-party dictatorship in Zaire broke down in 1991–1992; since that time the government has been trying to hang on to power through some grand transitional conference, as occurred in South Africa and some other smaller African states in the 1990s (see Chapter 3d). Some of Ethiopia's civil war–winning allies have shared governing responsibilities since 1991 in an assembly which established a system of ethnic-based autonomous regions; other party representatives of these regions were excluded from the initial power sharing, and then boycotted the first elections for the national assembly in 1995.

Table 6c
Moderating Military Regimes in Order of Institution-Building

State	Leader	Origin	Parties; Presidential and Assembly Election Information
Multiparty Experience (n=3):			
Peru	Fujimori '90/92/95	*mpr el./coup /mil^el.	*mpr history; but, parties & assy. suspended by Pres. in 1992; reinstated for 1993 con.assy., '95 gen. election.
Yemen	Saleh '78/90	coup/ /unification	4/93 mpe; but YSP later secedes; war to reunite ('94); YSP electoral status unclear.
Haiti	Aristide '91/94	mil^ el./coup	1st ever free mpr election in 1/91 followed by coup in 9/91 & US military intervention to restore mpe Pres. in 9/94.
Primarily militarized 1-party dominant (n=7):			
Indonesia	Suharto'66	coup	1pdom GOLKAR for 28 yrs. since 1966/69 assy els. 5x --->indir. Pres. el. 5x ('73,'78,'83,'88,'93)
Syria	Assad '70	coup	1pdom Ba'ath for 24 yrs. since 1970 assy. els. 3x--->Pres. el. 3x ('91,'85,'78) + 2 earlier refs.
Iraq	Saddam '69/79	coup	1pdom Ba'ath for 25 yrs. since 1969 assy els. only in '80,84,'89. 1st Pres. ref. ever in 10/95.
Burkina Faso	Campaore '87	coup	1pdom OPD-MT for 5 yrs. 12/91 Pres. 1 cand., 25% turnout; 5/92 assy. 78/102 seats
Ghana	Rawlings '81	coup	1pdom NDC. 11/92 Pres.el. (58%v); fraud claim----> 12/92 assy.el.boycott
Guinea	Conte '84	coup	1pdom minority (mil.) party win in '93 presidential suspicious; 6/95 assy. elections less important
Mozambique	Chissano '86	colonial war winning party	1pdom FRELIMO SG = Pres. in 1980s 1pdom els., 10/94 multi-party 5b(WAN) election win over RENAMO.
Power-Sharing Conferences (n=2):			
Zaire	Mobuto '65	coup	ex-1pdom (3 Pres. & assy. el. cycles) ended in 1991/92; since, rival national assemblies, uneasy power-sharing.
Ethiopia	Zenawi '91	cvw winner	multiparty 7/91 con. assy. of cvw winners; 5/95 elections for natl. assy. (heavily boycotted) confirms Pres. choice.
No Party (n=2):			
Uganda	Museveni '86	cvw winner	NO party *activity* allowed. Indep. cands. only for '94 con. assy. which opts for 5 more years of no party dem.,6/95.
Libya	Qaddaffi '69	coup	NO parties, after brief experiment with ASU in 1970s, local els. only; indirect assy. elections. NO Pres. ref.

Finally, parties have been effectively outlawed in Uganda (since 1986) and Libya (since 1976), and although each of these states has had elections (Libya only on the local level), only independent candidates have been allowed to run for office, with all the weaknesses vis-à-vis the ruling regime that that practice entails. Uganda cites tribalism and the unhappy, divisive history of ethnic-based politics in that country; the more homogeneous Libya does not even have that excuse, and the system seems to be a way of perpetuating the power of the charismatic leader, Muammar Qaddaffi.

Regarding direct elections, both a president and an assembly have been chosen in Syria (several times), Ghana, Guinea, Burkina Faso, and Mozambique (once each). Iraq's Saddam Hussein had a referendum on his tenure only in October 1995, twenty-six years after coming to power. Only an assembly election—and not even a one-candidate plebiscite for president—has been permitted in Yemen, Uganda, and Indonesia. Libya has elections just for local councils, which then (indirectly) elect the national assembly. The negotiated power-sharing arrangements of Zaire and Ethiopia seem to have precluded elections with the full participation of all significant parties for the time being. In Latin America, it is unclear whether the 1995 multiparty elections for president and assembly should result in a rise in the CGSS-status of Peru (arguable, based on its history) and Haiti (less justifiable, due to its previous record). Not enough time has passed to make a judgment to change CGSS placements at the time of publication of this book.

In summary, then, the 14 mil^s can be divided into the 4 Islamic zone states (Iraq, Syria, Yemen, and Libya) plus Indonesia (also Islamic, though not in the scheme of this work's geography), in which strong men who have ruled for long periods (Suharto since 1966; Qaddaffi, 1969; Saddam, 1969; Assad, 1970; Saleh, 1978) have adapted parties and political institutions to prolong regimes which originally began with violent takeovers (Hinnebusch, 1990; Kedourie, 1993); the 7 African countries, 3 of which are evolving from civil wars (Uganda, since 1986; Ethiopia, 1991; and Mozambique, 1992), and 4 from military coup regimes (Ghana, Guinea, Burkina Faso, and Zaire, in descending order of success in building transitional institutions [DeCalo, 1990]); and the 2 western Hemisphere states (Peru and Haiti) which had multiparty elections which were aborted and which are attempting to rebuild.

Each, in its own limited way, has attempted to replace the rule of blatant force and militarism with some minimal building of civilian governmental institutions, as can be seen in the mil^ Data Bank *Excerpts* at the end of subsection 6d, for Syria and Burkina Faso (surrogates, respectively, for coup-regimes in Iraq, Yemen, and Indonesia; Ghana, Guinea, and Zaire), Mozambique and Haiti (exemplars, respectively, for civil war–recovering Ethiopia and Uganda, and sometimes militarized multiparty Peru). Little such political activity, however constricted, can be seen in the 6d entrenched military regimes for which additional measures and concepts will be introduced next.

6d Entrenched Military Systems (mil°)

In the final category of military regimes, *entrenched military systems*, the political process has so broken down that civilian party activity and political institutions are practically nonexistent. All political space has been taken over by warring armed groups (Weinberg, 1993) or has been completely snuffed out by a military junta.

Referring again to **Table 6cd**, the high war scores and coup ratios of the entrenched military polities can be noted (especially as compared with the *mprs; 47.0 versus 28.2 for war experience, 0.590 versus 0.429 for coup-regime years, respectively). More to the point, few elections, parties, or representative assemblies are present in any of these entrenched military systems, as can be seen in **Table 6d**.

To highlight further the distinctiveness and the lack of institutions of the states in the mil° polity group, two new categories of analysis will be introduced here: the ex-Soviet republic beset by civil war, in which Russia plays a destabilizing role; and the contested, or collapsed, state. With these additional concepts, the 13 entrenched military states can be grouped in descending order of functioning institutions as follows: 5 traditional regimes of violent origin (Algeria and Myanmar, in the *Excerpts* at the end of this section, plus Nigeria, Rwanda, Sudan); 3 ex-Soviet republics enmeshed in civil war and dependent upon the Russian army for survival (Georgia, in the *Excerpts*; plus Azerbaijan and Tajikistan); and 5 contested states (Angola in the *Excerpts*, plus Somalia, Liberia, Afghanistan, and Cambodia).

Among the 5 polities in the first category, Nigeria does not even have the excuse of armed belligerent opposition, and is similar to the juntas in section 6c, except that it has not yet (mid-1996) begun to build any political institutions. The fifty-year civil war against the non-Burman tribal groups is hardly an excuse for Myanmar's military rule; rather, the regime (like Nigeria's) represents a failure of politics among fellow Burmans at the center (see *Excerpt*). In Rwanda, the Patriotic Front routed the forces of the previous Hutu Government to win the civil war in 1994, but it remains to be seen whether the latter regroup to return from exile as an rebel army, or come home to be integrated into a Tutsi-dominated government and society. Finally, the civil wars in Sudan and Algeria were related to the military seizures of power in 1989 and 1992, respectively; but the insurgency in Sudan is not a threat to the power of the state (the rebels want either autonomy or secession of a relatively small part of the country), whereas the war in Algeria could overthrow the government and be revolutionary in import (see *Excerpt*).

In the 3 ex-Soviet republics, Russia uses the presence of the former Red Army and membership in the new Commonwealth of Independent States to keep weak governments in power but also off balance by occasional tilts toward the opposition. This is the case not only in Georgia (vis-à-vis South Ossetians and Abhazians; see *Excerpt*) and in Azerbaijain (versus Ngorno-Karabakh and Armenia), but also in Tajikistan (where the permutations of ethnic [Tajik and Uzbek] and regional [north, center, and east] forces are too numerous to detail). (For more information, see Chapters 4 and 5.)

Tajikistan could also be considered a contested, or collapsed (Zartman, 1994) state, a term used to identify a 5b civil war state, in which the non-governmental side has more than 50 percent of the territory. This would describe the situations in Somalia, Liberia, and Afghanistan, where the writ of the nominal government holding minimal international recognition (e.g., a seat in the United Nations) does not extend much beyond the capital city. This category might also include Angola (where the government which won the election controls only about half the country), and possibly Cambodia. The latter has an ersatz power-sharing arrangement between King Sihanouk (the 1954–1970 leader), two Prime Ministers (one from the 1979–1992 Vietnam-installed government, the other the King's son), and the opposition Khmer Rouge (the 1975–1979 government) which controls 15 percent of the countryside. However, it is not clear that the three leaders at the center are united in their control of the remaining 85 percent of the state, or what will happen after the death of the King, who represents the only unifying political symbol of the nation.

The *Excerpts* from this section include Algeria and Myanmar (as representative of traditional coup regimes), Georgia (for the ex-Soviet republics now enmeshed in civil wars), and Angola (as an example of a contested, collapsed state).

Table 6d
Entrenched Military Regimes, by Descending Categories of Civilian Political Institutions

Traditional regimes of violent origin (n=5):

Nigeria	S. Abacha s '93	recent coup; NO political institutions restored as of Summer 1995.
Rwanda	P. Kagame '94	cvw winner 7/94; claims to want to restore 8/93 power-sharing instituts.
Sudan	O. Bashir '89	coup during cvw NO parties; indirectly elected assembly.
Algeria	Kh. Nazzar '92	coup due to cvw NO parties, assy. Election annulled, 12/91.
Myanmar	Th. Shwe '88/92	coup + cvw NO parties, assy. Election annulled, 5/90.

ex-Soviet Republics in destabilizing wars (n=3):

Georgia	E.Shevardnadze '92	ex-CP election winner among cvw winners, 5b(10%) +extl. pressures.
Azerbaijan	S.Guseinov '93	ex-CP cvw winner, 5b(25%) + extl. (Russian/CIS) pressures.
Tajikistan	I. Rakhmanov '92	ex-CP cvw winner, w/ extl. dependence in CONTESTED (50%) state.

Contested, Collapsed States (n=5):

Somalia	95% CONTESTED: USC Aideed v. USC ali Mahdi v. north Somilaland's Egil v. others.
Afghanistan	95% CONTESTED: Pres. Rabbani v. ex-PM Hekmytyar v. Uzbek Gen. Doestam v. Taliban Mvmt.
Liberia	95% CONTESTED: ECOMOG/IGNU v. NPLF Taylor v. ex-Doe AFL v. others
Angola	50% CONTESTED: between MPLA's dos Santos v. UNTA's Savimbi (since '74 independ.).
Cambodia	?15% CONTESTED: Khmer Rouge vs. divided 85% center of King Sihanouk plus 2 PMs.

Excerpts from Moderating Military Data Bank

Syria - mil^

i. 3/71 referendum (on 11/70 Col. Assad coup-regime); 3/73 referendum on constitution - both implicitly confirm Assad as leader/President. Subsequent 1-man Presidential elections:

2/78 - Assad, 99.6% vote; 2/85 - Assad, 97% vote; 12/ 91 - Assad 99.9% vote.

ii. Assy(=Peop.Coun.) results: 1981 - Ba'ath P. wins all 191 seats; then "Front" expands to bring in others:

	2/86 (t.o.=40%)	5/90	5/94(t.o.=61%)
Ba'ath Party	129 (66%)	134 (54% seats)	
Communist P. (in Cab. since'66)	9 (5%)	8	
Arab Soc. Union	9 (5%)	8	
Arab Soc. Union Movement	8 (4%)	7	
Arab Soc. Party	5 (2%)	5	
Arab Dem.Soc. Union Mvmt	n.a.	4	
(Natl.Prog.Front Subtotal)	(160 =82% f. Front)	(166=66% f. Front)	167
independents	35 (18%)	84 (34%, reserved)	83 (reserved)
Totals:	195	250	250

iii. ArabSocial Renaissance(Ba'ath) Party- SG Assad 3.6% pop. Ba'ath dominates flexibly-sized National Progressive Front wh. generally includes: Comm. Party, Arab Soc.Un., Arab Soc.Un. Mvmt, Arab Soc.P., & Arab Dem.Soc.Un. Mvmt. (n=6, w/ Ba'ath, in 1986; n=7 w/ Ba'ath + 2 w/ no seats, in 1990).

iv. mil^ bec. from '46-'70, 15 coups, successful (8) or attempted (7). Historic power of Army: in 1958-61 forced assy. to vote to form United Arab Republic w/ Col.Nasser's Egypt. In 1950s, Ba'ath was founded by civilian Christian M. Aflaq; by 1960s, party Mil. Cmtee of n=5 (3 Alawites incl. Assad, Jadid; 2 Ismailis) helped '63 coup, then emerged in it (Assad getting Air Force); in '66 bloodier Jadid coup, Assad rose to Def. Min. After Govt. hestitated to intervene in Black Sept. (PLO) War v. Jordan, Assad took full control in 11/70.

11/70 coup established present govt. structure, and was a military (& *Shia Alawi* sect) capture of party which had been governing since 1963; esp. w/ St.of Emerg. of 5/63 under which main opp. parties (including Communists & Muslim Brotherhood) were banned; other parties allowed into Ba'ath-controlled "Front"). Independent professional assocs. (medical, legal, & HR groups) also banned. Loyalty to Assad more impt. than to mil. or party, esp. in ~12 intelligence and paramil. party agencies, of wh. most impt. are: Army Cmdr. H. Shehabi(Sunni; de facto #2 and probable successor), Pres. Guard Head A. Makhlouf(Alawite), Chief of Mil.Intell. A. Duba (Alawite).

Further militarism: 30,000 troop deployment in Lebanon since 1975. 1982 massacre of Islamic Fundamentalist *Sunnis* @ Hama, dead = ~15,000. Wars with Israel in 1967 & 73. 4th largest army (408,000) in Islamic zone, despite having only 11th largest population; also, 6th in military spending ($2300/yr.), and 3rd in % mil.exp./CGE (26.2%) (ACDA's WMEAT '95 for 1993).

Burkina Faso - mil^

i. 12/91 Pres. election (7 yr. term): Campaore 86.6%, but only 27% turnout as opposition boycotted, protesting lack of independent transition group to supervise return to politics. 3/94: appoints loyalist PM.

ii. 5/92 Assy. (n=107) election: OPD/MT (Organization for Peoples Democracy-Labor Mvmt.) 78 seats (72.9% seats), in continued low turnout (35%) support of system.

iii. 1987 coup-Capt. Campaore; established Revolution Committee, 3/88; his OPD/MT party formed, 4/89. In 3/90, Coord. Cmtee. for Popular Front held congress with 3000 delegates to draft 12/90 constitution; approved in 6/91 referendum (93% Yes, 47% turnout). Then Govt. dissolved, and Campaore resigned from military to run for Pres. on OPD/MT ticket. Other parties "advised" to join OPD/MT in 1991. Opposition allowed to form Coordination of Democratic Forces (CDF) in 1992 and called for sovereign national conference for transition to return to civilian rule; ignored (see (i)).

iv. mil^ - due to severely controlled transition-to-civilian-politics process, not getting much support (27%, 35% in two main elections). Meanwhile, 9/89 coup attempt by members of earlier Govt. #s 2 & 3 (=Capt.Zongo, Maj.Ligani executed) & again in 12/89 (7 more executed). 2nd most coups (n=6) and coup years (29/35=.829) in Africa. #5 in Africa in mil.exp./CGE (17.1%; ACDA '95 for 1993.)

Mozambique - mil^

i. Indep.ldr.Pres. Samora Machel indir. elected by party Cent.Cmtee (1976); successor Joaquin Chissano by pop. referendum of C.Cmtee choice (1986); then by Peoples Assembly (1989). After war, 10/94 election (multi-party; 5 yr. term): Chissano - 53.3%; Dhlakama - 33.7%; n=10 others - 13.0%. (Turnout 89%.) Losers' call for "power-sharing" (S.Af. '94 model) rebuffed. Pres. appoints some Mins. fm. n. & c. to broaden base, but no RENAMO's, not even as province governors in areas where they're strong.

ii. Peop. Assy. els.: 12/77 - all 210 seats, single party list, no choice. 10/86, n=227, with some choice (20% more candidates on party list than seats); at least 15 non-party mbrs. elected, but so was entire C.Cmtee (n=130). 7/89, n=250, from 299 cands., all proposed by Frelimo, indir. elected at mtgs. of locally elected provincial delegates. Typical 1-party-other elections (little choice in 1977, 1986, 1989) during war, until... 10/94 (n=250): FRELIMO - 129 seats; RENAMO - 112; Dem. Union - 9.

iii. FRELIMO=Mozambique Liberation Front only legal party 'til11/90. SG: '62 fdr.S. Machel (until death), '86 J.Chissano. Union of 3 nationalist anti-Portugese parties for 1964-74 armed indep. struggle; esp. strong in south. Also, 1976-92 war vs. RENAMO=Mozmbq. Natl. Resistance Movement (ldr. ,Alfonso Dlakama), fd. 1970, aided after '76 by (white) Rhodesia, after '78 by S. Africa in effort to de-stabilize front-line anti-apartheid country; strong in center and north, esp. among chiefs, Ndau tribe, and Muslims.

iv. mil^ bec. country at war from 1964-74, 1976-92 with > 1 million deaths; otherwise, 1-party. Under 10/92 cease-fire, & 2-yr. transition, FRELIMO army of 75,000 and RENAMO army of 20,000 to be demobilized & integrated into Govt. army of 30,000 (see 5b [WAN] Data Bank.)

Haiti - mil^

i. Pres. - 12/90 election, 70% turnout, won by:

	100% vote
l:Rev.J-B.Aristide (endorsed by FNCD but his movement was Lavalas [Flood,Volcano] pop.org.)	68%
Other left: DeJoie (PAIN, 5%); Claude (PDCH, 3%); Theodore (Communist, 2%); Subtotal:	10%
c-r: M.Bazin (ANDP) - favored by international capital, US State Dept.	14%
Other right: n=6, incl. ex-'88 Pres. Manigat with total of:	8%

"Notorious Duvalierists" banned from campaign acc. to '87 cⁿnstitut. (aimed at: R.Lafontant [U.f.Natl.Reconcil. P., ex-Tontons head]; ex-Gen.Cl.Raymond; and 8 others of orig. 26 cands.); 16 left to run; 11 actually do. Pres. ousted in 9/91 coup, 3-yr. exile before return with help of 20,000 US troops in 10/94.

ii. Assy. el.-12/90-1/91 (turnout, Rds. 1,2(no Pres): 70%, 20%).   n=9+ w/ seats

	LH	UH	TOT
f-l:MRN=Movement f. National Reconstruction (R.Theodore; communist)	1	2	3
l:FNCD=Natl.Front f. Change & Dem. (11/90; Sen.Martinez, capital Mayor Evans Paul)	29	13	42
incl. CONACOM=Natl.Cong.o'Dem.Mvmts.(Benoit),Natl.Coop.Action Mvmt.(V.Joseph)			
lc:PDCH=Xtn.Dem. P. (Sylvio Claude, Baptist Rev.; assass. in 9/91 coup; J. Douze)	7	1	8
cl:PAIN=Natl.Agric.&Industry P. (de Joie)	6	2	8
r:ANDP=Natl.All.f.Dem. & Progress (fd. 8/89; ldr. World Banker Bazin of MIDH)	17	6	23
r:RPND=Rally o'Progress.Natl.Dem. (Manigat)	6	1	7
r:MDN=Movement f. Natl. Development (DeRonceray)	5	0	5
r:PNT=National Party of Labor (Desulme)	3	1	4
r:MODELH=Dem.Movement f. the Liberation of Haiti (LaTortue)	2	0	2
independents, vacancies, etc.	7	1	8
TOTALS	83	27	110

6/95 assy. el. - under UN/US peacekeepers (n=5000); 10,000 cands. from 28 parties, for 2200 natl. & local offices incl. 133 mayors. Lavalas Political Org., split of more leftist Aristide supporters (incl. ldr. G. Pierre-Charles, Ch. Jean-Baptiste) from FNCD wins most seats. Losers (esp. capital mayor E. Paul) claim fraud.

12/95 pres.el. - Aristide/Lavalas candidate Rene Preval wins with ≥67% vote; main opp. parties boycott.

iii. Parties - generally weak (see par. iv); 1st free els. in '90; Aristide was not a member of a party when elected. 6/95 el. has onerous candidate qualifications (land ownership; mbr. of "recognized profession"; birth certificate; higher registration fees for parties with few candidates; etc.) to discourage small parties.

iv. mil^: due to militarized (5,000 outside troops) post-10/94 transition from 9/91 coup regime; plus ..... mil° historically due to 186-year history of authoritarian, or military, rule before first free election in 1990. 8.5 coups, 100% years since 1945 (5c Data Bank); 29 coups or pres. assassinations since 1804. During 1957-86, 40,000 dead, 1 mil. refugees under Duvaliers & their private *Tontons Macoutes* army. Their sympatizers remained in Army of 7000, w/ 30% CGE. Also, 535 rural "section chiefs"=police/tax collector/ judge w/ ~50,000 in private armies controlled daily lives in totally militarized countryside. 9/91-9/93 coup regime of Def.Min.Gen.R.Cedras, Police Chief Col.M.Francois, & Army Chief Col. P. Biamby caused ~4500 dead (incl. Aristide Justice Min. G.Mallery), 300,000 internal refugees, 1 mil. external, 40-80,000 asylum-seekers via boats etc. Their CIA-supported Front for Advancement of Progress (FRAPH), n=500 armed, leaders E. Constant, J.Chamblain still at large after return of Aristide.

Excerpts from Entrenched Military Data Bank

Algeria - mil° (coup regime, civil war)

i. **Coup**, 1/11/92, ousted Pres. Chadli, & aborted assy. election which govering NLF party was losing. Its new Mil.Coun. (n=5, incl. Def.Min.Gen.Khalid Nizar) > existing High State Council (n=7, new Chm.=Pres. returning exile Boudiaf, assassinated 6/92; replaced by ali Kafi, who names new Def.Min. L. Zeroual) whose mandate expired 12/93. Replaced by mil-apptd. Transition Council which called 1/94 Natl. Conf. which, though boycotted by all main parties, named Def.Min. Zeroual to 3-yr term as new, one-man, <u>Pres.</u> In 11/95, Pres. Zeroual was reconfirmed with 61 percent of vote in election (75% turnout) from which main Islamic opposition was barred from contesting.

ii. **assy.**, 12/91 elections (n=430 seats): opposition FIS=Islamic Salvation Front won outright (>50%) 188 seats (& was leading in 150 others twd. the 216 needed to form govt., twd. the 287 2/3 needed for constit.amndmt. wh. could switch to parl.*mpr system & control over NLF Pres.); vs. Govt. NLF's 15 seats, FSF Berber party 25 seats, in Round 1, before Round 2 aborted by 1/93 coup. Turnout 60%.

iii. **Party** activity outlawed; 1/92 coup ended 10/88ff democratic opening of mil^ state with 65 parties of which 40 were creations of ~200 elites in power structure since 1962. Result: only well-organized FIS (Isl.Fndmtlsts) & FSF (Berbers) won seats. Since coup, only NLF even talks to mil. govt. about transition.
   NLF (Natl.Liberation Front),1954-62 rev. indep. party, split into spprtrs. (ex-PM Sid) & opponents (ex-Pres. Chadli, SG Mehri) of coup. NLF was challenged after1989 esp. by ex-outlawed FIS=Islamic Salv.Front (ldrs. Abassi Madani & Ali bel Hadj, jailed 6/91@ time of orig. sked. assy. el.) which won 65%v.,55% seats in local els. in 6/90, but this power lost when mil. govt. dissolved all local govts., 3/92. Moderate Isl. parties (Hamas & Ennadha) received no votes in 12/91 Round 1.

iv. **mil°** - due to 1/92 coup after which FIS turned to arms and started 5b civil war as well. ~40,000 dead as of mid-1995; 10,000s of FIS cadre political prisoners in desert camps. Also, history of military rule (30 of 33 independence years = .909, 2nd highest 5c.ii in islamic zone), + military had to step in to protect NLF rule from riots and demonstrations in 10/88 & 6/90 States of Emergency before complete take-over in coup of '92.

Myanmar - mil° (coup regime; civil wars)

i. **exec.** = SLORC=State Law & Order Restoration Council, coup-regime of Army Gens. Saw Maung (9/88), Than Shwe (4/92), & esp. Intelligence Chief Gen. Khin Nyunt (who still defer to 1962 coup leader Gen. Ne Win, age 85+). Since 1990, junta has tried to legitimate its rule and its future role via national conferences of SLORC-picked representatives of "approved" parties (n=10, incl. main opposition National League for Democracy) and ethnic, peasant, & professional groups. e.g.,1993/94 convention of ~700 reps to approve SLORC constitution draft which would keep Army role in all three branches of govt. (see par. iv). Acting NLD Chm. Aung Shwe & Shan NLD leader Khun Tun Oo among those objecting, walking out of national conference.

ii. **assy.** - 5/90 election: SLORC's Natl. Unity Party wins only 10 (of 489) seats, with about 30% of vote; vs. Natl. League of Democracy 392 seats, 67% vote, despite detention of its leaders (Mrs. Daw Aung San Suu Kyi, house arrest ,7/89-7/95, (Nobel Peace Prize, 12/91). This assembly never allowed to convene.

iii. **parties** - NUP=National Unity P., junta-renamed Burma Socialist Program P., formed in '74 to legitimize '62 coup. After arrests of NLD's acting leaders (SG Chit Khaing; also U Tin OO, U Kyi Maung), other (tamer) parties agree to give army right to draft new constitution, 1993-95.

iv. **mil°** because military rule since 1962 (5c=.723 coup years, 4.5 coups), with '62 coup leader Gen. Ne Win still behind-scenes power. Since '88 coup (with 3,000 dead), 5d army size has increased from 180,000 to nearly 300,000, & mil.expenditures estimated as high as 60% CGE (NY Times, 1995; vs. ACDA WMEAT '95 for '93 of 22.2%, 7th in zone). 5a war score of 46.5 from nearly constant fighting vs. tribal insurgents since 1948 independence (still 5b vs. Karens and "tolerated" druglords in 1995). In addition, pro-democracy movements among Burman majority population violently suppressed in '62,'74,'88. 3/95 constitution ensures military retains all political power.: fixed # of seats in assy., requirement that president to be indirectly elected (by "stacked" assy.), & of military background, military power to declare State of Emerg., etc. (see: Thailand,Indonesia,Chile Data Banks).

Georgia - ex-com--->mil° (coup; cvw)

ex-com transition - 5/89: declares sovereignty in USSR. 10/90: 1st free multiparty elections in USSR; n=11 parties for 250 assy. seats, indep. leader Zviad Gamsakhurdia's Ga.Pop.Front w/ 155 seats (62% vote) over Communists' 64, others' 31. 11/90: assy. elects Zviad president 232-5. 5/91: Pres. directly elected (1st in USSR, 1 month before Russia); Zviad wins w/ 87% vote, then opts his Natl. Guard (n=3000) out of Soviet Army. 9/91 (after Soviet putsch): PM T.Sigua, & Natl.Guard Head T.Kitovani (& ~1/2 Guard, n=1500) move into opposition. In12/91 (after USSR dissolves) these move into rebellion (5b) along with J.Ioseliani's Horseman (Mkhedrioni) paramilitary group (n=500).

. **cvw/coup,** 12/22/91-1/9/92: Military Council of Kitovani/Ioseliani drives Pres. Zviad out. 90 dead,600 wounded. Rename Sigua PM, bring home (fm. ex-SU) Shevardnadze as Chm. State Coun.(=Pres.)until 10/92 el. **3cb- - ->6d** interpretation: Pres. Zviad 1st natlst./populist dissident to come to power in ex-SU; backed by masses; then 1st to be overthrown by ex-Communist Party elites who resorted to force.

i. **assy.,** 10/92 el. 1st ex-Soviet republic to hold 2nd natl. multiparty election-Type A=assy.only. But assy. candidate Shevardnadze ran (nationally & unopposed) for "Assy.Spkr." (=~Pres.); got 93% vote in 85% turnout. He renames Sigua PM, estabs. a 2c.ii Military Council (n=8 w/ martial law powers to fight three civil wars (see par. iv)), uniting 2 militias (Def.Min. Kitovani's n=1500, State Council Dpty.Chm. Ioseliani's n=500; essentially disarming the latter). By 8/93, Shevardnadze has greater legitimacy, both militias & their leaders under his control, and his own PM (O.Patsatsian). 9/93 Shevardnadze becomes Head of "Natl.Emergency Council" with State of Emergency power, assy. suspended under 3-pronged civil war (see par. iv). Saved by Russia in return for joining Commonwealth of Independent States.

ii.#1 **party,** 10/92 el: Shevardnadze's Mshvidoba (=Peace) Bloc. Others: Round Table, NDP, NIP, CP, etc.

v. **mil°** because government of ex-communists came to power via force (+ legitimating election which coup-govt. ran under wartime conditions), and is still beset by three civil wars: vs. ex-Pres. Zviad supporters in w. Mingrelia region (he suicided in 12/93); vs. S.Ossetians in north-central area; vs. Abkhazians in northwest (see 5b). Georgia needs (ex-communist) Russian "peacekeeping" troops in Abkhazia to keep all these insurgent forces repressed.

Angola - mil° (contested, collapsed state/civil war)

. **exec.** - MPLA-PT Party Secy.Genl. Jose E. dos Santos elected Pres. in 9/79 (upon death of independence Pres. A. Neto), 12/80, 12/85, and 12/90 by MPLA party congress, to which delegates indirectly elected by lower levels of party organization. In first contested election, 9/92, dos Santos got 49.6% over 12 opponents in Round 1 (90% turnout); Round 2 (needed because <50% achieved) cancelled when 2nd place loser Jonas Savimbi of UNITA party (40.1% vote) returned to civil war.

i. **assy.**- n=223; in only general election during war, 1980, single MPLA-PT party list with no choice, approved overwhelmingly; then assy.'s term was renewed by indirectly elected party congress, until 1st multiparty (n=~18 parties), Prop.Rep. election, 9/92: MPLA 129 seats (56% vote), UNITA 70 seats (30% vote), others 24 seats (14% vote). Turnout 90%.

ii. **parties** - MPLA-PT = Popular Movement for the Liberation of Angola-Workers Party, elite vanguard revoltionary party (<30,000 members) founded in 1956 to fight for independence vs. Portugal. Tightly controlled by SG, Politburo, Central Committee until 1990 promise of multiparty elections once war ended. 1992: dropped PT-tag (too Marxist-Leninist), opened up membership to 300,000 in one year; allowed other parties including old revolutionary groups:

UNITA=National Union for the Total Independence of Angola, leader Jonas Savimbi, especially popular among Ovimbundu in south; FNLA=Natl.Liberation Front of Angle, leader Holden Roberto, popular among BaKongo in the north, supported by Zaire; FLEC=Front for the Liberation of the Cabindan Enclave, oil-rich, in north-west, separated from Angola by strip of Zaire.

v. **mil°** because almost constant war since 1961: vs. Portugal until 1974 independence; vs. UNITA *Ovimbundu* (35% population) since, except for ceasefires 6/89-8/89, 5/91-9/92, 11/94ff? (see 5b-WAN). Otherwise a 1-party polity.

6e MONARCHIES (mon°)

The final polity type on the Comparative Government Spread Sheet is the *monarchy*, a political system in which the leader is chosen from and by members of a single (royal) family. The reason this polity type appears on the second page of the CGSS is that the roots of this family can generally be traced back to some military conquest. This anachronistic form of government is found in only 3 of this study's 100 significant states—Saudi Arabia, Morocco, and Jordan.

In monarchies, power is shared only minimally beyond the royal family. Nevertheless, within this restricted framework, some modern governmental institutions have sometimes been introduced. Because there are so few such states in today's world, **Table 6e** broadens the focus of comparative analysis of these institutions to include 4 other countries with more than 1 million people each; 3 of these have a political existence in the shadow of Saudi Arabia (Kuwait, Oman, and the United Arab Emirates); the other one is Lesotho (Gause, 1994; Peterson, 1988).

Section i of **Table 6e** ranks these 7 countries on the basis of the presence of five modern political institutions. First, the least restraining upon the power of a royal family, is the existence of a written constitution limiting some of its prerogatives. Since Saudi Arabia finally adopted such a "Basic Document" in 1992, the sixtieth year of its existence, all formerly "absolute" monarchs, except for the Sultan of Oman, now have some check upon their power, even if it is merely a codification of traditional practices. With respect to divided offices for the head of state and the head of government, 5 of the 7 states do this, even if in 2 of them the Prime Minister is typically another member of the royal family (generally the Crown Prince, successor to the throne). In the more advanced monarchies, this person may be a "civilian," appointed by the king subject to approval by the representative asembly. (In the one monarchy most recently moved up in the CGSS to *mpr, Nepal, the appointment–approval sequence was reversed; the prime minister had been selected by the assembly subject to approval by the king even before the polity change in 1991 [Sullivan, 1991: 391].)

Representative assemblies with independent powers exist in only 4 of the 7 monarchies, although purely advisory consultative councils can be found in the others. Direct national elections to such bodies have been held in 3 countries, where either tame "loyal-opposition" parties have been allowed to participate (Morocco), or parties which have historically operated behind the cover of independent candidacies have recently been legalized (Jordan). In Lesotho, the main opposition to the monarchy is not a political party in the assembly, but the military, which has periodically taken over the country and exiled the ruler; when assembly elections are allowed (as in 1993 and 1970), the monarchy has shared power with its leaders.

In contrast to the presence in Morocco, Jordan, and Lesotho of all five

Table 6e
Monarchies (n = 7, including 4 ministates with > 1 million population)

i - Summary of Modern Political Institutions

State	Constitution	Divided Heads	Rep. Assy.	Elections	Parties	Rating
Morocco	Yes	Yes	Yes	Yes	Yes	5.0
Jordan	Yes	Yes	Yes	Yes	Yes('92)	5.0
Lesotho	Yes	Yes	Yes	Yes	Yes	5.0
Kuwait	Yes	Yes	Yes('92)	limited suffrage	No	3.5
Saudi A.	Yes('92)	No	No	No	No	1.0
UAE	provisional	Yes	No	No	No	1.0
Oman	No	No	No	No	No	0.0

ii - ministate monarchies with < 1 million population

Europe	Islamic	Africa	Asia	W.Hemisphere
Luxembourg	Bahrain	Swaziland	Bhutan	none in W.Hemisph.
Liechtenstein	Qatar		Brunei	
Monaco				

iii - Legitimacy Based upon Date of Original Dynastic Accession

Islamic Zone   Africa

Jordan (Hashemites)1517
Morocco (Alawites) 1660
Saudi A. (Sauds) 1766
-Kuwait (al Sabahs) 1756
-Oman (Saids)1775   -Lesotho (Basotho) -1818
-UAE (Nahayans)1790s

iv - Monarchs with Head of State Roles in other CGSS Polities

Europe   Asia

Denmark -1448   Thailand - 1238
UK -1701(1589?)
Spain -1700/14   Malaysia (n=9; 1890s)
Netherlands-1795(1579?)   Nepal - late 1700s
Sweden -1818
Belgium -1831   Japan - 1867(660 B.C.?)
Norway -1905

Note: - small print = ministate

modern political institutions, Saudi Arabia, UAE, and Oman are the most reactionary, unrepresentative governments in the world. Until the drafting of the 1992 Basic Law, Saudi Arabia had no civilian institutions and all power was in the hands of the king and his family. Kuwait represents a point about halfway between zero and five modern political institutions. It has a sheikh who shares power with his son as prime minister, and an assembly which comes in and out of existence at his whim. When it is allowed to operate

Format for 6e Monarchy Data Bank

State - mon (# of modern political institutions)
i. evidence of shared power (constitutionally-mandated?) with a PM or a representative assembly (appointed or elected?).
ii. distribution of seats in representative assembly (not consultative council), especially where elections and parties exist.
iii. historic legitimacy data (***starting date** and name of dynasty*).   iv. other remarks.

Excerpts from Monarchy Data Bank

Saudi Arabia - mon (1.0/5.0; before 1992, 0.0 with NO written limits on monarch's power.)
i. 2/92 "basic law" (83 Articles), 1st ever written, on 60th anniversary of kingdom. King Fahd ibn Abdal-Aziz al Saud is Head of State & Govt. (6/82). Crown Prince (successor, not PM) Abdullah confirmed 3/92, but future ones will not automatically succeed.
ii. NO representative assembly (despite promise of one in 1970s),but a "Counsultative Council", n=60, 4-yr. terms, chosen by King from five religious establishments, Islamic scholars, military, Govt. bureaucracy, Shiites, tribal elites, etc.; to review his laws & policies; 1st meeting, 12/93. Also, King appoints 13 regional councils with 210 members. Still no parties allowed; and women are banned from all political activities despite embarrassing 1991 drive-through-capital-in-automobiles protest.
iii. Dynasty from Mohammed ibn *Saud,* King of Daraiyya (died, **1 7 6** 6); Kingdom of Saudi Arabia proclaimed in 1932 by Emir Abdul Aziz II ibn Saud (his family goes back to 1902). 2/92 Law expands pool of electors for next King to include grandsons (n=~500 of total royal family of ~6500) of founder. King has $18 billion personal wealth; ~4000 princes w/ easy access to Govt. central bank.
iv. legitimacy stems from defense of Islam, protection of its holy places (Mecca, Medina). 1994 law transfers implementation of Koran away from fundamentalist Council of Ulemas to more moderate "Supreme Council of Islamic Affairs" under brother/Defence Minister Prince Sultan; ends spying by Ulemas' religious police. But because of dubious domestic political legitimacy: highest military expenditures in Islamic zone ($20.4 bill./yr. in 1993, 9th in world!); 2nd highest mil.exp./CGE (41.0%); armed personnel of 172,000 are divided (among family members) into separate commands for Army, Navy, Air Force, and National Guard. (There are also external threats [Iraq, Iran, even Yemen].)

~Kuwait - mon (3.5 of 5.0; no parties, limited electorate).
i. Sheikh Jaber Al-Ahmad al Sabah, Emir since 1977 > Crown Prince PM Saad A. S. al Sabah (2/78;4/91; 10/92.)   King reappointed Crown Prince as PM despite rebuff in 10/92 election over 1990/91 national security unreadiness. Cabinet of 16, includes 6 from 10/92 assy. (other 10 appointees automatically added to assy., giving it a new total of 60; see par. ii).
ii. A sometimes functioning Natl. Assy. (1976-81; 1985-86; 1992ff), n=50 (2 ea. x 25 districts); dir. el. based on electorate restricted to approx. 81,400 (10/92) male descendants from 1920 Kuwaiti male citizens (= ~3.5% of 1.7 mill. population.; ~10% Kuw. citizens. NOT: n=40,000 2nd class citizens (not pre-1920); n=250,000 pre-'90 Bedoons (Arabs, esp. fm. Syr.,Iq., there for sevl.decades; down to 125,000 in '92); 20,000 Palestinians, down from once 350,000 during '48-91. Assy. has right to: initiate & veto Govt. legislation; question & remove Cabinet Ministers (but not appoint them).
10/92 assembly election results:
     80% turnout, n=278 candidates for 50 seats. No parties allowed, but some recognized "factions":
     19 pro-Government (especially from rural areas dominated by the 11 tribes);
     31 opposition in 6 or 7 blocs, incl. n=12 fm. left, including: Kuw.Dem.Front/Forum (ldr. A. al-Nibari, for women vote) , Constitutional Group (J. al-Saqur), & Parl. Bloc (A. al-Saadoun); n=19 fm. right Islamic Fundamentalists, including: one Shiite (30% population) group, Isl.Natl.Alliance (ldr. Adnan Sayed Abdul Samed Sayed Zaher); two Sunni (Isl.Constitut. Mvmt, Isl. Parl. Alliiance); and Isl. Pop. Group.
iii. In 1711-16, clans of Aniza tribe (Uteiba sect) migrated from Arabia; head of *al Sabah* family was selected Emir in **1 7 5 6**. Senior family members choose Crown Prince (successor) from either the al-Jaber or al-Salim branch of family; all are direct descendants of Mubarak the Great.
iv. Pre-8/90 populaton ~2.1 million; Kuw. citizens ~650,000 (only 31% population!); Kuwaiti workers 150,000; Kuwaiti Govt.workers 120,000; voters 60,000; "royals" 2000; King's children 72; King's wives 40+; his wives at one time 4 (with1 annual trade-in).
5/92 pop.: 1.2 m., of wh. 700,000 Kuw. citizens = 58% population; + policy of never again <50% pop. But 2/93 pop.: 1.4 m., of wh. 606,000 Kuw. citizens, .5m foreign wrkrs (36%), incl. .1m "needed" domestics.

(1976–1981, 1985–1986, 1993ff), it is formed by the votes of a highly restricted electorate of less than 5 percent of the population: adult males who can trace their citizenship in Kuwait back to ancestors who lived there in 1920 (when Kuwait emerged from the Ottoman Empire under British tutelage).

The lack of modern political institutional structure might seem to present a situation ripe for revolution; a closer look at these regimes, however, reveals that most monarchies are rather stable. (This is even more true for those ministate monarchies with less than 1 million in population noted in section ii of **Table 6e**.) The reason is that, in these systems, legitimacy stems from the long tradition of many years of rule by a single dynasty. Longevity—rather than elections, popular representation in an assembly, or participation in party activity—is the important political component in these regimes. Section iii of **Table 6e** lists the dates of origin for the seven ruling families studied here; they generally go back several generations and a couple hundred years.

Such families continue to play a role (head of state) in 11 other countries among the CGSS's 100, but because this role is subservient to other institutions (parties, the representative assembly, the military, etc.), these states are not counted among the monarchies. The identities of these states and the years to which the families of the head of state trace back their dynastic roots are listed in section iv of **Table 6e**.

The *Format* for 6e—Monarchy Data Bank appears preceding the *Excerpts*, which are presented for Saudi Arabia and Kuwait, the ministate for whose political institutions a worldwide alliance fought in 1991.

6f OTHER: COLONIES, ASPIRANT NATION-STATES

At the end of the Comparative Government Spread Sheet, 13 additional polities are listed which could be independent sovereign states some time in the future. Two of these entities (Hong Kong and Puerto Rico) were historic colonies (of the United Kingdom and United States, respectively), and most of the others would consider themselves to be aspiring nation-states in some sort of "colonial" situation. Because this state of oppression and/or dependence is still a real part of international political reality for significant numbers of people today (the total number of people in these 13 entities is more than 50 million), it would seem appropriate to consider these phenomena before finishing this survey of global political types. To do so will also complement the analysis of ethnic rebellion, begun in Chapters 4 and 5, in a way which focuses upon those few insurgent movements mentioned there which have the greatest chance of some success; that is, the ones with the largest populations or the most powerful international patrons.

A *colony* exists when one state has direct political control over a group of people who are not citizens within its territorial jurisdiction. Historically, military force had to be applied to create such a relationship, and the status is generally a matter of some dispute to this day, hence the reason for their presence on the second (i.e., militarized) page of the CGSS.

In 1945, more than half the people in the world lived in such dependent territories; in 1990, fewer than 0.5 percent did (Sullivan, 1991: 388), and Table 2d.i in Chapter 2 plotts their rise to independence. There are fewer than 50 such colonies remaining today, most small islands with fewer than 100,000 people on them, including 16 in the Pacific Ocean and 11 in the Caribbean; for a complete list, see "Related Territories" in *Freedom in the World* (Freedom House, 1994: 603–670). The major colonial powers are still the United Kingdom (with 14 possessions), France (9), and the United States (8, including Guam, the U.S. Virgin Islands, American Samoa, Northern Marianas, and the virtually empty Midway and Wake Islands and Johnston Atoll). Although the United Kingdom has the most colonies, after its return of Hong Kong (population 5.7 million) to China in 1997, the most people subject to foreign rule will be under the United States, mainly in Puerto Rico (population 3.7 million) whose official name and relationship to the United States was changed in 1952 to that of "commonwealth" for reasons of political correctness (Carr, 1984; Scott, 1989). France is notable for having six possessions of significant size (i.e., greater than 100,000 in population): Reunion, Guadeloupe, Martinique, French Polynesia, New Caledonia, and French Guiana.

The "aspiring nation-states" to be discussed next would be considered by some sources to exist in a related semicolonial status; for example, see Freedom House's coverage of Israeli Occupied Territories (i.e., Palestine), North Cyprus, Western Sahara, and East Timor. To these, Kurdistan, Ngorno-Karabakh, southern Sudan, Kashmir, Tamil Eelam, Tibet, and Quebec will be added here.

These 11 suppressed nations can be analyzed with an eye to assessing their chances of ever emerging independent and sovereign like the 121 "new" states identified in Table 2d.i as having come into existence since 1945. All 11 have cohesive ethnic bases; but their populations vary from the Kurds (who number 20 million) to Western Sahara, Northern Cyprus, Ngorno-Karabakh, and East Timor with fewer than 1 million each. Ten of the 11 appear on the current-conflict Table 5b, 3 as parties to civil wars controlling significant territory or population (the Tamils, southern Sudanese, and Turkish Kurds), 1 as an insurgency (Kashmir), 3 waning (Ngorno-Karabakh, Palestine, Western Sahara), 2 latent (East Timor, Iraq's Kurds), and 2 as "prospective candidates for inclusion" (Tibet, Quebec). The only one not listed in Table 5b is the ministate of Northern Cyprus, split from the ministate of Cyprus since 1974 by Turkey, and still dependent upon that patron to this day.

International recognition (and its legitimation) varies from that of Palestine (for which the PLO is recognized by the United Nations and more than 100 countries as the sole legitimate representative), and Western Sahara (which is recognized by about 70 states, including half the countries in Africa), to nations being sustained by one or two large neighboring governments or their citizens (Northern Cyprus, Ngorno-Karabakh, south Sudan, Kashmir, Tamil Eelam), to those whose support is more distant and moral (Iraqi Kurdistan,

Tibet, East Timor, Quebec).

The list of aspirant nation-states does not include other non-state parties mentioned in current-conflict Table 5b which either want to seize power in existing states (e.g., Liberia, UNITA's Ovambos in Angola); are the subject of irredentism vis-à-vis a neighboring state (e.g., Northern Irish, Krajina, or Bosnian Serbs); present no significant challenge (Myanmar's tribes); or whose situation is unclear at the present time (Afghanistan, Tajikistan). Mention of these 11 national movements, however, puts closure upon the CGSS's survey of 100 political types, by providing for the most likely possibilities of future expansion.

REFERENCES

Austin, D. (1994) *India's Violent Democracy.* Chatham House Papers Series. London: Pinter.

Ayittey, G. B. (1992) *Africa Betrayed.* New York: St. Martin's Press.

Baxter, C. (1985) "Democracy and Authoritarianism in South Asia," *Journal of International Affairs,* 38: 307–319.

Bedeski, R. E. (1994) *The Transformation of South Korea: Reform and Reconstitution in the Sixth Republic under Roh Tae Woo, 1987–92.* New York: Routledge.

Binnendijk, H. (ed.) (1987) *Authoritarian Regimes in Transition.* Washington: U.S. Department of State, Foreign Service Institute, Center for the Study of Foreign Affairs.

Bungbongkarn, S. (1988) *The Military in Thai Politics.* Brookfield, VT: Ashgate.

Carr, R. (1984) *Puerto Rico: A Colonial Experiment.* New York: New York University Press.

Caspar, G. (1995) *Fragile Democracies: Legacies of Authoritarian Rule.* Pittsburgh: University of Pittsburgh Press.

Choudhury, G. W. (1988) *Pakistan: Transition from Military to Civilian Rule.* London: Scorpion.

Clapham, C. and G. Philip (eds.) (1984) *The Political Dilemmas of Military Regimes.* London: Croom Helm.

Danopoulas, C. P. (ed.) (1987) *Military Dictatorship in Retreat: Comparative Perspective on Post-Military Regimes.* Boulder, CO: Westview Press.

Decalo, S. (1990) *Coups and Army Rule in Africa: Motivations and Constraints.* New Haven, CT: Yale University Press.

Deegan, H. (1994) *The Middle East and Problems of Democracy.* Boulder, CO: Lynne Rienner.

Diamond, L., J. J. Linz, and S. M. Lipset (eds.) (1987–1989) *Democracy in Developing Countries* Series. 4 vols. Boulder, CO: Lynne Rienner.

Freedom House (1994) *Freedom in the World: Political Rights and Civil Liberties 1993–1994.* New York: Freedom House.

Gause, F. G., III (1994) *Oil Monarchies: Domestic Security Challenges in the Arab Gulf States.* New York: Council on Foreign Relations Press.

Goldman, R. M. (1990) *From Warfare to Party Politics: The Critical Transition to Civilian Control.* Syracuse, NY: Syracuse University Press.

Hale, W. (1994) *Turkish Politics and the Military.* New York: Routledge.

Hinnebusch, R. A. (1990) *Authoritarian Power and State Formation in Ba'athist Syria: Army, Party, and Peasant.* Boulder, CO: Westview Press.

Kedourie, E. (1993) *Democracy and Arab Political Culture.* Portland, OR: Frank Cass.

Kennedy, G. (1974) *The Military in the Third World.* New York: Scribners.

Kessler, R. J. (1989) *Rebellion and Repression in the Philippines.* New Haven, CT: Yale University Press.

Maniruzzaman, T. (1987) *Military Withdrawal from Politics: A Comparative Perspective.* Cambridge, MA: Ballinger.

Mansour, F. (1992) *The Arab World: Nation, State, and Democracy.* Lanham, Md: United Nations University Press.

O'Donnell, G., P. C. Schmitter, and L. Whitehead (1986) *Transitions from Authoritarian Rule.* 4 vols. Baltimore: Johns Hopkins University Press.

Perlmutter, A. (1981) *Modern Authoritarianism: A Comparative Institutional Analysis.* New Haven, CT: Yale University Press.

Peterson, J. E. (1988) *The Arab Gulf States: Steps toward Political Participation.* Westport, CT: Praeger.

Pinkney, R. (1990) *Right-Wing Military Government.* Twayne's Themes in Right-Wing Politics and Ideology Series, No. 3. Boston: Twayne.

Pion-Berlin, D. (1990) "Retreat to the Barracks: Recent Studies on Military Withdrawal from Power," *Journal of Interamerican Studies and World Affairs,* 31(1): 137–145.

Rouquie, A. (1987) *The Military and the State in Latin America.* Berkeley: University of California Press.

Scott, I. (1989) *Political Change and the Crisis of Legitimacy in Hong Kong.* Honolulu: University of Hawaii Press.

Sprinzak, E. and L. Diamond (1993) (eds.) *Israel: Democracy under Stress.* Boulder, CO: Lynne Rienner.

Sullivan, M. J., III (1991) *Measuring Global Values: The Ranking of 162 Countries.* Westport, CT: Greenwood Press.

Thomas, C. Y. (1985) *The Rise of the Authoritarian State in Peripheral Societies.* New York: Monthly Review Press.

Weinberg, L. (ed.) (1993) *Political Parties and Terrorist Groups.* Portland, OR: Frank Cass.

Welch, C. W., Jr. (1987) *No Farewell to Arms: Military Disengagement from Politics in Africa and Latin America.* Boulder, CO: Westview Press.

Wendt, A. and M. Barnett (1993) "Dependent State Formation and Third World Militarization," *Review of International Studies* 19: 321–347.

Zagorski, P. (1992) *Democracy vs. National Security: Civil–Military Relations in Latin America.* Boulder, Co: Lynne Rienner.

Zartman, I. W. (ed.) (1994) *Collapsed States: The Disintegration and Restoration of Legitimate Authority.* Boulder, CO: Lynne Rienner.

7

The Quality of Life in Different Political Systems

This book has dealt primarily with governing institutions in the public arena. There are, however, other aspects of a society which contribute to the quality of one's life but are not in the purely political domain. Two of these areas, which will be covered in this concluding chapter, involve individual rights and economic well-being.

Obviously, the governmental institutions adopted by a citizenry will speak to these areas of life in the general, or "macro," sense. But individual rights and economic well-being are suitable subjects of analysis from their particular perspectives as well. In both cases, measures have been developed according to which state performance can be assessed and correlated with the political systems described in the first six chapters, if one is interested in how particular polity types, or specific states, are doing in achieving their policy goals in these areas (Andrain, 1994; Groth and Wade, 1984). This chapter will report on six such measures, and in so doing will update some of this author's earlier work on inquiries into the comparative quality of life around the world (Sullivan, 1991: 218–229).

7a INDIVIDUAL RIGHTS: HUMAN, CIVIL, POLITICAL

There are certain "rights" due to all individuals by virtue of their being human beings, irrespective of the governmental systems under which they might live. Respect for these rights is often considered one of the chief requisites for democracy, but this subject is beyond the scope of the institutions of power sharing among elite political actors covered in this book. This chapter will simply summarize human-rights issues in governance by reference to two of the many sources which regularly assess their presence in surveys of states throughout the world. For more information on the significance of human rights in politics, one might see An-Naim (1992), Claude and Weston (1989), Lawson, 1989, and Nanda, Scaritt, and Shepherd (1981).

Individual rights have been spelled out in the International Bill of Human Rights (IBHR), made up of the 1948 Universal Declaration of Human Rights (UD), the 1966 International Covenant on Civil and Political Rights (CP), and the 1966 International Covenant on Economic, Social, and Cultural Rights (ESC). One or more of these documents have been signed by more than 100 of the world's states and, as such, they provide a universal standard to which a large majority of the world community can be held, regardless of political ideology or regional culture (Henkin, 1981; Donnelly, 1989; Howard, 1990; Jabine and Claude, 1992). Indeed, all member states of the United Nations accept Article 55c of its Charter, which calls for "universal respect for and observance of human rights and fundamental freedoms" (Humphrey, 1984), and particularly egregious violators are cited each year in that organization's annual yearbook on the subject (United Nations, 1995b).

Civil and political rights are cited more often than the economic rights by policy makers and analysts concerned with democracy, freedom, and other aspects of humane governance. This focus reflects a western European cultural bias relating to individualism, as compared with the concerns of many developing nations and former communist states, which give equal or greater weight to the economic and social rights of particular groups (Eide, 1986; Franck, 1982). These latter issues will be discussed in the next part of this chapter. But first, this section will utilize the structure of the IBHR as a framework to analyze some issues most closely associated with individual human rights. The numbers in parentheses at the end of each of the following paragraphs which guide this inquiry refer, respectively, to the relevant articles in the UD or CP being cited.

1. Government respect for equality of treatment of individual human beings, especially as concerns discriminaton with respect to race, color, religion, national origin, cultural heritage, political opinion, and the like (UD 1–2, 15, 27; CP 2–3, 26–27).

2. Government policies pertaining to the integrity of the person, especially as relates to the death penalty, torture, or cruel and degrading punishment, as such practices might be applied to prisoners (especially political prisoners) and others in government custody (UD 3–5; CP 6–8).

3. Evidence of government respect for the rule of law, especially regarding arbitrary arrest and detention, due process, fair and public trials by independent judiciaries, and states of emergency (UD 6–11, 28; CP 9–11); and related rights pertaining to privacy, freedom of movement, and the status of women (UD 1–2, 13–14; CP 2–5, 12–13).

4. Government attitude toward such individual personal freedoms as thought, expression, and association, especially as they might be applied to situations relating to religion, the press, and workers' unions (UD 18–20, CP 18–21).

From the perspective of legal theory, these four topics could be said to relate, respectively, to equal rights, human rights, civil rights, and political rights. The matters covered under government respect for the integrity of the person (freedom from illegal execution, torture, and imprisonment) are owed to everyone by virtue of their basic humanity. Issues under the rule of law (due process, fair trials, freedom of movement, and privacy) ought to be enjoyed in normal times by all citizens in their states. The personal freedoms of thought, expression, and association, if respected by one's government, are potentially powerful political instruments. The way a society defines these concepts and whether they are implemented equitably upon all individuals and groups significantly determine the quality of justice that society will experience (Sullivan, 1991: 236–241; 264–265).

Many organizations such as the U.S. Department of State (1995), Amnesty International (1995), and the various regional branches of Human Rights Watch (1995) annually produce narrative reports detailing the status of rights in countries around the world, and attempts have been made to quantify some of their efforts (Claude and Jabine, 1986; Gillies, 1990; Stohl, 1986). This study, however, will focus upon the research of Charles Humana and Freedom House because their reports lend themselves more readily to a quantification methodology which is adaptable to what has been used elsewhere in this work.

Humana (1992) has devised forty questions based upon specific articles in the International Bill of Human Rights to assess whether these rights are being honored by 120 governments, including 85 of those in this study. He gives the answers to these forty questions in a disaggregated and weighted fashion (YES, yes, no, NO) which can easily be translated into a 1-through-4 scale for each of the forty measures. One of these measures (the independence of judicaries) was cited in Chapter 2c.i.

Humana has normalized his scores on the basis of 100 points for a state receiving the highest ranking (YES) for each of the forty questions. His summarized conclusions reveal Sweden, Denmark, Netherlands, and Germany with the highest rates of compliance with the International Bill of Human Rights (98%), and Iraq and Myanmar with the lowest (17%).

In general, the European states have the highest scores according to Humana, and the states of the Western Hemisphere the next best numbers. The Islamic and Asian zones are especially represented among the lowest tier of countries. Humana's complete list is not reproduced here, and no attempt is made to correlate his human-rights scores with polity types here, for as comprehensive as Humana's work is with respect to the IBHR, his survey is somewhat dated and its scope is not as extensive as the Freedom House survey to be discussed next. Freedom House's work is not only more recent (it comes out annually), but it covers, in 1995, fully 191 states and 58 "related territories." The results are reproduced here in **Table 7a.**

The focus of Freedom House's inquiry is not human rights per se but "political rights and civil liberties." But a look at the questions asked to generate ratings (on a scale of 1 to 7) in each of these two categories shows considerable overlap with articles in the International Bill of Human Rights (Freedom House, 1994: 672–673)

"Political rights" are defined as those which enable people to participate freely in the process which chooses their society's authoritative policy makers. Nine questions are asked of each country. In addition to concern for free and fair elections for head of state and/or government and for legislative representatives, the following other areas are covered: the right to organize competing political parties; the freedom of citizens from domination by the military, foreign powers, totalitarian parties, religious hierarchies, or economic oligarchies; and the right of cultural groups to reasonable self-determination, self-government, autonomy, or participation through informal consensus in the decision-making process.

"Civil liberties" are defined as the freedoms to develop views, institutions, and personal autonomy, apart from the state. Thirteen areas are on the checklist which covers such issues as independent media, literature, and cultural expression; open public discussion and free private discussion; freedom of assembly and demonstration; freedom of political or quasi-political organization; equality under the law; protection from political terror and from unjustified imprisonment, exile, or torture; free trade unions and peasant organizations; free professional and other private organizations; free businesses or cooperatives; free religious institutions; personal social freedoms relating to gender equality, property rights, freedom of movement, choice of residence, and choice of marriage and size of family; equality of opportunity, including freedom from exploitation by or dependency on landlords, employers, union leaders, or bureaucrats; and freedom from extreme government indifference and corruption.

For each of the nine items on the political checklist and thirteen items on the civil-liberties questionnaire, a state is awarded from 0 to 4 raw points, depending on the comparative rights or liberties present, for a maximum of 36 and 52 points, respectively. Depending on where on the scale between 0 and 36, or 0 and 52, a state falls, it receives a score between 1 and 7 for each of the two (civil liberties and political rights) categories.

Table 7a averages these two scores for the most recent survey year. It presents the results in a way which clusters countries into the three Freedom House–designated categories of "Free," for states with an average score of 2.5 or lower; "Partly Free," for states scoring between 3 and 5; and "Not Free," for states with scores 5.5 or higher. Among the 100 states on the CGSS, 30 fall into the top tier, 36 are in the middle range, and 34 are on the lowest level.

To check whether this book's CGSS polity types correlate with these Freedom House rankings, country scores on **Table 7a** are annotated with m for the 25 multiparty republics (regular and weak); 1 for the 25 one-party polities; * for the 20 militarized party states; and ^° for the 30 military or monarchical regimes. (This methodology is an expansion of the annotating system used in Chapter 5, where militarism was measured. It will be used at this

Table 7a
Freedom House "Freedom" Scores, 1994 (average of 1 through 7 scores for political rights and civil liberties)

Europe	Islamic Zone	Africa	Asia	West.Hemisph.
Free, n=30: 23m + 1 "1" + 6*				
mBelgium 1				mUSA 1
mDenmark 1			mAustralia 1	mCanada 1
mSweden 1				
mNetherlands 1				
mPortugal 1				
mSpain 1.5				mCosta Rica 1.5
mIreland 1.5				
mFrance 1.5			mJapan 2	*Chile 2
mGermany 1.5			*S. Korea 2	
mItaly 1.5				
mUK 1.5				
mCzech Rep. 1.5	*Israel 2			mJamaica 2.5
mHungary 1.5				mEcuador 2.5
mPoland 2				*Argentina 2.5
mGreece 2				*Bolivia 2.5
mBulgaria 2		1S. Africa 2.5		*Panama 2.5
Partly Free, n=36: 2m + 10 "1" + 14* + 10°				
			1Taiwan 3	*Brazil 3
		*Madagascar 3	*Bangladesh 3	mVenezuela 3
1Russia 3.5		1Zambia 3.5	*Phil. Is. 3.5	*El Salvador 3
1Romania 3.5			*Nepal 3.5	*Colombia 3.5
1Ukraine 3.5		^oMozambique 4	*Thailand 4	mDom.Rep. 3.5
	^oJordan 4		*India 4	1Mexico 4
		^oBurkina F. 4.5	*Pakistan 4	
		1Senegal 4.5	*Sri Lanka 4.5	^oPeru 4.5
		^oGhana 4.5	1Malaysia 4.5	*Nicaragua 4.5
	^oGeorgia 5		^oCambodia 4.5	*Guatemala 4.5
	^oMorocco 5	1Zimbabwe 5		
	*Turkey 5	^oUganda 5	1Singapore 5	^oHaiti 5
Not Free, n=34: 14 "1" + 20°				
	1Kazakhistan 5.5	1Cameroon 5.5		
	1Tunisia 5.5	^oEthiopia 5.5		
	^oYemen 5.5	1Ivory Coast 5.5		
	^oAzerbaijan 6	^oGuinea 5.5		
	1Egypt 6			
1Yugoslavia 6	1Iran 6.5	1Tanzania 6		
	^oAlgeria 7	1Kenya 6		
	^oTajikistan 7			
	1Uzbekistan 7	^oNigeria 6.5	^oIndonesia 6.5	
	^oSaudi A. 7	^oZaire 6.5		
	^oIraq 7	^oLiberia 6.5	^oAfghanistan 7	
	^oLibya 7		^oMyanmar 7	1Cuba 7
	^oSomalia 7		1China 7	
	^oSudan 7	^oRwanda 7	1N.Korea 7	
	^oSyria 7	^oAngola 7	1Vietnam 7	
n=20:16+3+1	n=20:1+4+15	n=20:1+8+11	n=20:3+11+6	n=20:9+10+1 (100)

Source: Freedom House, 1995.
Notes: m = Multiparty Republic, 1 = One-Party Polity, * = Militarized Party System, and ^o = Military Regime from Comparative Government Spread Sheet.

point, and then later in this chapter, for the most recent and comprehensive quality of life measure, to show the connection between high scores in these indicators and high standing in the Comparative Government Spread Sheet.)

In confirmation of this thesis, there is significant correlation between high Freedom House scores and the more open polity types described in this study. Of the 30 "Free" states, 23 are multiparty, 1 is single party, and 6 are militarized multiparty. Of the 34 "Not Free" countries, 14 are one-party polities and 20 are military regimes. In between these two extreme categories, the 36 "Partly Free" states show the greatest variation: 2 multiparty, 10 one-party, 14 militarized multiparty, and 10 military. Geographically, Europe has the best record (16 of 20 "Free"), and the Islamic zone the worst (15 of 20 "Not Free"), a finding consistent with that of the distribution of states by zone on the Comparative Government Spread Sheet, where all 20 European states were on page 1, and 15 of 20 Islamic countries were on page 2 (the highest of any zone).

7b ECONOMIC AND SOCIAL RIGHTS AND WELL-BEING

In the International Bill of Human Rights, there are some articles relating to explicitly economic rights, including the right to own property, to work reasonable hours (in safe conditions, with fair remuneration and opportunities), and, implicitly, the right to not work (i.e., to strike) (UD 17, ESC 6–7); also, the right to have social security in the workplace including unions, unemployment compensation, and special protection for women and children (UD 22–24, CP 22, ESC 8–10); as well as the right to "economic justice," as reflected in access to adequate food, shelter, clothing, education, medical care, and social services (UD 25–26, ESC 11–14).

The traditional (western) human rights organizations do not typically address these economic and (group) social rights, especially as far as equal opportunity to achieve them is concerned (Howard, 1983; Hakhijani, 1992; Mower, 1985; Moon, 1991). However, there have always been ample economic data available on the macro level to assess how individual states are performing from agencies such as the International Monetary Fund (1995), the World Bank (1995a, 1995b), the United Nations (1995a), the U.N. Conference on Trade and Development (1995), and the U.S. Central Intelligence Agency (1995).

The gross domestic product, the most commonly accepted general measure for the health of a society's economy, was discussed in Chapter 1 and displayed for the 100 CGSS states in Table 1b.iii. But this statistic is more a function of a state's size than of its form of government, and does not necessarily speak to the equitable distribution of this product or the quality of life within individual states, particularly for the 135 countries not in the core of the capitalist system (Shaikh and Tonak, 1994).

Table 7b shows gross national product (GNP) per capita, which, historically, has been used as the most conveniently available figure to indicate the

Table 7b
Gross National Product per Capita, 1993

Europe	Islamic Zone	Africa	Asia	West.Hemisph.
-Switz.(#1) $36,410				
Denmark 26,500			Japan $31,450	
Sweden 24,830				USA $24,750
Germany 23,560				
France 22,360				Canada 20,670
Belgium 21,210			Singapore 19,310	
Netherlands 20,710			#Hong Kong 17,860	
Italy 19,620			Australia 17,510	
UK 17,970	Israel $13,760			
Spain 13,650				
Ireland 12,580				
			Taiwan 10,460^	
Portugal 7820	Saudi A. 7780('92)			Argentina 7290
Greece 7390	Libya 6384^		S.Korea 7670	#Puerto Rico 7020
		S.Africa 2900		
Hungary 3330				Mexico 3750
Czech Rep. 2730	Syria 2963^		Malaysia 3160	Chile 3070
Russia 2350	Iran 2230('92)			Brazil 3020
Poland 2270	Turkey 2120			Venezuela 2840
Ukraine 1910				Panama 2580
	Tunisia 1790			Costa Rica 2160
	Algeria 1650		Thailand 2040	Cuba 1959^
Yugoslavia-n.a.	Kazakh. 1540			Peru 1490
				Colombia 1400
				Jamaica 1390
				El Salvador 1320

\--------------**$1200 cut-off: Top 49/Bottom 51 States**--------------/

Europe	Islamic Zone	Africa	Asia	West.Hemisph.
Bulgaria 1160	Jordan 1190			Ecuador 1170
Romania 1120	Morocco 1030		Myanmar 1018e^	Guatemala 1110
	Yemen 976^			Dom.Rep.1080
	Uzbek. 960		N.Korea 877e^	
	Iraq 913e^	Cameroon 770	Phil. I. 830	
		Senegal 730		Bolivia 770
	Azerbaijan 730	Ivory Coast 630	Indonesia 730	
		Zimbabwe 540		
	Egypt 660	Guinea 510	Sri Lanka 600	
		Liberia 494e^		
	Georgia 560	Angola 456e^		
		Ghana 430		
	Tajikistan 470	Zambia 420	China 490	
		Nigeria 310	Pakistan 430	
		Burkina F. 300		Nicaragua 360
		Kenya 270	India 290	Haiti 332e^
		Madagascar 240	Cambodia 224^	
		Zaire 207e^	Bangladesh 220	
	Sudan 196^	Rwanda 200	Vietnam 170	
		Uganda 190	Afghanistan 169e^	
	Somalia 110e^	Ethiopia 100	Nepal 160	
		Tanzania 100		
		Mozambique 80		
=20 plus 1-	n=20	n=20	n=20 + 1#	n=20 + 1# (100)

 source: World Bank, *World Bank Atlas 1995;* plus ^U.S. Arms Control and Disarmament Agency, 1995.
otes: - = ministate (Switz.); # = colonies (Hong Kong, Puerto Rico); e = extrapolations (n = 16).

more general level of individual economic well-being. Gross national income per capita would be a better measure, because it would relate more to how much each citizen, on average, receives from the economy than to how much he or she has produced, but it is not as frequently reported; in fact, many secondary sources citing income per capita are actually using the more readily available GNP per capita statistic. But either of these is just an "average" macroeconomic measure and does not reflect whether a society's wealth is being distributed justly among all its members. Nevertheless, because it is a commonly accepted rough approximation, GNP per capita will be displayed here as the first of two economic measures to address how individuals within a given state are affected.

The standings of states in **Table 7b** reveal a range of GNP per capita from ministate Switzerland, highest in the world at $36,410 for each person, to Mozambique, the world's lowest at $80 for the latest year for which information is available. More than half the CGSS states (51 out of 100) have a GNP per capita of less than $1,200 per year, whereas the top 10 states average about $23,000, almost twenty times as much, providing additional testimony to the unfair distribution of the wealth of the world mentioned in Chapter 1b.

More to the point, with respect to issues of distribution of wealth *within* individual states, are two recently developed measures. Because of their novelty, however, the data are not as comprehensive or the measures as widely accepted (Mahler, 1989; Sen, 1992), and therefore they will be discussed here but not displayed.

The first, reported by the United Nations Development Program (UNDP) in its annual *Human Development Report* since 1990, identifies the percentage of population in absolute poverty, defined as the income level below which a minimum nutritionally adequate diet plus essential non-food requirements are not affordable (UNDP, 1994: 221). But the data gathered are spotty, drawn from various sources and years between 1980 and 1990. In addition, the term is not even applied to the 25 developed states, and so data are available for only 64 states in the CGSS, and of these, only for rural populations in 15 states.

Another potential measure for addressing the issue of distribution of wealth within states has been developed by the World Bank from national surveys on the percentage share of income or consumption accruing to groups of households ranked by total household income, per capita income, or per capita expenditures. Its most recent report (World Bank, 1995a: Table 30) had statistics for 69 states, including 60 of the CGSS countries. In general, the richer European states were the least stratified, with the top 10 percent of population accounting for about 22 percent of the income on average, and the Latin American countries the most so, with Brazil having the largest gap in the world, with 10 percent of the population getting 51 percent of the income. But there are comparability problems with these statistics: data vary from years spanning 1978 to 1993; primary sources differ in using income versus consumption expenditures as the living standard indicator; and finally, the surveys vary in using the household or the individual as their unit of observation. As a result, state rankings for this measure will not be presented here.

Rather, the second economic measure to be displayed will be "real" GNP per capita, a statistic developed by the United Nation's International Comparison Program in 1993, which presents GNP on an internationally comparable scale using purchasing-power parities rather than official exchange rates as conversion factors. The traditional method for converting national currency figures to U.S. dollars does not measure relative domestic purchasing power and understates the GNP for developing countries with many non-traded goods, cheap services, and subsidized housing and energy. Using "international dollars" converted at purchasing-power parities yields the number of units of a country's currency required to buy the same amounts of goods and services in the domestic market as one dollar would buy in the United States (World Bank, 1995a: 33).

In the resulting rankings, displayed in **Table 7b.i**, the gap between the highest country (now the United States, at $24,750) and the lowest (still Mozambique, now tied with Ethiopia, at $380) is not as vast as before. Moreover, the median cutoff for half the 100 CGSS states has almost tripled, to $3,500, a figure which is now only about one-fifth the average of the top 10 states. Although this is still an "average" macroeconomic measure, it is perhaps the best available for indicating the situation of the typical citizen in the economic environment of his or her particular state.

In the next and last section of this book, some non-economic measures, which more adequately encompass the issue of quality of life, will be introduced.

7c COMPOSITE QUALITY OF LIFE INDICATORS

Because of the inadequacy of purely economic statistics to reflect the status of well-being throughout varying strata of society, a number of other indicators have been developed to provide a more appropriate measure for the quality of life in a given country (Sen, 1987; Nussbaum and Sen, 1993; Goldstone, 1993). Several of these are composite indicators, and each has its own justification as to why the particular measure proposed correlates best with the standard the respective creator of the index is attempting to address.

This concluding section of this book will discuss five of the more significant quality-of-life indicators, presenting for three of them the most recent state rankings for the 100 CGSS states. For each of these measures, states scoring highest are generally in higher positions in the Comparative Government Spread Sheet, leading to the conclusion that the more open, participative forms of government generally correlate with a more congenial standard of living for their citizens.

The oldest composite measure displayed here was developed by Ruth Sivard in 1974 and has been updated regularly in her annual *World Military and*

Table 7b.i
"Real" GNP per Capita, Purchasing-Power Parity Dollars, 1993

Europe	Islamic Zone	Africa	Asia	West.Hemisph.
-Switzerland $23,620				USA $24,750
Germany 20,980			Japan $21,090	
France 19,440			Singapore 20,470	
Denmark 18,940				Canada 20,410
Belgium 18,490				
Italy 18,070				
Netherlands 18,050			Australia 18,490	
UK 17,750				
Sweden 17,560				
Spain 13,310	Israel $14,890			
Ireland 11,850			Taiwan-n.a.	
Portugal 9890	Saudi A.-n.a.		S.Korea 9810	
	Libya-n.a.			Argentina 9130
Greece 8360			Malaysia 8630	Chile 8380
Czech Rep. 7700				Venezuela 8130
	Syria-n.a.			Mexico 7100
Hungary 6260	Iran-n.a.		Thailand 6390	
				Panama 5940
	Turkey 5550			Colombia 5630
Russia 5240				Costa Rica 5580
Poland 5010	Tunisia 5070			Brazil 5470
Ukraine 4030	Algeria 4390	S.Africa-n.a		Ecuador 4260
	Jordan 4010			Cuba-n.a.
Bulgaria 3730	Kazakh. 3770			
	Egypt 3530			

\------------**$3500 cut-off: Top 49/Bottom 51 States**------------/

Europe	Islamic Zone	Africa	Asia	West.Hemisph.
	Morocco 3270			Guatemala 3390
	Yemen-n.a.		Indonesia 3140	Dom.Rep.3240
Romania 2910	Uzbekistan 2580	Ghana $2160	Sri Lanka 3030	Peru 3130
Yugoslavia-n.a.	Iraq-n.a.	Cameroon 2060	Phil. I. 2660	Jamaica 3000
		Zimbabwe 1900	Myanmar-n.a.	Bolivia 2400
	Azerbaijan 2230			El Salvador 2360
		Senegal 1640	China 2120	
			Pakistan 2110	Nicaragua 2070
		Nigeria 1480		
		Ivory Coast 1420		
	Tajikistan 1430	Kenya 1310		
	Georgia 1410	Angola-n.a.	Bangladesh 1290	
		Guinea-n.a.	India 1250	
		Zambia 1170	Nepal 1150	
		Uganda 840	Vietnam 1010	
		Burkina F. 800		
		Liberia-n.a.	N.Korea-n.a.	Haiti-n.a.
		Madagascar 700	Cambodia-n.a.	
		Zaire-n.a.		
	Sudan-n.a.	Rwanda 640		
		Tanzania-n.a.	Afghanistan-n.a.	
	Somalia-n.a.	Ethiopia 380		
		Mozambique 380		
n=19/20 plus Switz.	n=12/20	n=14/20	n=15/20	n=18/20 (100)

Source: World Bank, *World Bank Atlas 1995*.
Note: n.a. = not available (n = 22)

Social Expenditures publication. It is the "Economic and Social (ECOSOC) Rank," which lists states in an order (from 1st to 140th in the latest ranking) based upon ten variables—four relating to health (public expenditures per capita, population per physician, infant mortality, and life expectancy), five to education (public expenditures per capita and per student, school-age population per teacher, primary school-age population in school, and literacy rate), and GNP per capita. The method of averaging gives equal importance to each of the three elements. For education and health, this means that a summary rank—a simple average—is first obtained for each of the indicators. The measures chosen represent a mix of both input of national effort (the expenditures, etc.) and output of result (literacy, life expectancy, etc.). The latest scores (from Sivard, 1993) appear in **Table 7c.i.**

Morris D. Morris developed a "Physical Quality of Life Index" (PQLI) for the Overseas Development Council, which rates countries on a scale of 1 to 100 in accordance with three indicators: infant mortality, life expectancy, and level of literacy. His 1979 book, *Measuring the Condition of the World's Poor,* justifies the parsimony of using only these three measures. The figure was updated regularly for the Overseas Development Council's publications on U.S. foreign policy toward less developed countries during the 1980s. The most recent statistics available, based on Morris's 1995 revisions, are reproduced here as **Table 7c.ii.**

Two other measures will be mentioned here but not displayed, for they have not been updated since 1992. Richard Estes's "Index of Social Progress" (1984) combines forty-six indicators across ten categories—education, health, status of women, defense, economics, demography, geography, political participation, cultural diversity, and welfare—and compares them against an earlier base line to measure progress in these areas. The Population Crisis Committee (1992) has developed a "Human Suffering Index" in an effort to show that human misery was highly correlated with high rates of annual population increase (see also Anand, 1994). The measure combines ten factors: life expectancy, daily calorie intake, percentage of people with access to safe water, infant immunization, secondary school attendance, GNP per capita, inflation, level of communications technology, political freedom, and civil rights.

Finally, the most recently developed and probably the best composite figure to address the quality of life around the world is the "Human Development Index" (HDI), created by the United Nations Development Program in 1990, and refined in annual publications of its *Human Development Report* ever since. It purports to measure the "process of enlarging people's choice" and combines indicators of longevity (life expectancy), knowledge (education attainment), and income. The educational factor was originally measured only through adult literacy rate but has since been broadened to incorporate mean years of schooling, at one-third weighting, as well.

For income, the HDI initially used a specific dollar amount, beyond which a marginal increase in income was heavily discounted. Since 1994, this threshold value has been the current average global value of real GDP per capita,

Table 7c.i
Sivard's Economic and Social Rank (ECOSOC) (scale of 1 to 140)

Europe	Islamic Zone	Africa	Asia	West.Hemisph.
Sweden 1				
Denmark 3T				
France 7T			Japan 7T	
Netherlands 9T				USA 9T
Belgium 12				Canada 11
Germany 14				
UK 16T			Australia 16T	
Spain 16T	Israel 20			
Ireland 21T				
Italy 21T				
Greece 26T				
Portugal 26T				
!Czech. 28			Singapore 31	Cuba 39
			Taiwan 33	
!USSR 34				Argentina 46
Hungary 35			S. Korea 41	Panama 47
Bulgaria 36	Libya 47			Jamaica 49
Poland 43	Saudi A. 50			Venezuela 51T
!Yugo. 44	Jordan 57			Costa Rica 51T
Romania 51		S. Africa 63	Malaysia 60	Chile 57
	Iran 65T		N. Korea 67	Mexico 61
Ukraine-na	Syria 68T			Brazil 65T
	Algeria 68T		Thailand 71	Ecuador 73T
	Tunisia 68T			Colombia 73T
			Sri Lanka 77	Peru 73T
	Iraq 78T	Zimbabwe 80		
	Turkey 78T		Philippines 83T	Nicaragua 82
			Indonesia 83T	Dom.Rep. 83T
	Egypt 86T		China 86T	
		Cameroon 96T		El Salvador 91
		Kenya 99	Vietnam 96T	Guatemala 93
	Morocco 94	Ivory Coast 101		Bolivia 95
		Senegal 105T	India 103T	
	Yemen 103T	Angola 109T	Myanmar 105T	
		Zambia 109T		
		Ghana 109T		
		Guinea 113T	Pakistan 112	
		Liberia 113T		Haiti 115
	Sudan 117T	Madagascar 117T	Cambodia 117T	
		Uganda 121T		
		Zaire 121T		
	Ga.,Azerb.-n.a.	Nigeria 124T		
	Kazak.,Uzbek.-n.a.	Tanzania 124T		
	Tajikistan-n.a.	Rwanda 126	Bangladesh 128	
		Burkina Faso 132	Nepal 131	
	Somalia 138T	Mozambique 138T	Afghanistan 136	
		Ethiopia 140		
n=19/20	n=15/20	n=20	n=20	n=20 (100)
with !=ex-SU, Yugo.,Czech.				

Source: Sivard, 1993 , Table III.
Notes: ECOSOC is based on GNP per capita, plus four health measures and five education measures.
    n.a. = 6 CGSS states not available.
    T = Tied for this rank.

Table 7c.ii
Morris's Physical Quality of Life Index (PQLI) (scale of 100 to 0)

Europe	Islamic Zone	Africa	Asia	West.Hemisph.
Sweden 93.1			Japan 94.0	
Netherlands 92.9				Canada 92.7
France 92.3			Australia 92.3	
Denmark 91.8				USA 91.7
UK 91.7				
Spain 91.5				
Belgium 91.4				Cuba 90.0^
Germany 91.4				Jamaica 89.0
Italy 91.2	Israel 90.6		Taiwan 88.8	Costa Rica 88.5^
Ireland 91.0			Singapore 86.8	
Greece 89.8				
!Czech. 88.6				Chile 86.1
Poland 88.0			S. Korea 85.6	Argentina 85.3
Hungary 87.7			N. Korea 84.6^	Panama 84.6
!USSR 87.1			Sri Lanka 83.3	
Bulgaria 87.0				Venezuela 81.8
!Yugo. 86.4	Jordan 76.5		Thailand 81.3	Mexico 80.9
Romania 85.7	Turkey 73.0		Malaysia 79.7	Colombia 80.1
Portugal 85.5				
	Tunisia 70.7		China 77.4	Ecuador 76.1
	Syria 70.3		Philippines 77.4	Dom.Rep. 75.7
			Vietnam 74.4^	Brazil 74.2
	Iran 66.7			Nicaragua 73.9
	Saudi A. 66.7	S. Africa 67.0	Myanmar 70.4	Peru 71.8
	Iraq 66.4	Kenya 65.0		El Salvador 70.7
Ukraine - n.a.	Algeria 65.3	Zimbabwe 64.8		
	Libya 64.3			Guatemala 64.4
		Zambia 61.5		
	Morocco 59.7	Madagascar 60.5^		Bolivia 60.9
	Egypt 59.2	Zaire 59.9	India 55.4	
		Ghana 57.0		
		Tanzania 56.4		Haiti 54.6
		Cameroon 53.5		
	Ga.,Azerb.,- n.a.	Ivory Coast 53.0		
	Kazak.,Uzbek.- n.a.	Nigeria 49.7	Pakistan 49.1	
	Tajikistan - n.a.	Uganda 49.5		
		Ethiopia 47.4		
		Rwanda 46.5		
		Liberia 45.3		
	Yemen 44.5	Senegal 44.6	Bangladesh 43.7	
			Cambodia 41.0^	
	Sudan 41.0	Angola 36.3^	Nepal 40.0	
		Mozambique 34.3		
	Somalia 34.2	Burkina Faso 33.4		
		Guinea 30.8	Afghanistan 29.3	
n=19/20	n=15/20	n=20	n=20	n=20 (100)
w/ !=ex-SU,Yugo,Cz.				

Source: Morris, 1995.
Notes: PQLI, created by Overseas Development Council in 1978, is a composite of infant mortality, life
    expectancy, and literacy, normalized so that 0 = worst state in 1950, and 100 = best projected state in
    year 2000.
^ = supplemented by extrapolations from Tucker and Philips, 1991.
n.a. = 6 CGSS states not available.

adjusted for the local cost of living (purchasing-power parity). Once a country gets beyond the world average, any further increases in per capita income are considered to make a diminishing marginal contribution to human development. The threshold for 1994 was $5,120, and the spectrum of scores, after discounting, was from $330 (Ethiopia) to $5,371 (United States).

For each indicator, the range of values is put on a scale of 0 to 1 where, for the highest and lowest scores in the spectrum, fixed normative values, based upon the most extreme levels observed over a thirty-year period, were selected. This permits meaningful comparisons across countries and over time. The placements for the 174 states surveyed are then adjusted on the basis of 1,000, resulting in the display of the most recent scores, shown in **Table 7c.iii**.

This measure is the most recent (1992 data) and most complete (98 of 100 CGSS states; all except Yugoslavia and Taiwan) of the five composite indicators surveyed. Accordingly, and following the system introduced in section 7a, each state is annotated m, 1, *, or ^°, depending on which of the four major polity types (multiparty, one-party, militarized-party, military regime) it has been designated on the Comparative Government Spread Sheet.

Again, the basic thesis of this study is confirmed. Of the states in the high human development tier (according to the UNDP, with scores greater than 800), 77 percent are on page one of the CGSS (civilian polities); 86 percent of the 28 states in the lowest human development category (with scores under 500) are on page two (militarized polities). The 37 countries with medium HDI scores (between 500 and 800) ared divided roughly 50–50 between the two CGSS pages. As the United Nations Development Program has concluded, there definitely is a connection between good governance and human development (Transparency International, 1993).

Table 7c.iii
United Nations Human Development Index

Europe	Islamic	Africa	Asia	West.Hemisph.
"High" (>800), n=35 of which 27 (77.1%) are on CGSS, p. 1 (= m,1)				
mNethrlds. 936				mCanada 950
mFrance 930			mJapan 937	mUSA 937
mSpain 930				
mSweden 929			mAustralia 927	
mBelgium 926				
mGermany 921				
mDenmark 920			1Taiwan - n.a.	
mUK 916				
mIreland 915				
mItaly 912				mCosta Rica 883
mGreece 907	*Israel 907		*S.Korea 882	*Argentina 882
mPortugal 874			1Singapore 878	*Chile 880
mCzech.Rep.872				mVenezuela 859
mHungary 856				*Panama 856
mPoland 855				1Mexico 842
1Russia 849			*Thailand 827	*Colombia 836
1Ukraine 842			1Malaysia 822	*Brazil 804
"Medium" (500-800), n=37 of which 18 on CGSS, p.1, 19 on CGSS, p. 2				
mBulgaria 796	1Kazakhstan 798			
	*Turkey 792			mEcuador 784
	1Iran 770			
1Romania 729	^°Libya 768			1Cuba 769
	1Tunisia 763			
	^°Saudi A. 762			
	^°Syria 761			
	^°Jordan 758			
	^°Algeria 732		1N. Korea 733	mJamaica 721
	^°Georgia 709	1S. Africa 705	*Sri Lanka 704	^°Peru 709
1Yugo.-n.a.	1Uzbekistan 706			mDom.Rep. 705
	^°Azerbaijan 696		*Phil. I. 677	
	^°Tajikistan 643		^°Indonesia 637	*Nicaragua 611
	^°Iraq 617			*Guatemala 591
	1Egypt 613	1Zimbabwe 539	1China 594	*Bolivia 588
	^°Morocco 554	1Cameroon 503	1Vietnam 539	*El Salvador 579
"Low" (<500), n=28 of which 24 (85.7%) are on CGSS, p. 2 (= *,^°)				
		^°Ghana 482	*Pakistan 483	
		1Kenya 481	^°Myanmar 457	
		*Madagascar 432	*India 439	
	^°Yemen 424	1Zambia 425		
		^°Nigeria 40€		
		^°Zaire 384		
	^°Sudan 379	1Ivory Coast 369		
		1Tanzania 364	*Bangladesh 364	^°Haiti 362
		1Senegal 340	*Nepal 343	
		^°Rwanda 332	^°Cambodia 337	
		^°Uganda 329		
		^°Liberia 325		
		^°Angola 291		
	^°Somalia 246	^°Mozambique 246		
		^°Guinea 237		
		^°Burkina Faso 228	^°Afghanistan 228	
		^°Ethiopia 227		
n=20	n=20	n=20	n=20	n=20 (100)

Source: U.N. Development Program, 1995. n.a. = 2 (Yugo., Taiw.)
Notes: HDI is based on life expectancy, educational standards, and individual purchasing power.
   m = Multiparty Republic, 1 = One-Party Polity, * = Militarized Party System, and ^° = Military Regime from
      Comparative Government Spread Sheet.
   n.a. = not available (Yugoslavia, Taiwan), relative positions estimated.

REFERENCES

Amnesty International (1995) *Annual Report 1995*. London: Amnesty International.
Anand, S. (1994) "Population, Well-Being, and Freedom," in *Population Policies Reconsidered*, edited by G. Sen, A. Germain, and L. C. Chen. Cambridge, MA: Harvard University Press.
Andrain, C. F. (1994) *Comparative Political Systems: Policy Performance and Social Change*. Armonk, NY: M. E. Sharpe.
An-Naim, A. B. (ed.) (1992) *Human Rights in Cross-Cultural Perspectives: A Quest for Consensus*. Philadelphia: University of Pennsylvania Press.
Claude, R. P. and T. B. Jabine (1986) "Symposium: Statistical Issues in the Field of Human Rights, Editors' Introduction," *Human Rights Quarterly*, 8: 551–566.
Claude, R. P. and B. H. Weston (eds.) (1989) *Human Rights in the World Community*. Philadelphia: University of Pennsylvania Press.
Donnelly, J. (1989) *Universal Human Rights in Theory and Practice*. Ithaca, NY: Cornell University Press.
Eide, A. (1986) "The Human Rights Movement and the Transformation of the International Order," *Alternatives*, 11: 367–402.
Estes, R. J. (1984) *The Social Progress of Nations*. Westport, CT: Praeger.
Franck, T. M. (1982) *Human Rights in Third World Perspective*. Dobbs Ferry, NY: Oceana.
Freedom House (annual) *Freedom in the World: Political Rights and Civil Liberties*. New York: Freedom House.
Gillies, D. W. (1990) "Evaluating National Human Rights Performance: Priorities for the Developing World," *Bulletin of Peace Proposals*, 21(1): 15–27.
Goldstone, L. (1993) "The Use of Composite Indexes for Ranking Countries by Their Level of Development," Washington, DC: World Bank Working Paper.
Groth, A. J. and L. L. Wade (1984) *Comparative Resource Allocation: Politics, Performance, and Policy Priorities*. Beverly Hills, CA: Sage.
Hakhijani, A. (1992) *From Global Capitalism to Economic Justice: An Inquiry into the Elimination of Systemic Poverty in the World Economy*. New York: Apex Press.
Henkin, L. (ed.) (1981) *The International Bill of Human Rights*. New York: Columbia University Press.
Howard, R. (1983) "The Full-Belly Thesis: Should Economic Rights Take Priority over Civil and Political Rights?" *Human Rights Quarterly*, 5: 467–490.
——— (1990) "Monitoring Human Rights: Problems of Consistency," *Ethics and International Affairs*, 4: 33–52.
Humana, C. (1992) *World Human Rights Guide*. 3rd ed. New York: Oxford University Press.
Human Rights Watch (1995) *Human Rights Watch World Report: Events of 1994*. New York: Human Rights Watch.
Humphrey, J. P. (1984) *Human Rights and the United Nations: A Great Adventure*. Ardsley, NY: Transnational Publications.
International Monetary Fund (1995) *Government Finance Statistics Yearbook*. Washington, DC: International Monetary Fund.
Jabine, T. B. and R. P. Claude (eds.) (1992) *Human Rights and Statistics: Getting the Record Straight*. Philadelphia: University of Pennsylvania Press.
Lawson, E. H. (ed.) (1989) *Encyclopedia of Human Rights*. New York: Taylor and Francis.

Mahler, V. A. (1989) "Income Distribution within Nations: Problems of Cross-National Comparison," *Comparative Political Studies*, 22(1, April): 3–32.

Moon, B. E. (1991) *The Political Economy of Basic Human Needs*. Ithaca, NY: Cornell University Press.

Morris, M. D. (1979) *Measuring the Condition of the World's Poor*. New York: Pergamon Press.

——— (1995) *Measuring the Changing Condition of the World's Poor 1960–1990*. Providence, RI: Brown University World Hunger Program.

Mower, G. A. (1985) *International Cooperation for Social Justice: Global and Regional Protection of Economic and Social Rights*. Westport, CT: Greenwood Press.

Nanda, V. P., J. R. Scaritt, and G. W. Shepherd, Jr. (eds.) (1981) *Global Human Rights: Public Policies: Comparative Measures*. Boulder, CO: Westview Press.

Nussbaum, M. and A. Sen (eds.) (1993) *The Quality of Life*. New York: Oxford University Press.

Population Crisis Committee (1992) *The International Human Suffering Index*. Washington, DC: Population Crisis Committee.

Sen, A. K. (1987) *The Standard of Living*. Cambridge: Cambridge University Press.

——— (1992) *Inequality Reexamined*. Oxford: Clarendon Press.

Shaikh, A. M. and E. A. Tonak (1994) *Measuring the Wealth of Nations: The Political Economy of National Accounts*. New York: Cambridge University Press.

Sivard, R. L. (1993) *World Military and Social Expenditures, 1993*. Leesburg, VA: World Priorities.

Stohl, M. (1986) "State Violation of Human Rights: Issues and Problems of Measurement," *Human Rights Quarterly* 8: 592–605.

Sullivan, M. J., III (1991) *Measuring Global Values: The Ranking of 162 Countries*. Westport, CT: Greenwood Press.

Transparency International (1993) "Good Governance and Third World Development," with Contributions from Ulrich Albrecht et al., Background Paper for UNDP, *Human Development Report 1994*.

Tucker, S. K. and R. Philips (1991) *U.S. Foreign Policy and Developing Countries*. Washington, DC: Overseas Development Council.

United Nations (1995a) *World Economic Survey 1995*. New York: United Nations Publication.

——— (1995b) *Yearbook on Human Rights*. New York: United Nations Publications.

——— Conference on Trade and Development (UNCTAD) (1995) *Trade and Development Report 1995*. New York: United Nations Publications.

——— Development Program (UNDP) (annual) *Human Development Report*. New York: Oxford University Press.

United States Central Intelligence Agency (1995) *Handbook of Economic Statistics*. Washington, DC: U.S. Government Printing Office.

U.S. Arms Control and Disarmament Agency (ACDA) (1995) *World Military Expenditures and Arms Transfers (WMEAT) 1993–94*. Washington, DC: U.S. Government Printing Office.

United States Department of State (1995) *Country Reports on Human Rights Practices for 1994*. Washington, DC: U.S. Government Printing Office.

World Bank (1995a) *World Bank Atlas 1995*. Washington, DC: World Bank.

——— (1995b) *World Development Report 1995*. New York: Oxford University Press.

Glossary

civilian polity Political system in which most political power is in the hands of civilians. *See also* **militarized polity**.

civil war (CVW) Violent domestic political conflict in which the non-governmental side controls some identifiable percentage of territory or population, and in which the deaths involved are more than 1000 per year. *See also* **insurgency**.

coup A rapid blow against the state, perpetrated by the government's own soldiers, which generally leaves most of society's basic structures untouched and changes only the top administrative strata of government. *See also* **revolution**.

entrenched military regime (mil°) Political system which has so broken down that civilian party activity and institutions are practically nonexistent, and all political space has been taken over by warring armed groups or snuffed out by a military coup regime.

ethnic-conflict state A state where an ethnic group is involved in a civil war or an insurgency against the government.

ethnic group A group in a state which draws its political significance from its ethnicity.

ethnicity That aspect of self-identity (e.g., race, language, religion, cultural tradition) which gives a person membership in a politically significant group.

ethnic minority-rule state A state in which the government is controlled by members of a minority ethnic group.

ethnically interesting state A state with a minority ethnic group worthy of some political notice to the group(s) typically controlling the government.

ethnically problematic state A state in which a minority ethnic group creates significant policy problems for the government.

ex-communist political system (ex-com) A former one-party communist state (i.e., one vanguard party directing the government, economy, and cultural life) now in transition to another form of political system.

government The political machinery of a state created to organize and enforce (via the law) the public behavior of members over which it has jurisdiction. *See also* **state**.

insurgency (NSG)   Violent domestic political conflict in which the non-governmental side does not hold significant territory for any length of time, and the deaths involved are less than 1000 per year at the present time. *See also* **civil war.**

latent conflict (LAT)   Violent domestic political conflict which waxes or wanes over the years with occasional periods of intense fighting alternating with periods of comparative quiet but no affirmative moves toward resolution.

militarized multiparty republic (*mpr)   A multiparty republic with a high degree of military influence over the system due to either a history of military coup rule, the impact of civil war or lesser forms of insurgency, or both; although there is multiparty civilian political activity, it is deemed not as significant in determining governmental power sharing as in (civilian) multiparty republics (mpr).

militarized one-party dominant (*1pd)   A one-party dominant political system with a high degree of military influence.

militarized party system (MILP*)   A transitional category of political systems between the civilian and the military categories; there are two types, militarized multiparty (*mpr) and militarized one-party dominant (*1pd).

militarized polity   Political system in which the key political actors are military (or former military) officers, and where there is a record of governance by society's institutional military forces, or a history of civil warfare against some important segment of the population; a system characterized by a high degree of military influence to the point where civilian political institutions are of lesser importance. *See also* **civilian polity.**

military regime (MIL°)   A political system in which the influence of force and violence overwhelms that of political parties or other civilian institutions of government; there are two types: moderating military (mil^) and entrenched (mil°).

minority ethnic group   Any ethnic group which is not the largest one in a political system.

mixed presidential/parliamentary system   A political system where a directly elected head of state is chosen separately from the representative assembly and sometimes vies for power with a head of government who comes out of that representative body.

moderating military regime (mil^)   Political system in which the military controls the executive branch of government but allows parties to compete in elections and be represented in a weak representative assembly.

monarchy (mon°)   Political system in which the leader of the state is chosen from and by members of a royal family whose roots go back to some past military conquest.

multiparty republic (mpr)   Political system in which two or more political parties participate, and more than one has a credible chance of gaining power in a free and fair election; it has civilian political structures including a (generally divided) executive sharing power with an independent representative assembly with law-making power, an independent judiciary to enforce this rule of law, and legitimation from regularly scheduled elections.

multiparty systems   Political systems in which more than one significant party operates; there are three types: multiparty republics (mpr), weak multiparty republics (~mpr), and militarized multiparty republics (*mpr).

nation   An ethnic group with an explicit organizational apparatus dedicated to the purpose of maintaining the consciousness of its members precisely as members of the group in the most public of settings. *See also* **state.**

nation-state Extremely homogeneous state where 90 percent or more of the population belongs to the same ethnic group. *See also* **state-nation**.

one-party dominant (1pdom) Political system in which two or more parties participate and have representation in the non-administrative branch of government but which is structured so that only one party has a credible chance of gaining executive power in an election.

one-party other (1p-oth) Political system with extremely limited civilian party rule because opposition parties are either not allowed or are so restricted that they achieve only minimal representation in the non-executive branch of the government.

one-party polities (1PP) Political systems in which opposition parties are either not allowed or are so severely restricted they have no real chance of coming to power even though they may participate in an electoral exercise; there are two types, one-party dominant (1pdom) and one-party other (1p-oth).

parliamentary political system Political system in which the leading ministers of the government must be nominated by a representative assembly of the people and come from its membership.

political system The system according to which power is allocated in a state. *See also* **polity**.

polity The political system of a state.

presidential political system Political system in which the head of state is the most significant actor in determining the composition of the government, either serving also as the head of government or appointing a prime minister to serve at his or her pleasure.

region A smaller geographic division of the world than the zone, chosen for purpose of making comparisons of more closely related countries; fifteen regions are defined in this work, three in each zone. *See also* **zone**.

revolution Violent domestic struggle against the state in which the non-governmental side has as its goal not only the replacement of the government but a rapid and complete transformation of society. *See also* **coup**.

state Institutional machinery created to embody and organize members of a group within a defined territory. *See also* **government** *and* **nation**.

state-nation Relatively homogeneous state with betwen 71 and 89 percent of the population belonging to the main ethnic group. *See also* **nation-state**.

waning conflict (WAN) Violent domestic political conflict in which a peace process has been started, generally including a ceasefire, regrouping of forces, demobilization of troops, and preparation for elections.

weak multiparty republic (~mpr) A political system in which two or more political parties participate and have a credible chance of gaining power, but the structure of the system is weak because either one party nearly always rules or the state is relatively new to the mpr category, having been recently moved in from a militarized-party (*MILP) or one-party (1PP) category.

zone A broad geographic division of the world of roughly continental size; five zones are defined in this work: Europe, Africa, Asia, Western Hemipshere, and the Islamic zone. *See also* **region**.

Subject Index

Advisory councils, 43, 47, 176
All-party national conference, 49, 93, 161, 167
Annotating methodology, 133, 145, 186, 196
Arbitrariness, of numbers of selections, 1, 22, 109, 134
Autonomy,13, 49–51, 113, 123, 167, 170, 186

Bureaucracy, 46, 47, 51

Cabinet, 42, 47, 49, 70, 113
Capitalism, 26–31, 33, 87, 188
Civilian political system/polity, 14, 19–24, 69–104, 122, 141, 153–161 passim, 169–170, 196
Civil rights, 70, 183–185, 193
Civil war, 24–25, 85, 87–88, 109–111, 131–133, 134–141, 147, 153–155, 160, 165–171 passim, 180
Clustering methodology, 2, 5–6, 13, 186
Coalitions, in government, 70, 72, 74, 156, 161
Cold War, 1, 6, 8, 9, 13, 15, 22, 25, 52, 69, 80, 85, 121
Collapsed state, 141, 170–171
Colony, 9–10, 50–51, 53–54, 85, 119–120, 133, 179, 180

Communism, 27–30, 69, 82, 85–90, 92
Comparative government, 2, 8, 13, 15, 19–23
Comparative Government Spread Sheet, 13, 19–25, 69, 91, 153–155, 155–161 passim, 176–178, 188
and annotating methodology, 133, 145, 147, 186, 196
movements and placements within, 40, 80, 82, 96, 113, 165, 169, 180
Confidence, vote of, 40, 70, 76
Conflict, violent and domestic, 1, 14, 105, 122, 134–148, 158, 167, 168, 180–181
Conservative, 26–29
Constitution, 39, 43–47, 141, 153, 154, 176
Consultative council, 43, 176
Corporation, multinational and transnational, 26–27, 33, 51
Coup (violent origins) measures, 141–145, 165, 167, 170
Coup d'état, 25, 85, 131, 138–145, 147, 154, 155, 158, 165, 167
Coup regime, 96, 139, 141, 153, 154, 158, 160, 161, 165–171 passim
Courts, 43–48
Culture, 8–10, 25, 28, 46, 49, 52, 53, 105, 131, 184, 193

Index of States

ABOUT THE AUTHOR

Michael J. Sullivan III is Professor of Political Science at Drexel University. He is the author of *Measuring Global Values: The Ranking of 162 Countries* (Greenwood, 1991).

ISBN 0-313-29395-3

EAN

9 780313 293955

90000>

HARDCOVER BAR CODE